VOLUME TWO

DIAGNOSTIC ULTRASOUND

SECOND EDITION

Edited by

John P. McGahan
Department of Radiology
University of California, Davis Medical Center
Sacramento, California, USA

Barry B. Goldberg
Department of Radiology
Thomas Jefferson University
Philadelphia, Pennsylvania, USA

informa
healthcare

New York   London

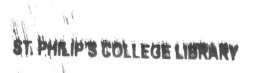

Informa Healthcare USA, Inc.
52 Vanderbilt Avenue
New York, NY 10017

© 2008 by Informa Healthcare USA, Inc.
Informa Healthcare is an Informa business

No claim to original U.S. Government works
10 9 8 7 6 5 4 3 2 1

International Standard Book Number-10: 1-4200-6978-0   (Hardcover: Volume 1)
International Standard Book Number-13: 978-1-4200-6978-5 (Hardcover: Volume 1)

International Standard Book Number-10: 1-4200-6979-9   (Hardcover: Volume 2)
International Standard Book Number-13: 978-1-4200-6979-2 (Hard cover: Volume 2)

International Standard Book Number-10: 0-8493-3076-9   (Hardcover: Set)
International Standard Book Number-13: 978-0-8493-3076-6 (Hardcover: Set)

International Standard Book Number-10: 1-4200-6742-7 (Hardcover: Set)
International Standard Book Number-13: 978-1-4200-6742-2 (Hardcover: Set)

This book contains information obtained from authentic and highly regarded sources. Reprinted material is quoted with permission, and sources are indicated. A wide variety of references are listed. Reasonable efforts have been made to publish reliable data and information, but the author and the publisher cannot assume responsibility for the validity of all materials or for the consequence of their use.

Library of Congress Cataloging-in-Publication Data

Diagnostic ultrasound / edited by John P. McGahan, Barry B. Goldberg.
  – 2nd ed.
    p. ; cm.
  Includes bibliographical references and index.
  ISBN-13: 978-1-4200-6742-2 (set : hardcover : alk. paper)
  ISBN-10: 1-4200-6742-7 (set : hardcover : alk. paper)
  ISBN-13: 978-1-4200-6978-5 (v. 1 : hardcover : alk. paper)
  ISBN-10: 1-4200-6978-0 (v. 1 : hardcover : alk. paper)
  ISBN-13: 978-1-4200-6979-2 (v. 2 : hardcover : alk. paper)
  ISBN-10: 1-4200-6979-9 (v. 2 : hardcover : alk. paper)
  1. Diagnosis, Ultrasonic. 2. Ultrasonics in obstetrics. I. McGahan,
John P. II. Goldberg, Barry B., 1937-
  [DNLM: 1. Ultrasonography–methods. WN 208 D536 2007]
  RC78.7.U4D5145 2007
  616.07'543–dc22   2007023721

For Corporate Sales and Reprint Permissions call 212-520-2700 or write to:
Sales Department, 52 Vanderbilt, 16th floor, New York, NY 10017.

Visit the Informa Web site at
www.informa.com

and the Informa Healthcare Web site at
www.informahealthcare.com

Printed in India

Preface

Diagnostic ultrasound is recognized worldwide as the premier cross-sectional imaging modality. Although other imaging modalities have advantages over sonography in certain anatomical regions, none are more readily available or more widely used throughout the world than sonography. Therefore, there is a growing need in every country to learn ultrasound.

Our text is a practical, comprehensive teaching and reference work on ultrasound. Our aim has been for the text to include detailed coverage of all anatomical structures accessible to ultrasound, including obstetrical applications. We have also included thorough coverage of such topics as the physics of ultrasound, artifacts, invasive and intraoperative ultrasound, endoscopic ultrasound, and three-dimensional sonographic imaging. The prior edition folded pediatric chapters into other anatomical areas. This second edition includes dedicated pediatric ultrasound chapters on the head, neck, spine, chest, abdomen, pelvis, and musculoskeletal system. We included these chapters to make this text more comprehensive in all facets of sonography. This approach has been taken to reduce redundancy and foster unified, comprehensive analyses of the organ or system under discussion. Artifacts that occur in all anatomical regions are addressed in a separate chapter, but artifacts or pitfalls that occur in site-specific regions are presented to the reader in those site-specific chapters, so as to avoid errors that we or others already have encountered.

We felt that it was vital that the chapters exploring organs or organ systems assess normal anatomy and pathology by using the logic inherent in most ultrasound examinations. The way in which we approach ultrasound imaging is by deciding if a particular finding truly represents an abnormality. We then determine the best choice or best differential of possibilities of what this abnormality represents. We have organized the chapters on anatomical regions into explorations based on this logic, which is used by most experienced ultrasound practitioners. First, we take the reader through the normal sonographic anatomy of the region. We then examine artifacts and pitfalls that are uniquely site-specific to that region. We elaborate on disease entities occurring within each organ system, but place emphasis on how we encounter ultrasound abnormalities in our daily practice. For instance, if on an ultrasound examination we visualize a solid lesion in a parenchymal organ, it may have pathopneumonic features that are listed within this text. More often, we have a number of possibilities that may be considered in the different diagnosis. Such ultrasound features as solid or cystic, single or multiple lesions, location, and the Doppler features may all be helpful in establishing a most probable diagnosis. We emphasize utilization of numerous tables, flow charts, and figures to help the reader to logically approach a differential diagnosis. If no specific diagnoses can be made by ultrasound, we suggest other imaging modalities that may be useful. We conclude each chapter with presentation of the ultrasound features of pathological entities. We also show how ultrasound may be used to guide biopsy, aspiration, drainage, operative, or percutaneous therapy for a variety of abnormalities.

We have placed heavy emphasis on pedagogy in developing the chapters. You will find frequent use of tables and flow charts to summarize important decision-making processes, key comparisons and relationships, and vital factual data. The tables are highlighted for quick reference, and outlines are placed at the beginning of each chapter for easy access.

We have tried to produce a volume that will serve as an accessible reference tool and teaching aid for any application of ultrasound in widespread practice. We hope that readers find the discussion, tables, differentials, and numerous figures to be a good background and reference for a logical approach to the daily practice of ultrasonography.

John P. McGahan, M.D.
Barry B. Goldberg, M.D.

Acknowledgments

This book is a selection of chapters written by an outstanding group of international experts in the field of diagnostic ultrasound, without whose efforts this book would not have been possible. We offer sincere thanks to each of these individuals for their contributions. Their years of hard work and experience have created both a valued reference text and a logical approach to the understanding of ultrasound.

We thank those individuals at Informa Healthcare USA, Inc., who were instrumental in the development of this textbook, especially Andrea Seils, who had the vision and gave us the encouragement and impetus to move forward on this text. Equally instrumental in the success of this endeavor was Vanessa Sanchez, who helped us with words of encouragement to produce high-quality work and to meet deadlines in spite of our busy work schedules.

In addition, we thank those individuals who are not often recognized but who contribute greatly in the development of any text by both transcribing and editing chapters. These individuals include, among others, Elisa Valenton, Angela Michelier, and Marilyn Lin-Kempeter.

Our many co-workers, including sonologists and sonographers, who provided case material for this text also deserve our sincere gratitude.

Finally, we thank our immediate and extended families for their patience while we were busy and, at times, distracted during the completion of this work.

Contents

Contributors

Andrei V. Alexandrov, M.D. ■ Comprehensive Stroke Center, Neurovascular Ultrasound Laboratory, University of Alabama Hospital, Birmingham, Alabama, U.S.A.

Sandra J. Allison, M.D. ■ Department of Radiology, Georgetown University Hospital, Washington, D.C., U.S.A.

John Amodio, M.D. ■ SUNY Downstate Medical Center, Brooklyn, New York, U.S.A.

Beryl R. Benacerraf, M.D. ■ Department of Radiology and Department of Obstetrics/Gynecology, Harvard Medical School, Boston, Massachusetts, U.S.A.

Carol B. Benson, M.D. ■ Department of Radiology, Harvard Medical School, Brigham and Women's Hospital, Boston, Massachusetts, U.S.A.

Lincoln L. Berland, M.D. ■ Department of Radiology, University of Alabama at Birmingham, Birmingham, Alabama, U.S.A.

Shweta Bhatt, M.D. ■ Department of Radiology, University of Rochester Medical Center, Rochester, New York, U.S.A.

William E. Brant, M.D. ■ Department of Radiology, Division of Thoraco-Abdominal Imaging, University of Virginia Health System, Charlottesville, Virginia, U.S.A.

Robert L. Bree, M.D. ■ Department of Radiology, University of Washington Medical Center, Seattle, Washington, U.S.A.

Étienne Cardinal, M.D. ■ Department of Radiology, Centre Hospitalier de l'Universite de Montreal, Pavillon Saint-Luc, Montreal, Quebec, Canada

Dru E. Carlson, M.D. ■ Department of Obstetrics and Gynecology, UCLA School of Medicine and Department of Reproductive Genetics, Cedars Sinai Medical Center, Los Angeles, California, U.S.A.

Frank A. Chervenak, M.D. ■ Department of Obstetrics and Gynecology, Division of Maternal Fetal Medicine, New York Hospital-Cornell Medical College, New York, U.S.A.

Rethy K. Chhem, M.D., Ph.D. ■ Department of Radiology and Nuclear Medicine, Schulich School of Medicine and Dentistry, University of Western Ontario, London, Ontario, Canada

W. K. Chooi, M.D. ■ Department of Radiology, University of British Columbia and St. Paul's Hospital, Vancouver, British Columbia, Canada

Terry L. Coates, M.D. ■ Department of Radiology, University of California, Davis Medical Center, Sacramento, California, U.S.A.

Dennis L. Cochlin, MB., BCh., FRCR ■ Radiology Department, University Hospital of Wales, Cardiff, U.K.

Peter L. Cooperberg, M.D. ■ Department of Radiology, University of British Columbia, and St. Paul's Hospital, Vancouver, British Columbia, Canada

Sidney M. Dashefsky, M.D. ■ Department of Radiology, University of Manitoba, Section of Diagnostic Ultrasound, Health Sciences Centre, Winnipeg, Manitoba, Canada

Greggory R. DeVore, M.D. ■ Fetal Diagnostic Center of Pasadena, Pasadena, California, U.S.A.

Vasudha Dhar, M.D. ■ Department of Gastroenterology New York-Presbyterian Hospital/Columbia University, New York, New York, U.S.A.

Vikram S. Dogra, M.D. ■ Department of Imaging Sciences, University of Rochester School of Medicine, Rochester, New York, U.S.A.

Peter M. Doubilet, M.D. ■ Department of Radiology, Harvard Medical School, Brigham and Women's Hospital, Boston, Massachusetts, U.S.A.

Harris J. Finberg, M.D. ■ Phoenix Perinatal Associates, Phoenix, Arizona and Department of Radiology, Mayo Medical School, Rochester, Minnesota, U.S.A.

Verlee L. Fines-Dailey, M.D. ■ Department of Obstetrics and Gynecology, Norton Maternal-Fetal Hospital, Louisville, Kentucky, U.S.A.

Flemming Forsberg, Ph.D. ■ Department of Radiology, Thomas Jefferson University, Philadelphia, Pennsylvania, U.S.A.

Wilbert Fortson, M.D. ■ Department of Obstetrics and Gynecology, Maternal-Fetal Medicine, Dekalb Medical Center, Decatur, Georgia, U.S.A.

Mary C. Frates, M.D. ■ Department of Radiology, Harvard Medical School, Brigham and Women's Hospital, Boston, Massachusetts, U.S.A.

Eugenio O. Gerscovich, M.D. ■ Department of Radiology, University of California, Davis Medical Center, Sacramento, California, U.S.A.

Marijo A. Gillen, M.D. ■ Department of Radiology, University of California, Davis Medical Center, Sacramento, California, U.S.A.

Barry B. Goldberg, M.D. ■ Department of Radiology, Thomas Jefferson University, Philadelphia, Pennsylvania, U.S.A.

Ruth B. Goldstein, M.D. ■ Department of Radiology, Obstetrics, Gynecology and Reproductive Science, University of California Medical Center, San Francisco, California, U.S.A.

Lawrence P. Gordon, M.D. ■ Department of Pathology, Crouse Hospital and Department of Pathology, Upstate Medical University, Syracuse, New York, U.S.A.

Lyndon M. Hill, M.D. ■ Department of Obstetrics and Gynecology, University of Pittsburgh School of Medicine and Magee-Women's Hospital of UPMC Health System, Pittsburgh, Pennsylvania, U.S.A.

Javine Horani, M.D. ■ Department of Obstetrics and Gynecology, Colorado Springs Health Partners, Colorado Springs, Colorado, U.S.A.

R. Brooke Jeffrey, M.D. ■ Department of Radiology, Stanford University Medical Center, Stanford, California, U.S.A.

Robert A. Kane, M.D. ■ Department of Radiology, Beth Israel Deaconess Medical Center, Boston, Massachusetts, U.S.A.

Mira L. Katz, Ph.D., M.P.H. ■ Division of Health Behavior and Health Promotion, The Ohio State University, Columbus, Ohio, U.S.A.

Ada Kessler, M.D. ■ Department of Radiology, Souraski-Tel Aviv Medical Center, Sackler School of Medicine, Tel Aviv University, Tel Aviv, Israel

Vijay P. Khatri, M.B.Ch.B.., FACS ■ Division of Surgical Oncology, University of California, Davis Cancer Center, Sacramento, California, U.S.A.

Viviane Khoury, M.D. ■ Department of Radiology, McGill University Health Center, Montreal, Quebec, Canada

Ercan Kocakoc, M.D. ■ Department of Radiology, Faculty of Medicine, Firat University, Elazig, Turkey

Ewa Kuligowska, M.D. ■ Department of Radiology, Boston University School of Medicine, Boston, Massachusetts, U.S.A.

Annabelle Lao, M.D. ■ Departments of Neurology and Psychiatry, University of Santo Tomas Hospital, Manila, Philippines and Department of Neurology, Barrow Neurological Institute, St. Joseph Hospital, Phoenix, Arizona, U.S.A.

Clifford S. Levi, M.D. ■ Department of Radiology, University of Manitoba, Section of Diagnostic Ultrasound, Health Sciences Centre, Winnipeg, Manitoba, Canada

Deborah Levine, M.D. ■ Department of Obstetric and Gynecologic Ultrasound, Beth Israel Deaconess Medical Center, Harvard Medical School, Boston, Massachusetts, U.S.A.

Anna S. Lev-Toaff, M.D. ■ Department of Radiology, Thomas Jefferson University, Philadelphia, Pennsylvania, U.S.A.

Ji-Bin Liu, M.D. ■ Department of Radiology, Thomas Jefferson University, Philadelphia, Pennsylvania, U.S.A.

Mark E. Lockhart, M.D., M.P.H. ■ Department of Radiology, University of Alabama at Birmingham, Birmingham, Alabama, U.S.A.

Edward A. Lyons, M.D. ■ Department of Radiology, Obstetrics and Gynecology, and Anatomy, University of Manitoba, Section of Diagnostic Ultrasound, Health Sciences Centre, Winnipeg, Manitoba, Canada

John P. McGahan, M.D. ■ Department of Radiology, University of California, Davis Medical Center, Sacramento, California, U.S.A.

Daniel A. Merton, B.S., RDMS, FSDMS, FAIUM ■ Department of Radiology, Thomas Jefferson University, Philadelphia, Pennsylvania, U.S.A.

Valdair Muglia, M.D., Ph.D. ■ Department of Radiology, Ribeiro Preto School of Medicine, Sao Paulo, Brazil

Laurence Needleman, M.D. ■ Department of Radiology, Thomas Jefferson University, Philadelphia, Pennsylvania, U.S.A.

Thomas R. Nelson, Ph.D. ■ Department of Radiology, University of California, San Diego, San Diego, California, U.S.A.

Matilde Nino-Murcia, M.D. ■ Department of Radiology, Stanford University School of Medicine, Stanford, California, U.S.A.

Suhas G. Parulekar, M.D. ■ Department of Radiology, The University of Texas, M. D. Anderson Cancer Center, Houston, Texas, U.S.A.

Catherine W. Piccoli, M.D. ■ Diagnostic Radiology, Turnersville and Voorhees, New Jersey; Philadelphia and Scranton, Pennsylvania; and Virginia Beach, Virginia, U.S.A.

Lawrence D. Platt, M.D. ■ Center for Fetal Medicine and Women's Ultrasound, Los Angeles, California, U.S.A.

Joseph F. Polak, M.D., M.P.H. ■ Department of Radiology, Tufts University School of Medicine, and Department of Cardiovascular Imaging, Tufts-New England Medical Center, Boston, Massachusetts, U.S.A.

M. Porto, M.D. ■ Department of Obstetrics and Gynecology, University of California-Irvine, Orange, California, U.S.A.

Myron A. Pozniak, M.D. ■ Department of Radiology, University of Wisconsin Clinical Science Center, Madison, Wisconsin, U.S.A.

Mladen Predanic, M.D. ■ Department of Obstetrics and Gynecology, Jamaica Hospital Medical Center, Jamaica, New York; and Department of Obstetrics and Gynecology of Weill Medical College of Cornell University, New York, New York, U.S.A.

Dolores H. Pretorius, M.D. ■ Department of Radiology, University of California-San Diego, San Diego, California, U.S.A.

John R. Richards, M.D. ■ Department of Emergency Medicine, University of California-Davis, Davis, California, U.S.A.

Ashley J. Robinson, M.D. ■ Department of Radiology, University of California Medical Center, San Francisco, California, U.S.A.

Henrietta Kotlus Rosenberg, M.D. ■ Department of Radiology and Pediatrics, Mt. Sinai School of Medicine, Mt. Sinai Medical Center, New York, New York, U.S.A.

Philip D. Schneider, M.D. ■ Department of Oncology, University of California-Davis, Davis, California, U.S.A.

Vijay K. Sharma, M.D. ■ Division of Neurology, National University Hospital, Singapore

Marilyn J. Siegel, M.D. ■ Mallinckrodt Institute of Radiology, Washington University School of Medicine, St. Louis, Missouri, U.S.A.

Beverly A. Spirt, M.D. ■ Oneida Medical Imaging Center, Oneida, New York; and Department of Radiology, Upstate Medical University, Syracuse, New York, U.S.A.

R. M. Steiger, M.D. ■ Department of Obstetrics and Gynecology, University of California-Irvine, Orange, California, U.S.A.

Rebecca Stein-Wexler, M.D. ■ Department of Radiology, University of California, Davis Medical Center and U.C. Davis Children's Hospital, Sacramento, California, U.S.A.

Peter D. Stevens, M.D. ■ Department of Clinical Medicine, Columbia University, New York, New York, U.S.A.

James F. Stinchon, M.D. ■ Department of Radiology, Boston University Medical Center, Boston, Massachusetts, U.S.A.

Mitchell E. Tublin, M.D. ■ Department of Radiology, University of Pittsburgh School of Medicine, Pittsburgh, Pennsylvania, U.S.A.

Vijay Viswanathan, M.D. ■ Department of Radiology, Harvard Medical School, Brigham and Women's Hospital, Boston, Massachusetts, U.S.A.

Peter N. T. Wells, F.R.S. ■ The Institute of Medical Engineering and Medical Physics, Cardiff University School of Engineering, Cardiff, U.K.

Annina N. Wilkes, M.D. ■ Department of Radiology, Thomas Jefferson University, Philadelphia, Pennsylvania, U.S.A.

Sandra L. Wootton-Gorges, M.D. ■ Department of Radiology, University of California, Davis Medical Center and U.C. Davis Children's Hospital, Sacramento, California, U.S.A.

Retroperitoneum, Pancreas, Aorta, and Inferior Vena Cava ● *Marijo A. Gillen*

31

RETROPERITONEUM

Normal Anatomy

The retroperitoneum extends from the posterior peritoneum to the posterior body wall. It is bounded superiorly by the diaphragm, inferiorly by the extraperitoneal pelvic musculature, anteriorly by the posterior peritoneum, and posteriorly by the transversalis fascia.

The retroperitoneum at the level of the kidneys is subdivided into three compartments by the renal fascia: the anterior pararenal space, the perirenal space, and the posterior pararenal space (Table 1). The anterior pararenal space extends between the posterior peritoneum and the anterior perirenal fascia bilaterally. It extends across the midline and contains the pancreas, the anterior visceral branches of the aorta, and the retroperitoneal portions of the duodenum and ascending and descending colon.

The perirenal spaces bilaterally are formed by the anterior (Gerota's) and posterior (Zuckerkandl's) perirenal fascia. Classically these spaces were felt not to communicate (1). Several authors have recently suggested that there is a connection in the midline between the right and left perirenal spaces (2–4). The perirenal spaces contain the kidneys, proximal collecting systems, adrenals, and renal vessels. Laterally, the anterior and posterior perirenal fascia join to become the lateral conal fascia (1). The perirenal space is open inferiorly and communicates with the pelvis (2).

The right and left posterior pararenal spaces are located between the posterior perirenal fascia and the transversalis fascia and contain only fat and no organs. Laterally the posterior pararenal space is posterior to the lateral conal fascia.

The aorta and inferior vena cava (IVC) are located in the midline, in a space anterior to the spine, which is continuous with the posterior mediastinum superiorly. Lymph nodes are adjacent to the aorta and IVC. The upper portion of the abdominal aorta is enclosed by the diaphragmatic crura as it goes through the aortic hiatus.

There has been controversy into which compartment to place the aorta and IVC. The perirenal fasciae are felt to join in the midline by a thin, fibrous communication (2–4), which is anterior to the aorta and IVC (5). There is controversy as to whether or not this fascia merges with the connective tissue around the great vessels (6). It has been suggested that the great vessels are in an interfascial plane within the leaves of the retroperitoneal fascia (7–9). The presence of interfascial planes helps to explain how rapidly progressing fluid collections can communicate between compartments (8,9).

Posterior to the transversalis fascia is the posterior abdominal musculature, consisting of the psoas and quadratus lumborum muscles. There is uncertainty in which anatomic space to classify these muscles since by classical definition, they are posterior to the retroperitoneum. However, they are often involved in retroperitoneal processes, since the posterior renal fascia inserts on the psoas fascia (10).

TABLE 1 ■ Compartments of the Retroperitoneum at the Level of the Kidneys

Anterior pararenal space
- Pancreas
- Anterior visceral branches at the abdominal aorta
- Retroperitoneal portions of the duodenum
- Retroperitoneal portions of the ascending colon
- Retroperitoneal portions of the descending colon
- Lymph nodes

Perirenal spaces (bilaterally)
- Kidneys
- Proximal ureters
- Adrenals

Posterior pararenal spaces (bilaterally)
- Fat

Interfascial planes of the retroperitoneum
- Aorta
- Inferior vena cava
- Lymph nodes
- Nerves

Fascial plane posterior to the transversalis fascia
- Psoas muscle
- Quadratus lumborum muscle

Scanning Technique

Evaluation of the retroperitoneum on ultrasound (US) usually consists of evaluation of the various organs in each compartment of the retroperitoneum since the retroperitoneal fascial planes are not seen on US unless involved by disease processes. Spread of disease in the retroperitoneum occurs initially within the anatomic boundaries of the compartments; it is important to evaluate areas that may be slightly remote from an involved organ, if they are connected by fascial planes. However, as noted, spread in atypical locations may be secondary to interfascial planes (8). Infection around the kidneys can track into the pelvis since the perirenal fascia is open caudally.

Lymph nodes, nerves, fat, connective tissue, and small blood vessels also are in the retroperitoneum but are normally too small to visualize, unless pathologically enlarged.

Scanning of the retroperitoneum is usually started with the patient supine using the liver and spleen as acoustic windows and also scanning midline, using gentle pressure to move bowel loops out of the way. Decubitus and prone positioning of the patient may be also helpful.

Pitfalls and Artifacts

The retroperitoneum can be difficult to visualize on US because of bowel gas. Firm pressure on the transducer may be able to move the bowel out of the way, but decubitus or prone scanning may be necessary. If the patient is very large, evaluation of the retroperitoneum is limited and computed tomography (CT) is preferred.

The psoas muscle can be hypoechoic on US, as can the iliacus muscle in the pelvis. These can be mistaken for fluid collections or abscesses. Changing the gain settings may help in showing these are solid; visualization from different positions may demonstrate this appearance to be bilateral.

Pathology

The major categories of disease (other than in the organs) involving the compartments of the retroperitoneum (including the psoas and quadratus lumborum musculature) are hemorrhage, infection, lymphadenopathy, and neoplasm.

Hemorrhage

On US, acute blood is echogenic; with age the hemorrhage evolves, and can have various appearances including isoechoic, hypoechoic, or anechoic (if it liquefies). As it evolves, and liquefies, it may have debris, thick septa, or layering components. If there is calcification in the hematoma, echogenicities may be present which will shadow when of a sufficient size. Acute echogenic clot can be distinguished from solid masses by its posterior enhancement.

Retroperitoneal hemorrhage can be caused by trauma, hematologic disorders (hemophilia, thrombocytopenia), anticoagulation (iatrogenic or from liver disease), or neoplasms. Traumatic hemorrhage can occur from laceration of any of the retroperitoneal organs such as kidneys, ureters, adrenals, pancreas, or retroperitoneal bowel, or from rupture of the major blood vessels (aorta or IVC) or branches (including spinal branches) or from intramuscular hemorrhage into the psoas, iliacus, quadratus lumborum, or paraspinal muscles. Hemorrhage can track into the retroperitoneum from dissection of blood leaking from a femoral artery catheterization. Retroperitoneal hemorrhage can also occur from bleeding from neoplasms, particularly renal angiomyolipoma, adrenal cortical adenocarcinoma, Wilms' tumor, neuroblastoma (11,12). Retroperitoneal hemorrhage can also be caused by bleeding after a percutaneous renal (Fig. 1) or pancreatic biopsy after percutaneous nephrostomy placement, after translumbar aortography, or in patients with vasculitis.

On color Doppler images, acute extravasation in a retroperitoneal hemorrhage can be detected as flow within a hematoma. Microbubble contrast-enhanced ultrasound (CEUS) can show flow in an active extravasation.

Infection

Infection in the retroperitoneum generally extends from infection of adjacent organs. It can manifest as nonspecific fluid tracking in the retroperitoneal spaces or as a retroperitoneal abscess. A retroperitoneal abscess on US is usually a complex collection containing a combination of fluid, debris, septa, and solid components of varying echogenicity; it exhibits posterior acoustic enhancement and may have a thick rim and debris.

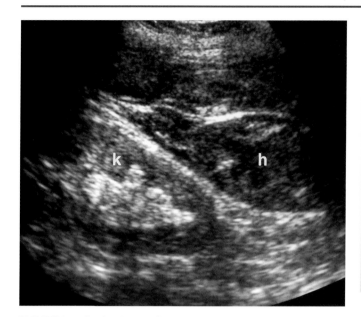

FIGURE 1 ■ Sagittal image of a patient with bleeding after a percutaneous renal biopsy shows a heterogeneous collection adjacent to the kidney (k) consistent with a hematoma (h). *Source*: Courtesy of A. Fried, University of Kentucky.

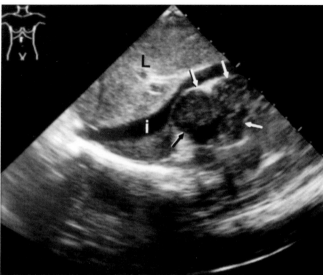

FIGURE 2 ■ Sagittal view of a child with Wilms' tumor and retroperitoneal lymphadenopathy causing anterior displacement of the IVC by a large lobular nodal mass (*arrows*). i, inferior vena cava; L, liver. *Source*: Courtesy of A. Fried, University of Kentucky.

Retroperitoneal abscesses usually require drainage, either surgical or percutaneous. Spread of infection usually occurs along compartmental planes.

Infection or inflammation from the pancreas (pancreatitis, pancreatic pseudocysts, pancreatic infection, or abscess), from the retroperitoneal portions of the duodenum (duodenal perforation or abscess), or from the retroperitoneal portions of the ascending and descending colon (colitis or diverticulitis) can extend across the midline in the anterior pararenal space. In the perirenal space infection developing in one kidney can spread to the other side across the midline.

Lymphadenopathy

On US, normal size lymph nodes (<1 cm in shortest diameter) are not usually identified. Enlarged lymph nodes are seen on US as hypoechoic or isoechoic round or ovoid masses; if lymph nodes are confluent, they appear as homogeneous, lobulated, hypoechoic masses, often with some posterior enhancement. Some pathological lymph nodes can appear anechoic and mimic cysts, especially if there is posterior enhancement.

Retroperitoneal lymphadenopathy often occurs along the IVC and aorta or in the retrocrural space. When the aorta or IVC are anteriorly displaced from the spine (except for the superior aspect of the IVC as it courses into the right atrium), a mass or lymphadenopathy should be suspected (Fig. 2). Causes include infection [AIDS or other immunodeficiency states (Fig. 3)] and neoplasm, either primary lymphoma or metastatic. Sources of metastases are commonly renal cancer [renal cell carcinoma, Wilms' tumor (Fig. 4)], adrenal cortical carcinoma, neuroblastoma (Fig. 5), and gynecologic and testicular neoplasms.

Retroperitoneal Cysts

Retroperitoneal cysts have been reported (13,14). Reported etiologies are urogenital, mesothelial, enteric, teratomas, parasitic, and lymphatic.

Retroperitoneal Neoplasms

Primary tumors of the retroperitoneum include lipoma, liposarcoma (Fig. 6), teratomas, myxoid liposarcoma, malignant fibrous histiocytoma, neurogenic tumors

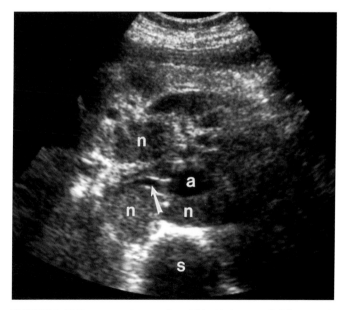

FIGURE 3 ■ Transverse image of a child with immunodeficiency with widespread retroperitoneal lymphadenopathy anteriorly displacing the aorta and anteriorly displacing and narrowing the IVC (*arrow*). a, aorta; n, lymphadenopathy; s, spine. *Source*: Courtesy of A. Fried, University of Kentucky.

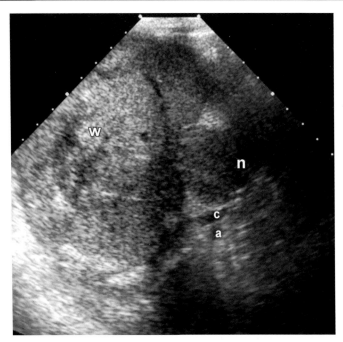

FIGURE 4 ■ Transverse image of a child with large retroperitoneal Wilms' tumor compressing the IVC and displacing it toward the right with a large nodal mass anterior to the IVC and aorta. w, Wilms' tumor; c, IVC; n, nodal mass; a, aorta.

(schwannoma, neurofibroma, ganglioneuroma, ganglioneuroblastoma, paraganglioma, malignant peripheral nerve sheath tumor), desmoid tumor, hemangiopericytoma, leiomyoma, leiomyosarcoma, malignant pericytoma, rhabdomyosarcoma, malignant mesenchymoma, lymphangiomas, lymphomas, primitive neuroectodermal tumor, or leiomyomatosis (15–25).

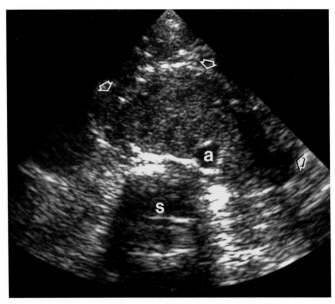

FIGURE 5 ■ Transverse image of a child with neuroblastoma with retroperitoneal spread causing a mass (*open arrows*) surrounding most of the aorta and displacing it to the left. a, aorta; s, spine. *Source*: Courtesy of A. Fried, University of Kentucky.

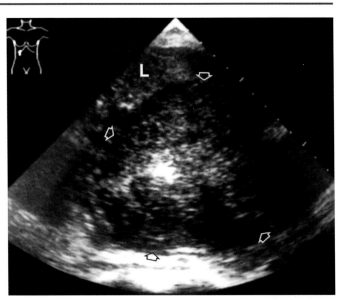

FIGURE 6 ■ A large heterogeneous retroperitoneal mass (*open arrows*) in a patient with a retroperitoneal liposarcoma. Central increased echogenicity was secondary to fat but could also be seen with hematoma. L, liver. *Source*: Courtesy of A. Fried, University of Kentucky.

On US, most of these appear as heterogeneous, sometimes complex, masses within the retroperitoneum. CT can be helpful in defining the overall extent of the mass as well as to distinguish certain characteristics such as fatty or myxoid elements (15), which may narrow the differential. However, a biopsy is usually needed.

PANCREAS

Embryology

The pancreas develops from two pancreatic buds—the dorsal bud and the ventral bud. The dorsal bud develops in the dorsal mesentery as a diverticula of the foregut. The ventral bud develops in the ventral mesentery as an invagination of the biliary-duodenal angle. With growth, the ventral pancreas rotates posterior to the duodenum to lie inferior to the dorsal pancreas. The two anlagen fuse to form the pancreas. The dorsal bud becomes most of the pancreas while the ventral bud becomes the uncinate process and the caudal portion of the pancreatic head. After fusion, a new duct connects the proximal and mid dorsal duct to the ventral duct to form the main pancreatic duct or duct of Wirsung, which enters into the duodenum at the major papilla. The distal part of the dorsal pancreatic duct is the duct of Santorini and can persist as an accessory pancreatic duct entering the duodenum at the minor papilla.

Normal Anatomy

The pancreas is mostly in the retroperitoneum, within the anterior pararenal space. There is a small bare area of the pancreas resulting from the reflection of two leaves of the posterior peritoneum forming the transverse

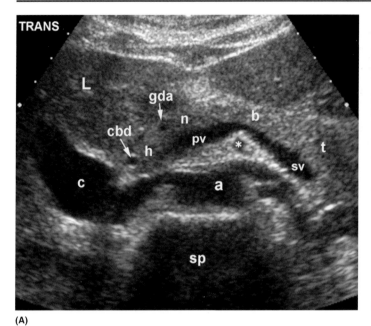

(A)

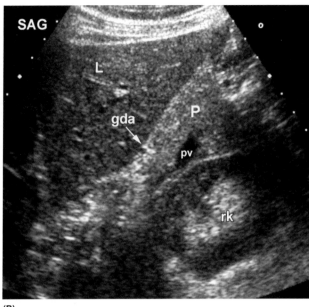

(B)

FIGURE 7 A AND B ■ Normal pancreas. Echotexture is coarse and homogeneous and slightly greater than that of the liver. (A) Transverse. (B) Sagittal. Most of the pancreas can be visualized on the transverse image, but only the pancreatic head is seen on the sagittal image. L, liver; P, pancreas; h, head of the pancreas; n, neck of the pancreas; b, body of the pancreas; t, tail of the pancreas; sv, splenic vein; pv, portal confluence; c, IVC; a, aorta; gda, gastroduodenal artery; cbd, common bile duct; rk, right kidney; sp, spine; sma, superior mesenteric artery; *, sma, surrounded by echogenic fat.

mesocolon (which is the posterior–inferior margin of the lesser sac) (26). The transverse mesocolon attaches to the anterior aspect of the head and body of the gland; the root of the small bowel mesentery is inferior to the pancreatic body but is contiguous with the transverse mesocolon. The tail of the pancreas is actually an intraperitoneal structure within the leaves of the splenorenal ligament. These relationships are important in the spread of disease from the pancreas.

In the adult, the pancreas measures approximately 15 to 25 cm in length, 3 to 5 cm in height, and 1.5 to 3.5 cm in thickness (26). The pancreas consists of a head, neck, body, and tail (Fig. 7). The right lateral aspect of the head of the pancreas is in a constant relationship to the "C" loop of the duodenum. The splenic vein forms the posterior margin of the pancreas, joining the superior mesenteric vein (SMV) at the level of the pancreatic head and neck to form the portal vein. The uncinate process projects medial from the pancreatic head, lying posterior to the portal confluence (Fig. 8). The neck is the thinnest portion and is posterior to the stomach pylorus and anterior to the junction of the SMV and splenic vein. The gland thickens slightly as it becomes the body.

The tail extends within the splenorenal ligament to the splenic hilum. The stomach antrum and body lie anterior to the pancreatic body and tail and are separated from the pancreas by the potential space of the lesser sac. The third and fourth portions of the duodenum are inferior and posterior to the pancreatic head and body. The

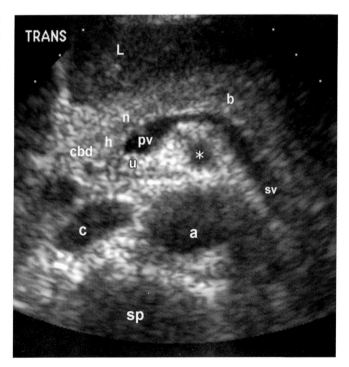

FIGURE 8 ■ Transverse image of a normal pancreas showing the uncinate process extending posteriorly to the portal confluence. L, liver; h, head of the pancreas; n, neck of the pancreas; b, body of the pancreas; u, uncinate process of the pancreas; sv, splenic vein; pv, portal conflunce; c, IVC; a, aorta; sma, superior mesenteric artery; cbd, common bile duct; sp, spine; *, sma, surrounded by echogenic fat.

right kidney is posterior and lateral to the pancreatic head, while the left kidney and adrenal are posterior and slightly inferior to the pancreatic tail. The celiac axis is superior to the pancreatic body, and the tortuous splenic artery lies superior to the body and tail. The aorta and the origin of the proximal portion of the superior mesenteric artery (SMA) are posterior to the pancreatic body. The SMA can be recognized by the echogenic mesenteric fat surrounding it. The IVC is posterior to the pancreatic head.

On US, the pancreas can be recognized by anatomic landmarks. The gastroduodenal artery (GDA) is at the anterior aspect of the pancreatic neck. The common bile duct is located in the posterior aspect of the pancreatic head (or close to the posterior border). On a transverse image of the pancreatic head on gray scale, two circular anechoic structures are seen: the anterior is the GDA and the posterior is the common bile duct (Fig. 9). On color Doppler, flow will be seen in the anterior structure, the GDA. The portal confluence and splenic vein are posterior.

The pancreatic duct can often be seen in normal patients. This is seen either as a thin echogenic line in the middle of the gland or as a tubular structure with echogenic walls and an anechoic lumen (Fig. 10). The walls of the lumen should be parallel and the internal diameter of the lumen can measure up to 2.5 mm (not including the walls) or 3 mm including the walls. Arterial supply to the pancreas is from branches of the celiac

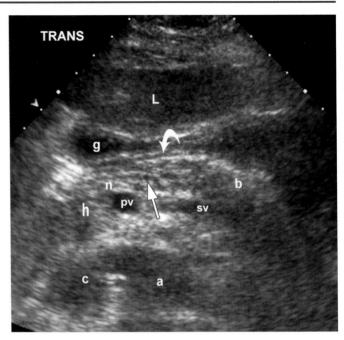

FIGURE 10 ■ Transverse scan of the pancreas showing a normal size pancreatic duct seen as a tubular structure with echogenic wall (*arrow*) and an anechoic lumen. Note also the hypoechoic posterior wall of the stomach (*curved arrow*) which could be mistaken for the pancreatic duct. L, liver; h, head of the pancreas; n, neck of the pancreas; b, body of the pancreas; sv, splenic vein; pv, portal confluence; c, IVC; a, aorta; g, gastric antrum.

artery and SMA. Venous drainage is by the SMV, splenic vein, and portal vein.

On US, the normal pancreas is homogeneous and slightly coarse, with an echogenicity equal to or greater than that of the liver in adults (Fig. 11). In infants or young children, the echogenicity of the pancreas can be less than that of the liver (since there is less pancreatic fat). The pancreas is larger in young patients and decreases in size with age. With age (starting at the fifth decade) there is gradual fatty involution of the pancreas with some fibrosis that causes increased echogenicity (Fig. 12), sometimes causing the pancreas to be indistinct from the retroperitoneal fat.

The pancreas can have varying shapes: some of the more common are tadpole shaped, dumbbell shaped, and sausage shaped (26). The contour of the pancreas is smooth with homogeneous echotexture; this can be distinguished from masses or enlargement from neoplasm or infection, which have a more abrupt transition and change in texture (more hypoechoic) than the remainder of the gland.

The uncinate process can have varying contours but should be tapered and sharply pointed or convex. If the uncinate is rounded, enlarged, blunted, or concave, a mass should be suspected.

The size of the pancreas also varies with age and shape of the pancreas. Maximum anteroposterior (AP) diameter of the pancreas ranges from 2.5 to 3.5 cm for the head, 2.0 to 2.5 cm for the body, and 2.2 to 3.5 cm for the tail (27).

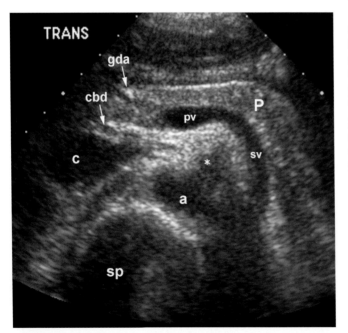

FIGURE 9 ■ Normal transverse image of the pancreas showing the two circular anechoic areas in the head. The anterior one is the gastroduodenal artery and will show flow on color Doppler images. The posterior anechoic area is the common bile duct and will not show flow on Doppler. P, pancreas; sv, splenic vein; pv, portal confluence; c, IVC; a, aorta; sma, superior mesenteric artery; gda, gastroduodenal artery; cbd, common bile duct; sp, spine; *, sma, surrounded by echogenic fat.

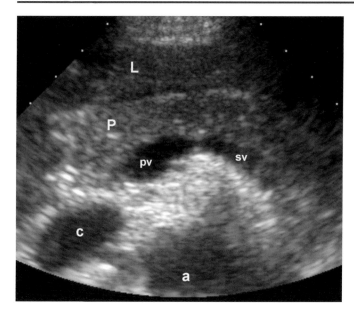

FIGURE 11 ■ Transverse image of a normal hypoechoic pancreas in a young patient. L, liver; sv, splenic vein; pv, portal confluence; c, IVC; a, aorta; P, pancreas.

Scanning Technique

Scanning of the pancreas is started in the supine position with the highest frequency transducer that provides adequate penetration. In adults, this is generally 3 to 4 MHz but in children or thin adults, a 5 MHz transducer can be used. The spine and great vessels should be identified to ensure good penetration. Scans are performed in transverse, sagittal, and oblique planes to adequately visualize the entire gland. The left lobe of the liver is a good acoustic window for the pancreas. Portions of the liver should be included so comparison of pancreatic echotexture to that of the liver can be made. The pancreatic tail may be visualized using the left kidney posteriorly or the spleen as an acoustic window.

Microbubble contrast agents have been used to evaluate the pancreas. The pancreas shows bright homogeneous enhancement with prompt washout (28).

Pitfalls and Artifacts

If the left lobe of the liver is small, visualization of the pancreas may be difficult. Bowel gas interferes with visualization of the pancreas. Sometimes this can be overcome by firm pressure on the transducer to move the gas out of the way; curved array transducers may help. Giving the patient water to drink (8–12 oz) can displace air from the stomach and duodenum. Initially, this can cause increased echogenicity because of microbubbles but after a few minutes the bubbles disappear leaving a good acoustic window. Imaging the patient during ingestion of water in a semi-upright position or moving the patient to a right lateral decubitus position (to fill the second portion of the duodenum) may also be helpful.

The posterior wall of the stomach can be mistaken for the pancreatic duct; the posterior wall has a hyperechoic mucosal layer with a hypoechoic muscularis layer that can look like the interface of the pancreatic duct. However, there is pancreas on both sides of the pancreatic duct but only posterior to the posterior wall of the stomach (Figs. 10 and 13).

Although the pancreas is usually homogeneous in echotexture, it does originate from two different buds: the dorsal and ventral. The ventral bud gives rise to the caudal

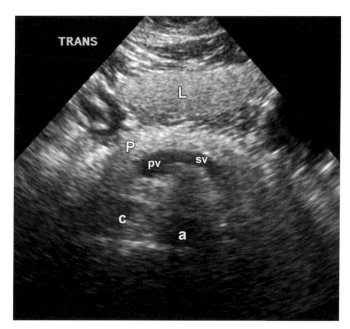

FIGURE 12 ■ Transverse image of an echogenic pancreas that can be seen with age and fatty involution. Note also that the liver is echogenic consistent with fatty infiltration. L, liver; sv, splenic vein; pv, portal confluence; c, IVC; a, aorta; P, pancreas.

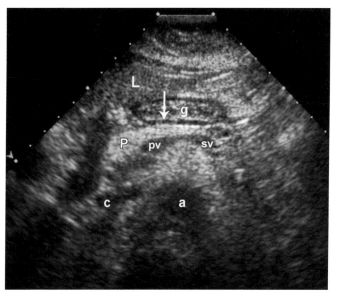

FIGURE 13 ■ Transverse image of the pancreas showing a normal gastric antrum anteriorly. Note the hypoechoic wall of the stomach (*arrow*); the posterior wall has pancreas only at its posterior aspect, whereas a normal pancreatic duct will be surrounded on both sides by pancreas (Fig. 10). L, liver; sv, splenic vein; pv, portal confluence; c, IVC; a, aorta; g, gastric antrum; P, pancreas.

portion of the head and the uncinate process; this has decreased fat content and may appear hypoechoic. This could be mistaken for a mass; however, the contour of the gland is normal and there is no compression of the common bile duct (29).

If the liver has increased echogenicity, as can be seen with fatty infiltration, the pancreas can appear hypoechoic in comparison. In these cases, when comparison of the liver echogenicity is made to the right kidney, the liver is seen to be very echogenic and the portal triads of the liver are not well seen.

If the liver is very hypoechoic, as can be seen in viral hepatitis, the pancreas can appear too echogenic. This can be suspected by evaluating the portal triads of the liver, which would be unusually bright ("starry night" appearance).

Variants

Fusion abnormalities of the ventral and dorsal pancreatic buds lead to pancreas divisum, annular and semiannular pancreas, heterotopic pancreatic tissue, and other anomalies such as a bifid pancreas (30).

In pancreas divisum, the dorsal and ventral ducts do not fuse. The pancreatic head and uncinate process are drained by the duct of Wirsung through the major papilla, and the pancreatic body and tail are drained by the duct of Santorini through the minor papilla; there is no communication between these ducts. This can lead to recurrent pancreatitis.

Annular pancreas occurs when pancreatic tissue persists on the lateral side of the duodenum, forming a ring around the duodenum, which can obstruct. On US, this can be seen as a nonspecific enlargement of the pancreatic head (31).

Pathology

Pancreatitis

Acute Pancreatitis ■ Pancreatitis can be classified into acute and chronic. Acute pancreatitis is separated into mild acute pancreatitis and severe acute pancreatitis.

Causes of acute pancreatitis are alcohol abuse, cholelithiasis, peptic ulcer disease, postoperative [including post endoscopic retrograde cholangiopancreatography (ERCP), posttrauma, postbiopsy], hyperparathyroidism, pregnancy, hyperlipidemia, hypercalcemia, hereditary pancreatitis, infection, or autoimmune. Some drugs can cause pancreatitis; these include azathioprine, thiazide diuretics, sulfonamides, estrogens, and corticosteroids (Table 2) (32).

In mild acute pancreatitis, the symptoms are predominately pain, vomiting, and abdominal tenderness. Laboratory results show elevated amylase and lipase. On US in early or very mild pancreatitis, the pancreas may appear normal. Subsequently, the pancreas can become diffusely enlarged and edematous with diffusely decreased echogenicity (Fig. 14). Focal enlargement can also occur, usually involving the head and proximal body (Fig. 14). Isolated enlargement of the pancreatic tail is unusual in acute pancreatitis and is suspicious for a neoplasm.

TABLE 2 ■ Causes of Pancreatitis

Biliary disease
  Cholelithiasis
  Choledocholithiasis
  Choledochocele

Drugs
  Alcohol
  Azathioprine
  Thiazide diuretics
  Sulfonamides
  Estrogens
  Corticosteroids
  Tetracycline
  Phenformin
  Procainamide
  Asparaginase
  Procainamide
  Furosemide
  Ethacrynic acid
  Narcotics

Infection
  Viral (mumps, measles, mononucleosis, AIDS, CMV)
  Parasites (ascariasis, clonorchis)

Pancreatic etiology
  Autoimmune
  Hereditary pancreatitis
  Annular pancreas
  Trauma
  Papillary stenosis
  Cystic fibrosis
  Tropical pancreatitis

Systemic processes
  Hypercalcemia (hyperparathyroidism, sarcoidosis, amyloidosis)
  Hyperlipidemia
  Hypercholesterolemia
  Alcohol abuse
  Peptic ulcer disease
  Hyperparathyroidism
  Kwashiorkor
  Vasculitis such as polyarteritis nodosa

Injury
  Trauma
  ■ Blunt trauma
  ■ Penetrating trauma
  ■ Penetrating gastric ulcer
  Iatrogenic
  ■ Post-ERCP or endoscopy
  ■ Postbiopsy
  ■ Postsurgery
  ■ Postbiliary stenting
  ■ Percutaneous transhepatic cholangiopancreatography
  ■ Cardiac catheterization (from emboli)

Neoplasms
  Pancreatic neoplasm
  Duodenal neoplasm
  Invasion by tumor in adjacent organs
  Ampullary neoplasm
  Lymphoma

Idiopathic

Abbreviations: CMV, cytomegalovirus; ERCP, endoscopic retrograde cholangiopancreatography.
Source: From Ref. 32.

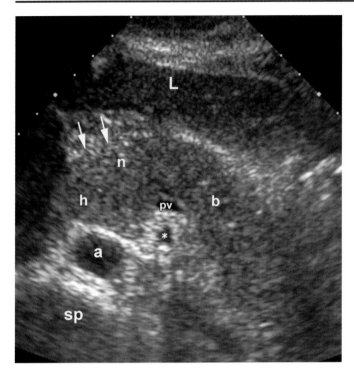

FIGURE 14 ■ Transverse image of patient with acute pancreatitis showing a hypoechoic edematous pancreas with an enlarged head and neck and an indistinct ventral margin (*arrows*). L, liver; h, head of the pancreas; n, neck of the pancreas; b, body of the pancreas; pv, portal confluence; a, aorta; sp, spine; sma, superior mesenteric artery; *, sma, surrounded by echogenic fat.

Patients with mild acute pancreatitis recover without complications or other organ involvement. Progression to severe acute pancreatitis is rare.

Severe acute pancreatitis manifests with more severe symptoms such as hypotension, gastrointestinal (GI) bleeding, pulmonary insufficiency, renal failure, and ecchymotic areas of the flank (Grey Turner's sign) or in the periumbilical region (Cullen's sign). Patients with severe acute pancreatitis have multisystem failure, pancreatic necrosis, or other complications such as hemorrhage, abscess, or pseudoaneurysm formation.

Associated sonographic findings in acute pancreatitis are peripancreatic fluid collections, pancreatic inflammation, mild dilatation of the pancreatic duct, heterogeneous echogenicity of the pancreas, perivascular inflammation (some fluid near the SMV, splenic vein, or confluence), an indistinct ventral margin of the pancreas (Fig. 14), a left pleural effusion, and venous thrombosis (33). Finstad et al. (33), in a study of 71 patients, found that the three most common sonographic findings in acute pancreatitis were hypoechoic extrapancreatic inflammation (60%), pancreatic parenchymal inhomogeneity (56%), and decreased gland echogenicity (44%).

In acute pancreatitis, US is useful to detect biliary abnormalities as an etiology for pancreatitis, to evaluate for signs of more severe pancreatitis such as necrosis that may be better evaluated by CT, and later to follow up complications such as pseudocysts. CT has been found to accurately stage acute pancreatitis, detect complications, and detect pancreatic necrosis. Balthazar (34) has developed a CT severity index which is superior to previous classification systems such as Ranson and Acute Physiology, and Chronic Health Evaluation (APACHE) II in predicting outcomes (35).

Complications of Acute Pancreatitis ■ Pancreatic necrosis is best seen at CT; it can become secondarily infected. Pancreatic hemorrhage can be detected as focal areas of increased echogenicity; it can be complicated by infection. Peripancreatic inflammation is seen as decreased echogenicity in the surrounding fat and as hypoechoic densities in the fat.

The mild peripancreatic fluid densities in acute pancreatitis may resolve but can persist and develop into pseudocysts after six weeks when a fibrous lining develops (Fig. 15A). Pseudocysts are also seen in chronic pancreatitis. They are of varying sizes, are round to ovoid, and have a visible wall. They can be anechoic or may have debris or septa. Some can spontaneously resolve but drainage may be required, either percutaneously (Fig. 15B) or with surgery.

Fluid collections and pseudocysts can be found commonly adjacent to the pancreas, within the pancreas, around the spleen, lesser sac, perirenal areas, or in the mesentery, but can also occur in the mediastinum or pelvis. These can become infected, develop into an abscess, rupture, or cause a pseudoaneurysm.

Pseudoaneurysms occur when an arterial wall is disrupted from digestion by pancreatic enzymes. Common sites are the splenic artery, GDA, pancreatoduodenal arteries, or left gastric artery. Doppler images show pulsatile flow in a cystic mass.

Venous thrombosis can occur in the adjacent vessels, usually in the SMV, in the splenic vein, or in the portal vein or branches. This can be detected by color Doppler.

Rupture of a pseudocyst into the abdomen causes pancreatic ascites and can cause peritonitis.

Pancreatic abscesses can develop from infected peripancreatic fluid or infection of a pseudocyst; air within the abscess can be seen on US as echogenic areas with "dirty shadowing." These require drainage either percutaneous or surgical.

Chronic Pancreatitis ■ After repeated episodes of pancreatitis, there is progressive parenchymal destruction. Etiologies are alcohol abuse, hyperlipidemia, hereditary, autoimmune, or hyperparathyroidism. The pancreas commonly decreases in size, the duct becomes dilated, and calcifications are seen in the gland.

On US, the pancreas shows heterogeneous echotexture, irregular margins, ductal dilatation, and echogenic foci representing calculi in the pancreatic tissue or pancreatic duct. Echogenicity can be increased, normal, or decreased (especially with acute episodes). The pancreatic size may be small, normal, or focally or diffusely enlarged (36).

Focal pancreatic enlargement in chronic pancreatitis can be secondary to a fibrotic mass (36) or secondary to an acute episode of pancreatitis. These can be difficult to

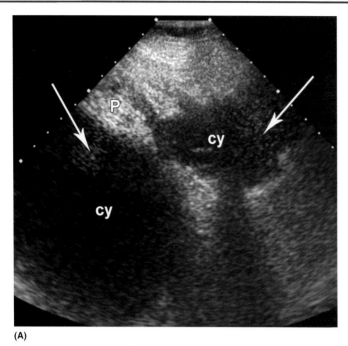

(A)

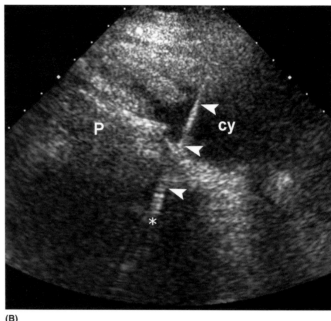

(B)

FIGURE 15 A AND B ■ Transverse image of a large bilobed pancreatic pseudocyst replacing most of the pancreatic body and tail. This contains echogenic material consistent with debris. (**A**) Predrainage. (**B**) Image obtained during percutaneous drainage shows the catheter containing an echogenic stilette placed with the pseudocyst. P, pancreas; cy, pseudocyst. *Arrows*, debris; *arrowheads*, catheter; *, tip of stilette.

distinguish from a neoplasm with ductal dilation, particularly in the pancreatic head, since chronic pancreatitis predisposes to carcinoma. Biopsy may be necessary.

Pancreatic ductal dilatation is often seen in chronic pancreatitis; the duct can be smooth, irregular, or beaded. A beaded or irregular appearance is most common and characteristic since smooth ductal enlargement can also be associated with obstruction from a carcinoma (37). Pseudocysts may be present and pseudoaneurysms and venous thrombosis can also occur.

In many cases, chronic pancreatitis can be difficult to distinguish from carcinoma of the pancreatic head, since both can show ductal dilatation, a focal mass, cyst-like areas, calcifications, and venous thrombosis (38). Calcifications are less likely in pancreatic adenocarcinoma (39). Koito et al. evaluated patients with inflammatory pancreatic masses and patients with ductal carcinoma with carbon dioxide microbubble enhanced US and found that 95% of the inflammatory pancreatic masses were isovascular and 91% of the ductal adenocarcinomas were hypovascular (40).

Groove Pancreatitis ■ Groove pancreatitis is a form of segmental chronic pancreatitis occurring at the space between the head of the pancreas, the duodenum, and the common bile duct (41).

In the pure form of groove pancreatitis only the groove is involved and the pancreatic parenchyma and main pancreatic duct are normal. It is caused by a scar plate in the groove. The scar plate causes abnormal duodenal motility, duodenal stenosis, and tubular stenosis of the common bile duct.

In the segmental form of groove pancreatitis, the pancreatic head is involved as well as the groove and there is stenosis of the duct of Santorini but sparing of the duct of Wirsung (42). It can be associated with abnormalities of the duct of Santorini, including pancreatic heterotopia (43). US shows a hypoechoic mass in the groove.

Pancreatic head carcinoma can also occur in this groove and the distinction between groove pancreatitis and groove pancreatic adenocarcinoma is difficult; biopsy is often necessary (44).

Autoimmune Pancreatitis ■ Autoimmune pancreatitis is a chronic inflammatory condition of the pancreas that can be associated with other autoimmune diseases (45). On US, there is diffuse, sausage-like pancreatic enlargement or focal enlargement (46); the pancreatic duct is irregular and narrowed with areas of stricture and strictures of the common bile duct (47). There is lymphoplasmacytic (48) infiltration of the pancreatic parenchyma. Other autoimmune diseases that have been associated include Sjogren syndrome, primary sclerosing cholangitis, primary biliary cirrhosis, ulcerative colitis, and systemic lupus erythematosus. Cases have been reported of associated retroperitoneal fibrosis (49). Autoimmune pancreatitis usually responds to steroid therapy.

Cystic Fibrosis

Cystic fibrosis causes diffuse fatty replacement of pancreatic parenchyma. This causes diffuse increased echogenicity on US. This is especially noted in children, in whom the pancreas is normally hypoechoic (50). Pancreatic cysts are more common in patients with cystic fibrosis (51).

Pancreatic Neoplasms

Pancreatic neoplasms can be divided into exocrine, endocrine, and nonepithelial origins (Table 3) (52).

Pancreatic Adenocarcinoma ■ Pancreatic adenocarcinoma arises from ductal epithelium and accounts for approximately 90% of all pancreatic neoplasms. It is twice as common in men and the age of occurrence is usually between 60 and 80. Location is more frequent in the pancreatic head (up to 60%) (52) than in the body or tail but can be diffuse. Those in the head of the pancreas are often detected earlier because of symptoms of common bile duct obstruction. On US, adenocarcinomas present as focal masses, often hypoechoic although some are hyperechoic, isoechoic, or heterogeneous (Fig. 16) (53). Other US findings include smooth dilatation of the pancreatic duct (more common in malignancy than beaded or irregular), the "double duct" sign (Fig. 17) (with dilation of both the common duct and pancreatic duct by masses in the head of the pancreas or ampulla), focal distortion of pancreatic contour, convex rounded borders of the uncinate process, or pancreatitis. Involvement of the fat in the mesentery around the SMA can be seen with carcinoma. It can be difficult to distinguish a mass from pancreatic adenocarcinoma from a mass produced by focal pancreatitis, by either clinical or radiologic means and biopsy is often necessary.

CEUS helps to increase visibility of hypoechoic tumors; adenocarcinomas show less enhancement than adjacent parenchyma but some inflammatory masses can also show the same enhancement (54).

Doppler US can be used to detect complications of adenocarcinoma including thrombosis of the SMV, splenic vein, or portal vein. US can also detect adjacent lymphadenopathy and liver metastases.

Serous (Microcystic) Pancreatic Neoplasm ■ Serous (microcystic) pancreatic neoplasm occurs more frequently in women, with age approximately 60 years. It appears as a well-circumscribed mass, round or oval, and contain multiple small cysts. Procacci et al. (55) identified three subtypes: microlacunar, macrolacunar, and mixed. The microlacunar type has multiple small cysts with septa, a central scar, and calcifications. This appears on US as an echogenic mass (since the cysts are too small to be resolved) (Fig. 18) with occasionally an echogenic scar, which may calcify. In the macrolacunar pattern, large cysts are seen which can be unilocular or multilocular and are difficult to distinguish from mucinous tumors. US shows a large cyst with or without septa which may be multilocular. The mixed type shows both large and small cysts. Serous tumors are usually benign but a few malignant cases have been reported (56).

Mucinous (Macrocystic) Pancreatic Neoplasm ■ Mucinous (macrocystic) neoplasm of the pancreas occurs most often in females, who are younger than those with pancreatic adenocarcinoma and in an age group of approximately 40 to 60 years. Location is more common in the pancreatic tail and lesions tend to be large at the time of diagnosis. US shows a well-circumscribed cystic mass which can be unilocular or multilocular, can be thick walled, and may have septa or mural nodules (Fig. 19). Calcification can be seen in the septa or mural nodules. Cysts are usually larger than 2 cm. These tumors do not communicate with the pancreatic duct or branches. Distinction between benign and malignant can be difficult. There is a continuum between benign, dysplastic, and invasive malignant (57). These should be considered malignant until proven otherwise. Invasion of adjacent structures or papillary projections into the cysts suggest malignancy. If these are unilocular, they can mimic simple cysts.

Intraductal Papillary Mucinous Tumors ■ Intraductal papillary mucinous tumors (IPMTs) can be classified into main branch type and side branch type or a combination.

TABLE 3 ■ Pancreatic Neoplasms

Exocrine

Ductal cell origin
  Ductal adenocarcinoma
  Ductectatic mucinous tumor
  Cystic neoplasm
    Serous (microcystic) neoplasm
    Mucinous (macrocystic) neoplasm
  Solid and papillary epithelial neoplasm

Acinar cell origin
  Acinar cell carcinoma
  Acinar cell cystadenocarcinoma

Indeterminate origin
  Pancreatoblastoma

Endocrine

Nonfunctioning islet cell tumor
Functioning islet cell tumor
  Insulinoma
  Glucagonoma
  Gastrinoma
  Somatostatinoma
  VIPoma

Nonepithelial origin

Lymphoma
  Primary
  Secondary

Metastases
  Melanoma
  Renal cell
  Lung
  Breast
  Ovarian
  HCC
  Sarcoma

Abbreviations: HCC, hepatocellular carcinoma; VIPoma, vasoactive intestinal polypeptide.
Source: From Ref. 52.

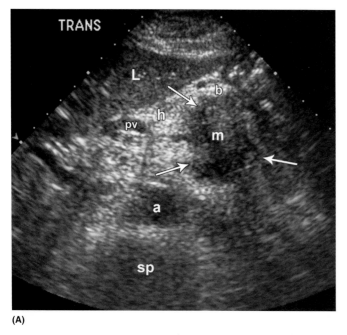

(A)

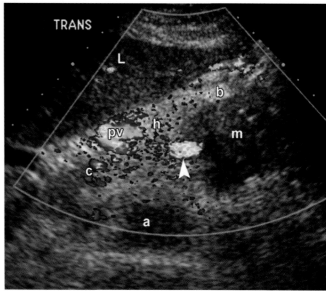

(B)

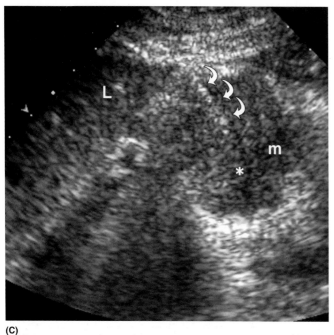

(C)

FIGURE 16 A–C ■ Transverse oblique image showing a 5 cm mass in the body of the pancreas, which is hypovascular on color Doppler images. Note that the intrahepatic ducts are not dilated since this mass is in the body of the pancreas, not in the head. (**A**) Gray scale image. (**B**) Color Doppler image. (**C**) Gray scale image during biopsy of the mass showing the needle (*curved arrows*) within the mass; this was proven to be pancreatic adenocarcinoma. L, liver; h, head of the pancreas; b, body of the pancreas; pv, portal confluence; a, aorta; sp, spine; c, IVC; IVC, inferior vena cava; m, mass; *, needletip; arrows, outline of margins of the mass; *arrowhead*, branch of hepatic artery.

These are more common in men, with age 60 to 70 years (58). In main duct tumors, US shows segmental or diffuse dilatation of the pancreatic duct and pancreatic atrophy. Echogenic filling defects correspond to mucin but, because they fill the duct, may be difficult to distinguish from the pancreatic parenchyma (59).

With branch duct tumors, US shows a focal cystic mass with some septae and occasional echogenic material (corresponding to mucin). They are commonly located in the uncinate process or pancreatic head but can occur elsewhere (60). The main duct can be dilated. They are histologically a spectrum from benign to dysplastic to malignant. Diagnostic distinction from chronic pancreatitis can be difficult. ERCP aids in the diagnosis (61).

Endocrine Tumors ■ Endocrine tumors of the pancreas are functional (islet cell) or nonfunctional. Functional tumors produce hormones and include insulinoma, glucagonoma, somatostatinoma, vasoactive intestinal polypeptide (VIPoma), and gastrinoma. Nonfunctioning tumors usually do not produce clinical symptoms until they become very large. A tumor secreting pancreatic polypeptide, a PPoma, is usually nonfunctional.

Functional tumors tend to be small (<2 cm) and are hypoechoic or isoechoic with the remainder of the pancreas. CEUS shows increased enhancement of the islet cell tumor as compared with the remainder of the pancreas (54). Interoperative US can be helpful in locating the tumor (Fig. 20). Some islet cell tumors (between 4% and

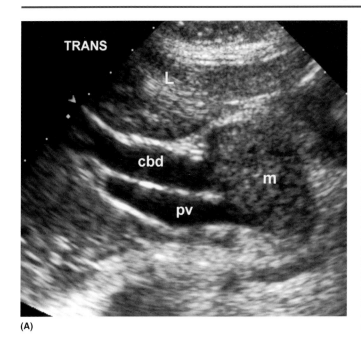

(A)

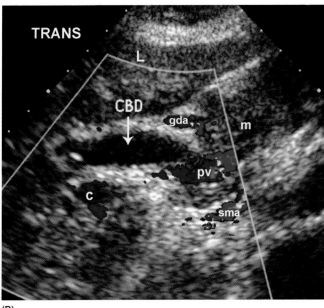

(B)

FIGURE 17 A AND B ■ Transverse images through the head of the pancreas show a 3.5 × 2.0 cm hypoechoic mass in the head of pancreas dilating the common bile duct. The mass is hypovascular and was found to be pancreatic adenocarcinoma. There was intrahepatic ductal dilatation and dilatation of the proximal pancreatic duct. (**A**) Gray scale images. (**B**) Color Doppler images. L, liver; pv, portal vein; c, IVC; gda, gastroduodenal artery; cbd, common bile duct; m, mass; sma, superior mesenteric artery. *Source*: Courtesy of A. Fried, University of Kentucky.

30%) are cystic. They are usually larger than the solid type and have associated calcifications (62).

Solid and Papillary Epithelial Neoplasm ■ Solid and papillary epithelial neoplasms of the pancreas is an uncommon

tumor usually seen in young women. It can be located in the pancreatic head, body, or tail. There is a low malignant potential. The tumor presents as a large heterogeneous mass with variable areas of cystic change. It is often surrounded by a thick pseudocapsule that enhances with CEUS (63).

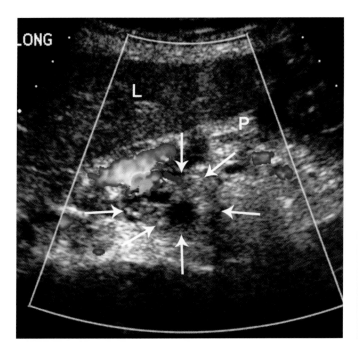

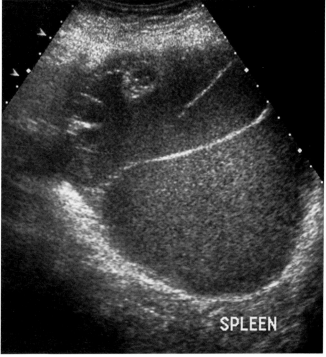

FIGURE 18 ■ Sagittal color Doppler image of the uncinate process showing a small microcystic adenoma (*arrows*), which shows no flow. L, liver; P, pancreas.

FIGURE 19 ■ Transverse image through the tail of the pancreas showing a large macrocystic adenoma with a thick rim, debris, and septations. *Source*: Courtesy of Philip Ralls, MD.

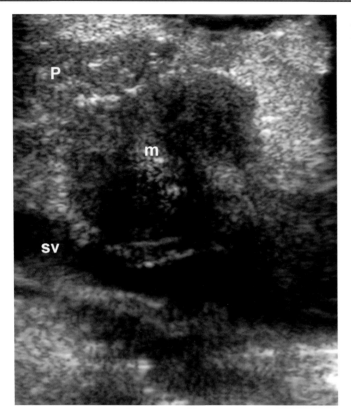

FIGURE 20 ■ Sagittal intraoperative image through the body of the pancreas shows a heterogeneous mass which is hypoechoic to the remainder of the pancreas. It is immediately anterior to the splenic vein. On CT this showed dramatic enhancement on arterial phase imaging; this was an insulinoma; the patient had symptoms of hypoglycemia. CT, computed tomography; sv, splenic vein; m, mass; P, pancreas.

Pancreatic Lymphoma ■ Pancreatic lymphoma presents as a hypoechoic mass, single or multiple within the pancreas (Fig. 21). It can present as lobular enlargement of the pancreas. Adjacent lymphadenopathy is often seen. Pancreatic lymphoma can narrow the pancreatic duct or displace it.

Pancreatic Metastases ■ Metastases to the pancreas can occur from local invasion by gastric, duodenal, or colonic neoplasm. Hematogenous spread can occur, most commonly from melanoma, breast, lung, or renal cell. Leukemia can also involve the pancreas (52).

Trauma

Pancreatic injury is uncommon in blunt abdominal trauma, but occurs in up to 2% to 12% (64). Isolated injury to the pancreas is rare. Most pancreatic injuries occur in the body (two-thirds) with the rest in the head, neck, and tail (64). Injuries include lacerations, contusions, and transection; complications include hematomas, pseudocysts, and abscesses. Evaluation is best made with CT but focused abdominal sonogram for trauma (FAST) scans can detect the more severe pancreatic injuries (65). US is useful in following the complications of trauma including hematomas and pseudocysts.

Pancreatic Calcifications

Pancreatic calcifications are commonly seen in chronic pancreatitis, hereditary pancreatitis, and hypercalcemic states but can also be seen with neoplasms (serous cystadenoma, mucinous cystadenoma, adenocarcinoma, or islet cell tumors) (Table 4). Since pancreatic adenocarcinoma occurs in patients with chronic pancreatitis, it is uncertain whether the calcifications arise in the adenocarcinoma or are from the chronic pancreatitis.

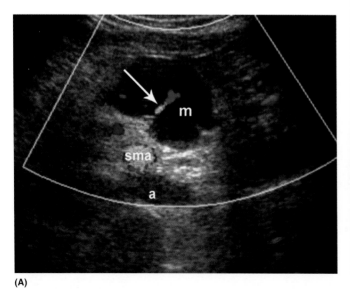

(A)

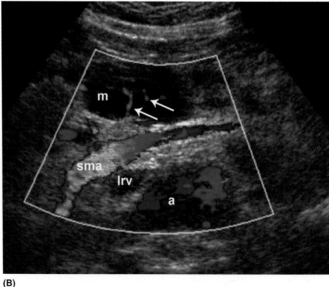

(B)

FIGURE 21 A AND B ■ Transverse sagittal color Doppler images of a homogeneous lobular hypoechoic mass (m) in the body of the pancreas proven to be lymphoma; this has some vessels within it (*arrows*). Note that the Doppler sensitivity is optimized for arterial flow and that some of the venous structures (lrv) do not show color. (**A**) Transverse. (**B**) Sagittal. lrv, left renal vein; m, mass; a, aorta; sma, superior mesenteric artery.

TABLE 4 ■ Pancreatic Calcifications

Pancreatitis
  Chronic

Prior injury
  Hematoma
  Infection
  Abscess

Systemic disease
  Hyperparathyroidism
  Hypercalcemia
  Cystic fibrosis
  Hemachromatosis

Neoplasm
  Microcystic (serous) adenoma—in central scar
  Macrocystic (mucinous) adenoma—peripheral
  Adenocarcinoma
  Hemangioma
  Metastases (colon)

Vascular
  Splenic artery calcifications
  Pseudoaneurysms

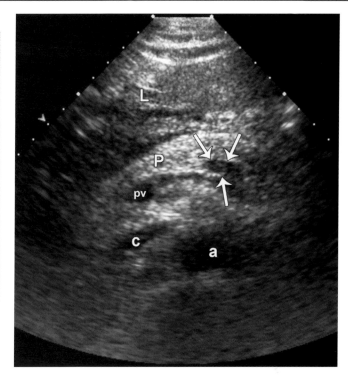

FIGURE 22 ■ Transverse image of a small hypoechoic lesion in the body of the pancreas (*arrows*), stable over time, consistent with a small cyst. L, liver; P, pancreas; pv, portal confluence; c, IVC; a, aorta.

Pancreatic Cysts

Two types of cysts are seen in the pancreas—true (epithelial lined) cysts and pseudocysts (without a true epithelial lining). True cysts can be either parasitic or nonparasitic cysts. Infections from amebiasis or echinococcus are causes of parasitic cysts. Nonparasitic cysts (Fig. 22) can be congenital (such as a foregut cyst) (66) or can be seen in association with systemic diseases such as adult polycystic kidney/liver disease and von Hippel-Lindau disease (Fig. 23) (67). Other manifestations of von Hippel-Lindau disease in the pancreas are microcystic adenomas and pancreatic islet cell tumors.

Other causes of pancreatic cysts are cystic neoplasms and cystic metastases (Table 5). In addition, lymphoma can appear hypoechoic and can mimic cysts in the pancreas if the gain is too low. Cysts within the pancreas need followup or additional studies such as magnetic resonance imaging (MRI) since cysts can often not be differentiated from an IPMT or a cystic neoplasm.

AORTA

Normal Anatomy

The abdominal aorta is located anterior to the spine, posterior to the diaphragmatic crus, and to the left of the IVC. The abdominal aorta enters the abdomen at the aortic hiatus and extends caudal to its bifurcation into the common iliac arteries at the level of L4. The thoracic aorta is not usually visualized on US. With US, the abdominal aorta can usually be visualized from the diaphragm to the bifurcation; the proximal iliac arteries are usually seen. Posterior to the aorta the lumbar spine is visualized as a series of inverted "U" shapes echogenicity with posterior shadowing (Fig. 24). The diaphragmatic crus is visualized as a thin, curvilinear, hypoechoic structure anterior to the aorta on both sagittal and transverse images (Fig. 24). In one study of 160 patients without vascular disease, the average diameter of the distal aorta was 1.7 cm in men

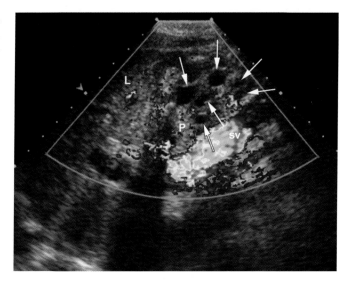

FIGURE 23 ■ Color Doppler transverse image through the pancreas show multiple cysts (*arrows*) in a patient with von Hippel-Lindau disease. L, liver; P, pancreas.

TABLE 5 ■ Cystic Masses of the Pancreas

True cysts
   Congenital
   Adult polycystic kidney disease
   von Hippel-Lindau disease
   Parasitic (amebiasis, echinococcus)

Pseudocysts
   Pancreatitis (acute or chronic)

Cystic neoplasms
   Serous cystadenoma or cystadenocarcinoma
   Mucinous cystadenoma or cystadenocarcinoma
   Solid and papillary epithelial neoplasm
   Ductectatic mucinous tumor of the pancreas
   ■ Main branch type
   ■ Side branch type
   Cystic metastases
      Renal cell carcinoma
      Melanoma
      Lung
      Breast
      Hepatocellular carcinoma
      Ovarian carcinoma

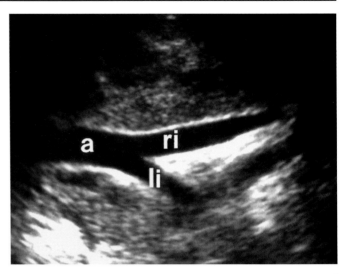

FIGURE 25 ■ Distal aorta and proximal iliac arteries on a coronal image. a, aorta; ri, right common iliac artery; li, left common iliac artery. *Source*: Courtesy of Dr. A. Fried, University of Kentucky.

and 1.5 cm in women and the average diameter of the proximal iliac arteries was 1.0 cm in men and 0.9 cm in women (68). The upper limit of the diameter of the proximal abdominal aorta is 3 cm; it tapers distally toward the bifurcation (Fig. 25) as it gives off the visceral branches.

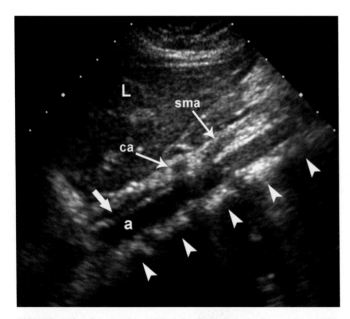

FIGURE 24 ■ Proximal to mid abdominal aorta in the sagittal plane showing origins of celiac artery and SMA (sma). *Arrowheads,* anterior margins of the vertebral bodies with posterior shadowing; *arrow,* right diaphragmatic crus. L, liver; a, aorta; ca, celiac artery; sma, superior mesenteric artery.

The major visceral branches are the celiac artery, the SMA, the renal arteries, the inferior mesenteric artery (IMA), and the gonadal arteries. On US, the celiac artery and SMA originate at the anterior aspect of the proximal aorta and can usually be identified on both sagittal and transverse planes (Fig. 24). The celiac axis branches close to its origin (branching is best seen on transverse images). Just inferior to the celiac artery, the SMA originates within 1 to 2 cm, at a more acute angle. The renal arteries can be difficult to identify, particularly in obese patients, but usually originate from the lateral or antero-lateral aspect of the aorta, within 1 to 2 cm of the origin of the SMA. The IMA and gonadal arteries are not usually seen on US.

It is important to distinguish the aorta from the IVC. The walls of the aorta are echogenic whereas the walls of the IVC are thin and not echogenic. The aorta remains in a posterior location, close to the spine, as it courses cephalad, whereas the IVC, as it courses cephalad, moves anteriorly, traversing the liver, to enter the right atrium.

Doppler interrogation easily distinguishes the two vessels. The aorta shows a single expansile pulsation without respiratory variation; the IVC shows a double pulsation consisting of "a" and "v" waves, which are lower in velocity. The aorta shows only minimal change in diameter with pulsation and no change with respiration; the IVC shows definite change in diameter with both pulsation and respiration.

Scanning Technique

US examination is usually started with the patient in the supine position with scanning in the sagittal and transverse planes although oblique and coronal views are usually necessary; decubitus positioning of the patient can also be helpful. The highest frequency transducer is used that will give adequate penetration to visualize the aorta; this is usually in the 3 to 4 MHz range, or higher if the patient is thin. The aorta is imaged in both sagittal and axial planes from the diaphragm to at least the bifurcation and proximal iliac arteries. Measurements should be obtained in AP and transverse planes of the proximal, mid, and distal portions of the aorta, of the proximal iliac arteries, and of any aneurysms. Color and duplex Doppler interrogation should be performed in all segments. The origins of the celiac artery and the SMA should be visualized as well as the origin of the renal arteries.

Pitfalls and Artifacts

If there is a large amount of abdominal bowel gas, it can be difficult to visualize the aorta. This is of particular concern in postoperative patients, who may have postoperative ileus or bowel obstruction. Obese patients may also be difficult to image. Firm, prolonged pressure with the transducer may push some of the bowel gas out of the way of the US beam. Placing the patient in a right lateral decubitus position and imaging through the left flank, spleen, or left kidney may be helpful.

If the aorta is tortuous from atherosclerotic change, scanning will need to be done in planes parallel and perpendicular to the axis of the aorta, which may not be the same as true sagittal and transverse planes of the abdomen. The diameter of the aorta can be overestimated on oblique views if the transducer is not aligned with the plane of the aorta. Also, if scanning in a sagittal plane with an ectatic aorta, occlusion of the aorta can be mimicked if the aorta wanders out of the plane of imaging; orienting the transducer to the plane of the aorta will confirm that it is just tortuous and not occluded.

Mural thrombus produces low-level echoes at the periphery of the vessel. If the gain is too low, the thrombus may not be visualized and if the gain is too high, reverberation artifact may obscure it. The gain should be set just below the level at which artifactual echoes appear in the IVC. Color or power Doppler images are useful to confirm the presence of mural thrombus. Mural calcification in the aorta produces curvilinear echogenicities that may shadow, obscuring portions of the lumen.

Retroperitoneal adenopathy may appear as low to intermediate echogenicity masses adjacent to the aorta. If extensive, these can mimic an aneurysm with thrombus. However, when evaluated in two planes, adenopathy can be shown to extend more laterally than would be expected for an aneurysm and does not conform to the shape of a vessel.

Pathology

Atherosclerotic Changes of the Aorta

Early changes of atherosclerotic disease in the aorta are intimal plaque, and later calcified intimal plaque. Intimal plaque is seen as irregular intermediate level echogenicities in the aortic lumen. When plaque calcifies, curvilinear echogenicities are noted with posterior shadowing which can sometimes obscure the lumen (Fig. 26). Mural thrombus is noted as a curvilinear crescent within the aortic lumen. Acute thrombus is more echogenic, heterogeneous, and convex. Chronic thrombus is hypoechoic, homogeneous, and concave although it can be heterogeneous with acute on chronic thrombus. On Doppler images, there is no flow within the thrombus.

Ulceration in plaques is seen as small hypoechoic areas within the plaque (69). Eventually, plaque may narrow the lumen sufficiently such that a thrombus or an embolus may narrow or occlude the vessel. With occlusion, US will show echogenic material filling the vessel lumen; Doppler interrogation will show no flow. Ectasia is another atherosclerotic change seen in the aorta.

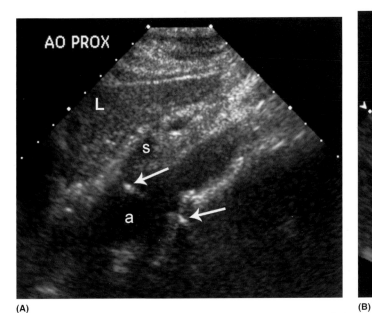

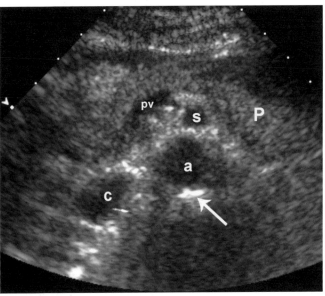

(A)

(B)

FIGURE 26 A AND B ▨ Atherosclerotic plaque in the aorta. (**A**) Sagittal. (**B**) Transverse. *Arrows*, calcified plaque in the aorta. s, superior mesenteric artery; P, pancreas; pv, portal vein; a, aorta; c, IVC.

Aortic Aneurysm

A true aneurysm is dilatation of all layers of the aortic wall with an intact wall; a false aneurysm is focal penetration of the aortic wall with hematoma contained by adventitia, connective tissue, and adjacent structures such as the spine (70). Aneurysms can be fusiform or saccular.

Most true abdominal aortic aneurysms (AAAs) are from atherosclerotic disease although other etiologies include infection (bacterial, syphilis), inflammation (Takayasu arteritis, giant cell arteritis, collagen vascular diseases, postradiation), trauma, aortic dissection, Ehlers-Danlos syndrome, and Marfan's syndrome. Aneurysms usually occur in older individuals (>50 years) and are more common in men (69). Risk factors for AAAs include smoking, hypertension, male gender, older age, hypercholesterolemia, family history, and chronic obstructive pulmonary disease (69,70).

The upper limit of normal for diameter of the abdominal aorta is 3 cm at the hiatus; it should gradually taper to the bifurcation. An AAA is defined as enlargement of the abdominal aorta greater than 3 cm or as a localized dilatation of at least 50% times the expected normal diameter (70). If there is a focal dilatation of less than 50% of the expected diameter, it is called a focal area of ectasia.

Measurement of the AP diameter of the aorta should be made on the sagittal image; on the transverse plane the AP diameter can be falsely increased or decreased by an oblique plane with angulation cephalic or caudal. The transverse measurement should be made on the transverse image. The cranial-caudal length of the aneurysm should be measured in the sagittal plane. The aortic diameter is measured from outer wall to outer wall; the luminal diameter is measured from inner wall to inner wall (Fig. 27).

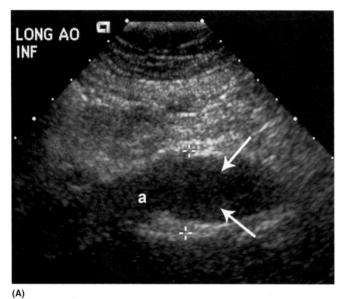

(A)

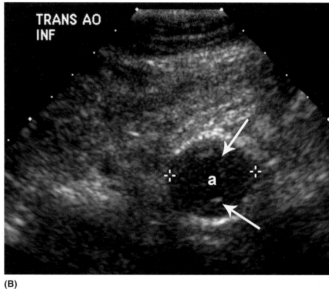

(B)

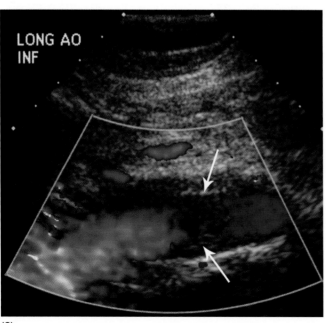

(C)

FIGURE 27 A–C ▪ Fusiform infrarenal AAA with mural thrombus. (**A**) Sagittal image showing widest portion of AAA measured at 3.0 cm. (**B**) Transverse image showing maximum transverse diameter of 2.8 cm. (**C**) Color Doppler image showing color flow in patent lumen and marginal mural thrombus. + *calipers* measuring AAA; *arrows*, outline the inner margin of the mural thrombus; a, aorta; AAA, abdominal aortic aneurysm.

More than 90% of AAAs are infrarenal with only 2% to 7% extending to the renal arteries or to the suprarenal abdominal aorta (69). Most extend to the bifurcation or proximal iliac arteries. Most are fusiform but some are saccular.

Aneurysms that involve the renal arteries or suprarenal aorta are more likely to be mycotic or posttraumatic (69).

It is important to visualize the renal arteries to determine whether the aneurysm is infrarenal since this affects surgical management. The renal arteries can be difficult to visualize on US especially in obese patients or in those with a large amount of bowel gas. Since the renal arteries originate within 1 to 2 cm of the SMA, if the aneurysm is at least 2 cm below the SMA, it can be inferred to be infrarenal.

AAAs tend to increase in size; mean growth is approximately 0.4 cm/yr (70), but growth is higher with larger aneurysms. Complications of AAA are rupture, leakage, fistula to adjacent structures (IVC, GI tract), distal embolization, infection, occlusion of the renal or mesenteric vessels, duodenal obstruction, or obstructive uropathy (69). Most of these are best visualized on CT.

The most life-threatening complication is rupture. The risk of rupture increases with the size of the AAA. For aneurysms less than 5.0 cm, the yearly rupture rate varies between 1% and 6%. For larger aneurysms, the risk of rupture is greater, up to 9% per year for an aneurysm of 6.5 cm and up to 12.5% per year for aneurysms of 7.5 cm (71). Although women have a lower prevalence of AAA than do men, the rate of aneurysm rupture is higher in women than in men (71). Brown et al. (72) showed in a recent paper that in male patients the average risk of rupture with aneurysms between 5.0 and 5.9 cm is 1.0% per year, but in female patients with aneurysms between 5.0 and 5.9 cm, the average risk of rupture is much larger, at 3.9% per year. In patients with an aneurysm size of 6.0 cm or greater, they found the risk of rupture in males to be 14.1% per year and in females to be 22.3% per year.

Treatment is by surgical repair or endovascular stent graft. The elective surgical repair of aneurysms less than 5.5 cm does not increase survival even when associated with low surgical mortality (73). The risk of rupture of aneurysms less than 5.0 cm is low. The Joint Council of the American Association of Vascular Surgery and Society for Vascular Surgery (74) reports that surveillance up to a diameter of 5.5 cm is safe unless the patient is symptomatic or the expansion of the aneurysm is rapid (>1 cm/ yr). A 5.5 cm diameter threshold for repair is recommended in the "average" male patient, but for women the threshold should be at a size of 4.5 to 5.0 cm (74).

Screening by US yearly has been shown to be safe in patients with AAA up to 4.5 cm (75).

Aortic Rupture

US can detect periaortic fluid as can be seen with leakage. Rupture of an AAA has a high mortality rate. CT is better for evaluation of rupture, since it is not compromised by bowel gas.

On US, with rupture of an AAA a large hypoechoic fluid collection can be seen in the retroperitoneum (69). Catalano and Siani (76) analyzed a series of patients with AAA and rupture and reported several US signs of rupture. These are deformation of the aneurysm, thrombus inhomogeneity, thrombus interruption, an intraluminal "floating thrombus" layer, aneurysm wall interruption, paraortic hypoechoic areas, retroperitoneal hematoma, and hemoperitoneum. The floating thrombus layer is an irregular flap detached focally from the thrombus only on one side and floating freely with the aneurysm; this is not the same as an intimal flap in dissection.

Aortic Pseudoaneurysm

Pseudoaneurysms, or false aneurysms, are usually from trauma or infection. They occur from a defect in the intima through which blood escapes but is contained by the surrounding tissue. Blood flows into the pseudoaneurysm during systole and out in diastole. This to and fro flow causes a "Ying-Yang" sign on color Doppler images. Pseudoaneurysms can occur after survival of an incomplete traumatic aortic rupture. Most occur in the thoracic aorta. Pseudoaneurysms of the abdominal aorta are usually from penetrating trauma or mycotic aneurysms. Penetrating trauma etiologies include stab or gunshot wounds or iatrogenic including surgery, vessel catheterization, or biopsy of adjacent structures.

Mycotic Aortic Aneurysms

Mycotic aneurysms are aneurysms of any type that have become infected. They are more common in patients younger than 50 years. These are rapidly progressive, surrounded by perivascular inflammation, and have a high incidence of rupture. Since they occur in younger patients, there may be less calcified plaque. Predisposing conditions to infection are the presence of atherosclerotic plaques or presence of grafts or stents in the aorta. Infection can be from hematogenous spread (endocarditis) or spread from adjacent organs or peritonitis (77). Diabetes, immunocompromise, chronic disease, and malignancy can be underlying conditions.

US demonstrates an aneurysm but is nonspecific. US may show lack of mural thrombus and lack of calcified plaque; a mycotic aneurysm is more likely to be saccular and irregular than fusiform. It has been reported that gas seen within an aneurysm may be an initial sign on US of a mycotic aneurysm (77). On US, small gas bubbles can be seen as echogenic foci with a "ring-down" artifact.

Inflammatory Aortic Aneurysm

Inflammatory aortic aneurysms are aortic aneurysms that have thickened walls with surrounding fibrosis and adherent visceral organs. Changes of atherosclerosis with plaque may also be seen. The fibrosis extends beyond the limits of the normal aortic adventitia. It may be part of the spectrum of inflammatory aortitis. Infection does not appear to be a cause and the etiology may be immunologic (78). US shows a thickened echogenic aortic wall which is surrounded at the anterior and lateral aspects (but limited posteriorly) by a thick hypoechoic area corresponding to the inflammatory fibrosis. This appearance can be confused with aortic dissection.

The periaortic inflammation or fibrosis may involve the ureters, duodenum, and IVC. Ureteral involvement ranges from narrowing to obstruction with proximal hydroureter and hydronephrosis (78). The extent of the fibrosis may be better evaluated with CT. Detection of an inflammatory aneurysm is important since surgical repair can be more complicated and associated with high morbidity and mortality (78).

Postsurgical Changes

During postsurgical or endovascular repair of AAA, US can be used for followup of aortic size; CT may be more sensitive for small endoleaks. After surgical repair, US will show a uniform caliber circumferential tubular echogenicity corresponding to the wall of the graft. A small amount of soft tissue around the graft is consistent with wrapping of the aneurysm around the graft. Some perigraft fluid can be seen around the grafts as normal postoperative appearance, for up to approximately three months. However, if fluid persists or occurs after a few months, bleeding or infection must be considered (79). If repair was done for a ruptured aortic aneurysm, hematoma can remain around the aorta postoperatively and may not indicate an acute postoperative problem (80). Endografts in the abdominal aorta will appear on US as tubular structures composed of multiple parallel echogenic struts within an aneurysm sac (Fig. 28).

Complications of surgical aneurysm repair include perigraft abscess, perigraft hematoma, retroperitoneal hemorrhage, pseudoaneurysm, aorto-enteric fistulas, lymphoceles, and ureteral obstruction. Complications of endograft repair include endoleaks, graft thrombosis, graft kinking, pseudoaneurysm, graft infection, graft occlusion, distal embolism, penetration of mural thrombus by the delivery system, colon necrosis, aortic dissection, and hematoma at the arteriotomy site (81). Most of these are best seen on CT but US also can detect many of these complications without the radiation exposure or nephrotoxicity of intravenous (i.v.) contrast.

The postoperative aneurysm repair patient should be followed for any evidence on US of increasing aortic diameter (representing a leak or endoleak), increasing periaortic tissue (representing abscess or hematoma), or any evidence of abnormal flow (representing an endoleak, pseudoaneurysm, or fistula).

Color and duplex Doppler US have been shown to be an accurate method for the detection of endoleaks (Fig. 29) (82–84). If a leak is detected, it can be further characterized by contrast enhanced CT (CECT). Microbubble CEUS has been shown to increase the sensitivity for detection of endoleaks over color and duplex Doppler US (85). Napoli et al. (86) showed that CEUS demonstrated endoleaks in several patients with very slow flowing leaks, which were not seen on CT angiography or Doppler US but were later confirmed with conventional angiography. In these patients, CEUS showed slow and diffuse enhancement in the sac around the endograft, occurring greater than two minutes after contrast administration (86).

Aortic Dissection

Aortic dissection is a progressive separation of the aortic wall layers that occurs from a tear in the intima or inner media. As the separation propagates within the layers of the media, two or more channels are formed. The true lumen is the original lumen, lined by intima. The false

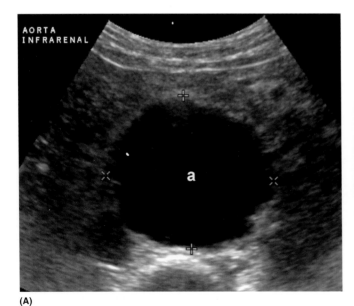

(A)

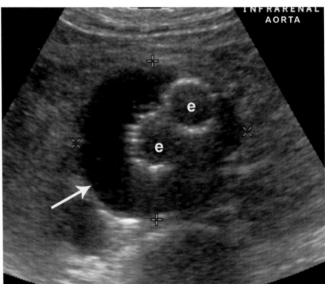

(B)

FIGURE 28 A AND B ▪ AAA pre- and postrepair with endograft. (**A**) Transverse image of AAA measuring 5.3 × 4.6 cm, without mural thrombus, preop. (**B**) Transverse image of endograft repair of AAA; two limbs of the echogenic endograft are within the aneurysm sac. *Arrow*, aneurysm sac; + and x *calipers*, measuring margin of AAA; a, aorta; e, limbs of endograft; AAA, abdominal aortic aneurysm.

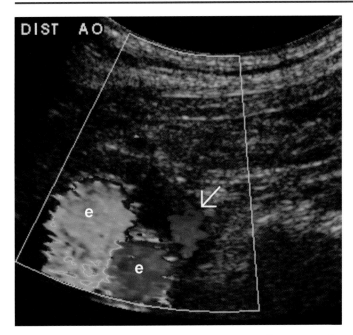

FIGURE 29 ■ Endograft repair of AAA with endoleak. Transverse color Doppler image shows flow in both limbs of the endograft with flow in the aneurysm sac (*arrow*) consistent with an endoleak. AAA, abdominal aortic aneurysm; e, limbs of the endograft.

lumen is the new channel within the layers of the media. A thin membrane, the dissecting membrane, separates the two lumens. Additional tears within the dissecting membrane form communications, re-entry sites, between the true and false lumens. The dissection can progress proximally or distally (87). Risk factors for aortic dissection are any condition that weakens the aortic wall such as general cardiovascular risk factors (smoking, hypertension, atherosclerosis, and hypercholesterolemia), connective tissue disorders (Ehlers-Danlos and Marfan syndromes and disease of the aortic media), aortitis, bicuspid aortic valve, pregnancy, drugs (cocaine and amphetamine), or iatrogenic (catheterization or surgery) (87). Classification is based on the portions of the aorta that are involved (Stanford and DeBakey classifications) as well as on the time elapsed (acute, subacute, or chronic). Most aortic dissections begin in the thoracic aorta.

Complications of aortic dissection include cardiac tamponade, disruption of flow to the coronary arteries, aortic valve injury, and compromised flow to branch vessels causing ischemia to organs, to the spinal cord, and to the bowel (87).

CT is best for evaluating a dissection and its extent, particularly in the thoracic aorta, which is not visualized on US. Distal aortic dissection is often managed medically. On US, a dissection in the abdominal aorta is seen as an intimal flap within the aortic lumen (Fig. 30). The intimal flap moves with arterial pulsation if both lumens are patent unless the flap is very thick; the lumens may be equal or unequal in size. Color Doppler shows antegrade flow in the true lumen, but the waveforms in both lumens can be abnormal with turbulent

flow and unusual waveforms (69). Flow in the false aneurysm is usually slower than in the true lumen and may not be detected with Doppler.

If flow is not seen in one of the lumens, this can represent very slow flow in a dissection, thrombosis of the dissection lumen, or mural thrombus in an aortic aneurysm mimicking a dissection. If an aorta with mural thrombus is imaged and the gain is too low, the thrombus could seem echolucent and mimic a dissection; however, no flow is seen in this "pseudodissection." Normally in AAAs which have mural thrombus, the thrombus is homogeneous in echotexture. There have been several reported cases of an anechoic crescent between more solid thrombus and the wall of the aorta on US in asymptomatic patients with AAA (Fig. 31). On CT, these patients were found not to have a dissection, but to have thrombus of varying density. It has been postulated that this appearance may be secondary to a portion of the thrombus liquefying (88).

INFERIOR VENA CAVA

Embryology

The IVC, the azygous vein, and the hemiazygos veins are mostly formed from development and regression of three paired veins (the posterior cardinal, subcardinal, and supracardinal veins). If there is interruption of any of these developmental phases, different anomalies will occur such as duplicated IVC, interrupted IVC with azygous or hemiazygous continuation, circumaortic left renal vein, retroaortic left renal vein, transposition of the IVC, or circumcaval ureter as well as rarer anomalies (Table 6) (89,90). Some of these anomalies can be visualized by US, but most are better appreciated by contrast-enhanced CT or MRI.

Interruption of the IVC with azygous or hemiazygous continuation can be isolated or can be associated with polysplenia and asplenia syndromes or cardiac abnormalities. Some of these venous anomalies have been detected prenatally (89–91); if detected, a search should be made for associated cardiac and other anomalies (91). Developmental anomalies of the IVC have also been associated with renal aplasia (92) and renal vein anomalies (93). Anomalies of the IVC may predispose to deep venous thrombosis (94–99). If a patient younger than 30, without any other known risk factors, presents with deep venous thrombosis, a search should be made for anomalies of the IVC (94,98,99).

Normal Anatomy

The IVC is located in the posterior right abdomen, to the right of the aorta and at the right anterior aspect of the spine. Inferiorly it is at the medial anterior aspect of the right psoas muscle; superiorly it is anterior and lateral to the crus of the right hemidiaphragm, anterior and medial to the right kidney and right adrenal, and at the posterior medial aspect of the liver. It forms as the confluence of the right and left common iliac veins at approximately the

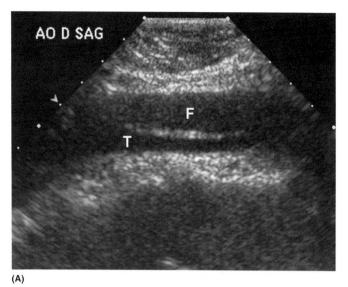

(A)

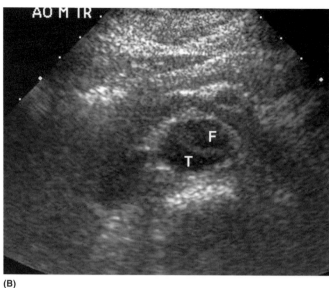

(B)

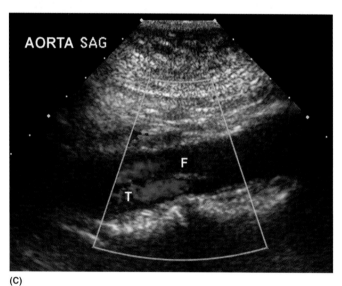

(C)

FIGURE 30 A–C ■ Aortic dissection. (**A**) Sagittal and (**B**) transverse images show a dissection flap in the mid aorta extending caudally. (**C**) Sagittal color Doppler image shows forward flow in the true lumen and retrograde flow in the false lumen. T, true lumen; F, false lumen; on gray scale images the false lumen is slightly more echogenic because of slower flow.

level of L5 and empties into the right atrium. It consists of subhepatic, intrahepatic, and suprahepatic segments. As it courses cephalad, veins draining into the IVC include the median sacral vein (which drains at the confluence of the common iliac veins but can also drain into the left common iliac vein), the lumbar veins, the right gonadal vein (the left gonadal vein drains into the left renal vein), the renal veins, the adrenal veins, the inferior phrenic veins, and the hepatic veins.

On US, the IVC is a thin-walled, tubular structure to the right of the aorta (Fig. 32). It can be distinguished from the aorta by a thin wall (vs. the thicker wall of the aorta), its more anterior position as it courses through the liver to join the right atrium (vs. the aorta, which remains in a posterior location), its change in diameter with breathing and pulsation (vs. minimal change in the aorta only with pulsation), and the double pulsation with "a" and "v" waves (vs. single pulsation with higher velocity in the aorta). On transverse plane the IVC can be round or ovoid, or even flat if there is sufficient pressure on the transducer.

After administration of microbubble contrast agents, the IVC densely enhances and then washes out (Fig. 33).

The IVC diameter changes with the patient's hydration status, respiration, abdominal pressure, and cardiac status. Diameter increases with Valsalva maneuver in normal patients. Diameter is increased with congestive heart failure, volume overload, and deep expiration (Table 7). The maternal IVC is enlarged in early pregnancy (100). IVC diameter is decreased with hypovolemia (101), elevated intra-abdominal pressure (102), and deep inspiration (Table 8) (103).

Cephalad, the hepatic veins can be seen draining into the IVC (Fig. 32). On US, the renal veins can often be visualized draining into the IVC with the left renal vein seen passing between the aorta and SMA as it joins the IVC.

Scanning Technique

The IVC is best visualized with the patient in the supine position either using the liver as an acoustic window or in

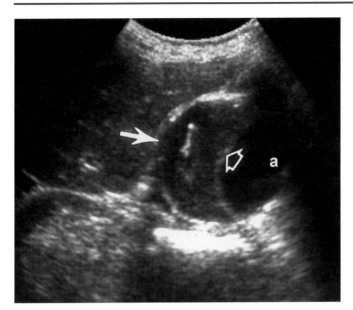

FIGURE 31 ■ Heterogeneous mural thrombus in AAA. Transverse image shows mural thrombus (*arrowhead*) at the margin of an AAA with more lucent clot near the wall (*arrow*) representing liquefying portion of the clot in this asymptomatic patient. This was not a dissection and no flow was seen with Doppler. AAA, abdominal aortic aneurysm; a, aorta. *Source*: Courtesy of A. Fried, University of Kentucky.

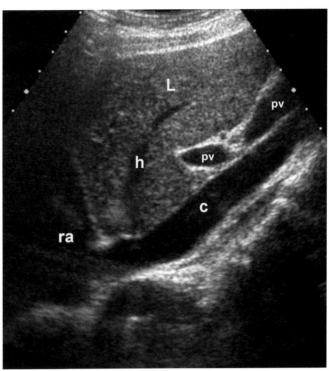

FIGURE 32 ■ Normal cephalic aspect of the IVC on sagittal image. Note the thin wall of the IVC and its course away from the spine to enter the right atrium. c, IVC; L, liver; h, hepatic vein; pv, portal veins; ra, right atrium.

the midline, inferior to the xiphoid, angling to the right. Placing the patient in a left lateral decubitus position may be helpful. Gentle pressure on the transducer is helpful especially in the midline approach to displace bowel loops.

Pitfalls and Artifacts

Portions of the IVC can be difficult to visualize if there is a large amount of bowel gas. It may be necessary to use pressure on the transducer to move bowel out of the way.

In a thin patient, pressure from the transducer may cause collapse of the IVC or it may appear flattened. Reduction of external pressure should increase the luminal diameter.

If flow is slow in the IVC, low level moving echogenicities can be seen in the lumen, from reflection of sound on aggregates of red blood cells (a "rouleaux" formation); this is not of pathologic significance.

IVC Catheterization

Catheters introduced into the IVC may originate inferiorly from the common femoral veins, superiorly from the superior vena cava, or from the umbilical vein in neonates. On US, a catheter appears as a curvilinear echogenicity

TABLE 6 ■ Anomalies of the IVC

- Duplicated IVC
- Right-sided, interrupted IVC with azygous continuation
- Right-sided, interrupted IVC with hemiazygous continuation
- Retroaortic left renal vein
- Circumaortic left renal vein
- Transposition of the IVC (left-sided IVC)
- Circumcaval ureter
- Left-sided, interrupted IVC with azygous continuation
- Left-sided, interrupted IVC with hemiazygous continuation

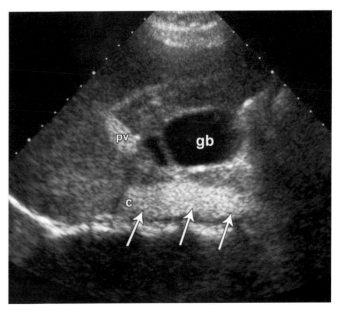

FIGURE 33 ■ Sagittal image of normal IVC after microbubble contrast administration. Note dense echogenic enhancement of the normal IVC and the portal vein. *Arrows*, dense enhancement of IVC. gb, gallbladder with fold; pv, portal vein with dense enhancement; c, IVC.

TABLE 7 ■ Increased Size of IVC

Congestive heart failure

Volume overload

Tumors

■ Leiomyosarcoma

■ Leiomyoma

■ Metastases

Deep expiration

Valsalva

Pregnancy—early stages

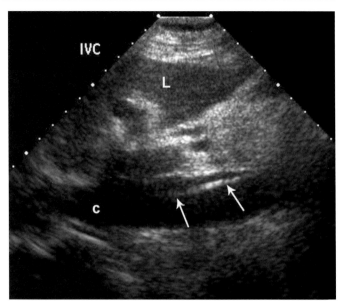

FIGURE 34 ■ Sagittal image of IVC with a Swan-Ganz catheter introduced via the right common femoral vein. *Arrows*, echogenic catheter in the IVC. c, IVC; L, liver.

within the IVC (Fig. 34) which moves with respiration and flow. It is important to document this appearance within the IVC; if the vessel were mistaken for the aorta, it could be mistaken for a dissection (although a catheter is usually thicker than a dissection flap). Prolonged catheterization can predispose to IVC thrombus.

Pathology

Thrombosis

Thrombosis in the IVC can occur from nontumoral (bland) or tumoral causes. Bland thrombus occurs from propagation of deep venous thromboses from the lower extremities or from septic thrombophlebitis. Predisposing conditions are prolonged immobilization, hypercoagulable states (such as nephrotic syndrome) (104), developmental abnormalities of the IVC (94–99), i.v. catheterization of the IVC or femoral veins, and postpartum (105).

Nonocclusive thrombus is seen on US as a filling defect in the IVC which can move with respiration and flow (Fig. 35). Acute thrombus is usually echogenic. If the IVC is totally occluded, there will be no flow; acutely, enlargement of the IVC can be seen. With chronic occlusion, Doppler US may detect venous collaterals around the IVC or in the azygous or hemiazygous system; a small, occluded IVC, which can be echogenic from calcifications, can also be seen.

Obstruction

Membranous or segmental obstruction of the IVC occurs in the hepatic or suprahepatic portions of the IVC and is a cause of chronic Budd-Chiari syndrome; it is common in

TABLE 8 ■ Small IVC

Congenital

Hypovolemia

Elevated intra-abdominal pressure—narrows the intrahepatic IVC

■ Massive ascites

■ Large intra-abdominal mass

Negative intrathoracic pressure (deep respiration) narrows the intrahepatic segment

Asia and South Africa. This is thought to be congenital (but usually manifests in adulthood) but one type may be acquired from prior thrombus. Obstruction can be from a thin membrane (membranous, in which the caliper of the IVC is normal) or by replacement of a segment of the IVC by a fibrous cord (segmental, in which the IVC is narrowed) (106–108). Focal elastic obstruction has also been reported (108).

US can visualize the membrane or fibrous cord and evaluate the relationship of the hepatic veins to the obstruction. These can be treated by angioplasty, stent, or surgical repair (109). After liver transplant there can be postsurgical narrowing of the IVC at the anastomosis; this can also cause hepatic vein stenosis (110), which can be treated with stenting (111). Other causes of obstruction or narrowing of the IVC are shown in Table 9.

Septic Thrombophlebitis

Septic thrombophlebitis in the IVC can occur as a result of an infected lower extremity venous catheter, propagation of pelvic infection from the gonadal veins, or by hematogenous spread from bacterial endocarditis. Septic emboli appear on US as filling defects within the IVC; echogenic foci with "dirty" shadowing may be seen within the thrombus, corresponding to air bubbles. Gonadal vein thrombosis on the left can propagate into the left renal vein and on the right can propagate into the IVC. Causes included postpartum endometritis, pelvic inflammatory disease, and postgynecologic surgery.

Tumor Thrombus

Tumor thrombosis extending into the IVC is commonly seen from extension of tumor in the renal veins from renal cell carcinoma (112), Wilms' tumor, neuroblastoma (113),

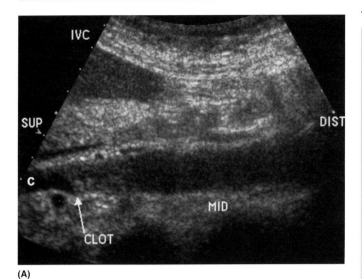

(A)

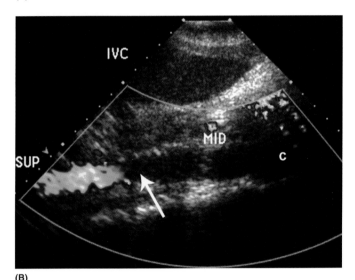

(B)

FIGURE 35 A AND B ■ Sagittal images showing clot in the IVC. (**A**) Gray scale images show an echogenic filling defect in the IVC, consistent with clot. The inferior aspect of the clot is more hypoechoic. (**B**) Color Doppler images show the lack of flow in the region of the clot and inferior to it. *Arrow,* superior margin of the clot. c, IVC.

adrenal cortical carcinoma, and pancreatic carcinoma; extension into the IVC from the hepatic veins can be seen with hepatocellular carcinoma (114) or hepatoblastoma (115). Tumoral thrombus can show flow within the thrombus on Doppler images and can enhance with microbubble contrast agents. Tumoral thrombus can also extend into the IVC from tumor in the gonadal veins (116) or left renal vein from malignant pelvic tumors. Extension of masses from uterine myomas (intravenous leiomyomatosis) has been reported (117–120). Renal angiomyolipomas (121) and lymphoma also have been reported to involve the IVC. If the IVC is separated from the spine (except in its most cephalic portion, as it enters the right atrium), causes such as lymphadenopathy or retroperitoneal masses should be considered.

TABLE 9 ■ IVC Obstruction

Intraluminal obstruction

Caval origin

  Congenital membrane

  Fibrous cord—segmental obstruction

  Neoplastic

    ■ Leiomyoma

    ■ Leiomyosarcoma

    ■ Fibrosarcoma

Noncaval origin

  Nonneoplastic

    ■ Thrombus

      ■ Coagulation disorders

      ■ Budd-Chiari syndrome

      ■ Dehydration

      ■ CHF

      ■ Extension from deep veins of pelvis and thigh

    ■ Infectious/inflammatory

      ■ Septic thrombophlebitis

      ■ Endocarditis

      ■ Pelvic inflammatory disease

      ■ Postpartum

    ■ Postoperative

      ■ Traumatic thrombophlebitis

      ■ Ligation

      ■ Clip

      ■ Cava filter

      ■ Prolonged catheterization

      ■ Anastomotic narrowing postliver transplant

  Neoplastic

    ■ Neuroblastoma

    ■ Renal cell carcinoma

    ■ Wilms' tumor

    ■ Adrenal carcinoma

    ■ Pheochromocytoma

    ■ Pancreatic adenocarcinoma

    ■ Hepatic cellular carcinoma

    ■ Metastatic disease

Extraluminal obstruction/compression

Nonneoplastic

  ■ Retroperitoneal fibrosis

  ■ Retroperitoneal hematoma

  ■ Hepatomegaly

  ■ Tortuous aorta

  ■ Aortic aneurysm

Neoplastic

  ■ Renal cell carcinoma

  ■ Wilms' tumor

  ■ Adrenal carcinoma

  ■ Hepatocellular carcinoma

  ■ Pancreatic tumors

  ■ Desmoplastic reaction from tumor (carcinoid)

  ■ Retroperitoneal lymphoma

  ■ Retroperitoneal lymphadenopathy

Functional obstruction

  ■ Pregnant uterus

  ■ Compression from a large abdominal mass in a supine position

  ■ Valsalva maneuver

  ■ Straining

  ■ Compression from elevated abdominal pressure such as sudden bleeding or ascites

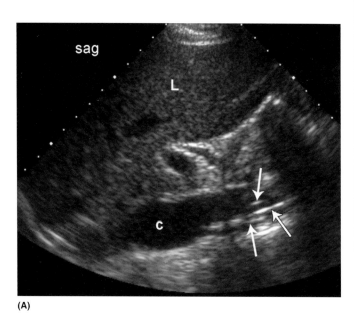

(A)

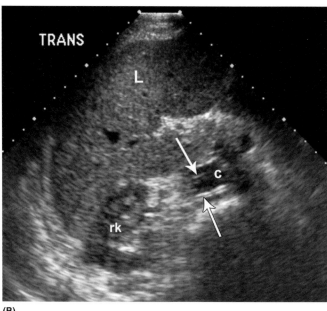

(B)

FIGURE 36 A AND B ▪ Gray scale images of a filter in the IVC. Note the curvilinear echogenicities (*arrows*) within the IVC which converge, corresponding to the filter. (**A**) Sagittal. (**B**) Transverse. c, IVC; L, liver; rk, right kidney.

IVC Filters

Filters have been placed in the IVC to prevent propagation of deep venous thrombosis from the lower extremities into the pulmonary circulation. Optimal location of the filter is inferior to the level of the renal veins. On US, a filter in the IVC appears as curvilinear echogenicities that converge (Fig. 36). Occasionally, clot can be detected within the filter (Fig. 37). Perforation of a portion of the filter through the wall of the IVC may be detected indirectly as a hematoma around the IVC, but is not well seen on US; CT is more sensitive for small leaks and is better to detect abnormalities of filter position.

Tumors

Focal collections of fat around the IVC have been reported (122); these are around the IVC, but not within the lumen. Cases of lipomas actually within the lumen of the IVC have been reported (123). These appear on US as echogenic intraluminal masses, narrowing the IVC lumen. Leiomyomas have been reported in the IVC and hepatic veins (124,125) as well as intravenous leiomyomatosis (117–120).

Primary leiomyosarcomas can occur in the wall of the IVC (126–128). These most commonly occur in older women and are most commonly located in the IVC between the renal veins and the diaphragm. Most have both intra- and extraluminal components but can be only intraluminal or only extraluminal. Fibrosarcoma has been reported in the IVC (129). Metastases can occur within the IVC [e.g., from nonseminomatous germ cell tumor (130)] as intraluminal filling defects. Tumor thrombus has already been discussed.

Vascular

Aneurysms of the IVC have been reported. These can cause obstruction of the IVC (131). IVC aneurysms can be saccular or fusiform. IVC aneurysms are at risk for developing fistulas to the GI tract or causing thrombus. Some of the reported cases have been associated with developmental anomalies of the IVC so that if an aneurysm of the IVC is seen, search should be made for a possible IVC anomaly (131).

FIGURE 37 ▪ Sagittal image through the IVC showing clot inferior to the IVC filter but IVC patent above the filter. Note the curvilinear echogenicities, which converge within the IVC (*arrows*), corresponding to the filter and the echogenic thrombus contained by the filter (*curved arrow*). c, IVC.

REFERENCES

1. Heiken JP, Aizenstein RI, Balfe DM, Gore RM. Peritoneal cavity and retroperitoneum: normal anatomy and examination techniques. In: Gore RM, Levine MS, eds. Textbook of Gastrointestinal Radiology. 2nd ed. Philadelphia: W.B. Saunders Company, 2000:1930–1947.

2. Kneeland JB, Auh YH, Rubenstein WA, et al. Perirenal spaces: CT evidence for communication across the midline. Radiology 1987; 164(3):657–664.

3. Lim JH, Kim B, Auh YH. Anatomical communications of the perirenal space. Br J Radiol 1998; 71(844):450–456.

4. Thornton FJ, Kandiah SS, Monkhouse WS, Lee MJ. Helical CT evaluation of the perirenal space and its boundaries: a cadaveric study. Radiology 2001; 218(3):659–663.

5. Mindell HJ, Mastromatteo JF, Dickey KW, et al. Anatomic communications between the three retroperitoneal spaces: determination by CT-guided injections of contrast material in cadavers. Am J Roentgenol 1995; 164(5):1173–1178. Comment in: Am J Roentgenol 1996; 166(3):722–723.

6. Korobkin M, Silverman PM, Quint LE, Francis IR. CT of the extraperitoneal space: normal anatomy and fluid collections. Am J Roentgenol 1992; 159(5):933–942.

7. Molmenti EP, Balfe DM, Kanterman RY, Bennett HF. Anatomy of the retroperitoneum: observations of the distribution of pathologic fluid collections. Radiology 1996; 200(1):95–103.

8. Aizenstein RI, Wilbur AC, O'Neil HK. Interfascial and perinephric pathways in the spread of retroperitoneal disease: refined concepts based on CT observations. Am J Roentgenol 1997; 168(3):639–643. Comment in: Am J Roentgenol 1997; 169(6):1748–1749. Am J Roentgenol 2001; 176(6):1601–1602.

9. Gore RM, Balfe DM, Aizenstein RI, Silverman PM. The great escape: interfascial decompression planes of the retroperitoneum. Am J Roentgenol 2000; 175(2):363–370. Comment in: Am J Roentgenol 2001; 176(6):1601–1602.

10. Feldberg MA, Koehler PR, van Waes PF. Psoas compartment disease studied by computed tomography. Analysis of 50 cases and subject review. Radiology 1983; 148(2):505–512.

11. Adriazola M, Ortiz Cabria R, Alonso A, Garcia Cobo E, Tejeda E, Romero F. Renal angiomyolipoma with arteriovenous fistula causing retroperitoneal hematoma. Case report. Arch Esp Urol 2004; 57(7):754–756.

12. Slapa RZ, Kasperlik-Zaluska AA, Polanski JA, Borowicz K, Serafin-Krol M, Jakubowski W. Three-dimensional sonography in diagnosis of retroperitoneal hemorrhage from adrenocortical carcinoma. J Ultrasound Med 2004; 23(10):1369–1373.

13. Yohendran J, Dias MM, Eckstein R, Wilson T. Benign retroperitoneal cyst of Mullerian type. Asian J Surg 2004; 27(4):333–335.

14. Konno K, Ishida H, Naganuma H, et al. Retroperitoneal cyst: sonographic findings. Abdom Imaging 2002; 27(6):680–684.

15. Nishino M, Hayakawa K, Minami M, Yamamoto A, Ueda H, Takasu K. Primary retroperitoneal neoplasms: CT and MR imaging findings with anatomic and pathologic diagnostic clues. Radiographics 2003; 23(1):45–57.

16. Sato M, Ishida H, Konno K, et al. Abdominal involvement in neurofibromatosis 1: sonographic findings. Abdom Imaging 2000; 25(5):517–522.

17. Gossios K, Zikou A, Stavropoulos N. Primary seminoma of the retroperitoneum. Eur Radiol 2000; 10(4):590–592.

18. Chaudhary A, Misra S, Wakhlu A, Tandon RK, Wakhlu AK. Retroperitoneal teratomas in children. Indian J Pediatr 2006; 73(3):221–223.

19. Vasudevan SA, Cumbie TA, Dishop MK, Nuchtern JG. Retroperitoneal hemangioma of infancy. J Pediatr Surg 2006; 41(1):e41–e44.

20. Nah YW, Suh JH, Choi DH, et al. Benign retroperitoneal schwannoma: surgical consideration. Hepatogastroenterology 2005; 52(66): 1681–1684.

21. Dursun P, Salman MC, Taskiran C, Yuce K, Ayhan A. Retroperitoneal leiomyomatosis: a case report. Int J Gynecol Cancer 2005; 15(6):1222–1225.

22. Ahmad GF, Athavale R, Hamid BN, Davies-Humphreys J. Pelvic malignant hemangiopericytoma mimicking an ovarian neoplasm: a case report. J Reprod Med 2004; 49(5):404–407.

23. Kawakami M, Koda M, Matsunaga N, et al. Adult-type neuroblastoma originated in retroperitoneum beginning with obstructive jaundice. Clin Imaging 2001; 25(4):284–287.

24. Kurosaki Y, Tanaka YO, Itai Y. Well-differentiated liposarcoma of the retroperitoneum with a fat-fluid level: US, CT, and MR appearance. Eur Radiol 1998; 8(3):474–475.

25. Pardalidis NP, Grigoriadis K, Papatsoris AG, Kosmaoglou EV, Horti M. Primary paratesticular adult ganglioneuroma. Urology 2004; 63(3):584–558.

26. Hoff FL, Gore RM. Pancreas: normal anatomy and examination techniques. In: Gore RM, Levine MS, eds. Textbook of Gastrointestinal Radiology. 2nd ed. Philadelphia: W.B. Saunders Company, 2000:1728–1745.

27. Haber K, Freimanis AK, Asher WM. Demonstration and dimensional analysis of the normal pancreas with gray-scale echography. AJR Am J Roentgenol 1976; 126(3):624–628.

28. Thorelius L. Contrast-enhanced ultrasound: beyond the liver. Eur Radiol 2003; 13(suppl 3):N91–N108.

29. Atri M, Nazarnia S, Mehio A, Reinhold C, Bret PM. Hypoechogenic embryologic ventral aspect of the head and uncinate process of the pancreas: in vitro correlation of US with histopathologic findings. Radiology 1994; 190(2):441–444.

30. Halpert RD, Shabot JM, Heare BR, Rogers RE. The bifid pancreas: a rare anatomical variation. Gastrointest Endosc 1990; 36(1): 60–61.

31. Orr LA, Powell RW, Melhem RE. Sonographic demonstration of annular pancreas in the newborn. J Ultrasound Med 1992; 11(7): 373–375.

32. Balthazar EJ. Pancreatitis. In: Gore RM, Levine MS, eds. Textbook of Gastrointestinal Radiology. 2nd ed. Philadelphia: W.B. Saunders Company, 2000:1767–1795.

33. Finstad TA, Tchelepi H, Ralls PW. Sonography of acute pancreatitis: prevalence of findings and pictorial essay. Ultrasound Q 2005; 21(2):95–104; quiz 150:153–154.

34. Balthazar EJ. Acute pancreatitis: assessment of severity with clinical and CT evaluation. Radiology 2002; 223(3): 603–613.

35. Leung TK, Lee CM, Lin SY, et al. Balthazar computed tomography severity index is superior to Ranson criteria and APACHE II scoring system in predicting acute pancreatitis outcome. World J Gastroenterol 2005; 11(38):6049–6052.

36. Alpern MB, Sandler MA, Kellman GM, Madrazo BL. Chronic pancreatitis: ultrasonic features. Radiology 1985; 155(1):215–219.

37. Bolondi L, Li Bassi S, Gaiani S, Barbara L. Sonography of chronic pancreatitis. Radiol Clin North Am 1989; 27(4):815–833.

38. Taylor B. Carcinoma of the head of the pancreas versus chronic pancreatitis: diagnostic dilemma with significant consequences. World J Surg 2003; 27(11):1249–1257. Epub 2003.

39. Patel B, Chenoweth J, Garvin P, et al. Role of imaging in the diagnosis of chronic pancreatitis and differentiation from carcinoma of the pancreas. Radiologist 1998; 5(6):245–255.

40. Koito K, Namieno T, Nagakawa T, Morita K. Inflammatory pancreatic masses: differentiation from ductal carcinomas with contrast-enhanced sonography using carbon dioxide microbubbles. Am J Roentgenol 1997; 169(5):1263–1267.

41. Becker V, Mischke U. Groove pancreatitis. Int J Pancreatol 1991; 10(3–4):173–182.

42. Shudo R, Obara T, Tanno S, et al. Segmental groove pancreatitis accompanied by protein plugs in Santorini's duct. J Gastroenterol 1998; 33(2):289–294.

43. Chatelain D, Vibert E, Yzet T, et al. Groove pancreatitis and pancreatic heterotopia in the minor duodenal papilla. Pancreas 2005; 30(4):e92–e95.

44. Gabata T, Kadoya M, Terayama N, Sanada J, Kobayashi S, Matsui O. Groove pancreatic carcinomas: radiological and pathological findings. Eur Radiol 2003; 13(7):1679–1684. Epub 2002.

45. Deshpande V, Mino-Kenudson M, Brugge W, Lauwers GY. Autoimmune pancreatitis: more than just a pancreatic disease? A contemporary review of its pathology. Arch Pathol Lab Med 2005; 129(9):1148–1154.

46. Hyodo N, Hyodo T. Ultrasonographic evaluation in patients with autoimmune-related pancreatitis. J Gastroenterol 2003; 38(12): 1155–1161.

47. Sahani DV, Kalva SP, Farrell J, et al. Autoimmune pancreatitis: imaging features. Radiology 2004; 233(2):345–352. Epub 2004. Comment in: Radiology 2005; 236(1):371; author reply 371–372.

48. Okazaki K. Autoimmune pancreatitis: etiology, pathogenesis, clinical findings and treatment. The Japanese experience. JOP 2005; 6(1 suppl):89–96.

49. Kamisawa T, Matsukawa M, Ohkawa M. Autoimmune pancreatitis associated with retroperitoneal fibrosis. JOP 2005; 6(3):260–263.

50. Daneman A, Gaskin K, Martin DJ, Cutz E. Pancreatic changes in cystic fibrosis: CT and sonographic appearances. Am J Roentgenol 1983; 141(4):653–655.

51. Dietrich CF, Chichakli M, Hirche TO, et al. Sonographic findings of the hepatobiliary-pancreatic system in adult patients with cystic fibrosis. J Ultrasound Med 2002; 21(4):409–416; quiz 417.

52. Chezmar JL. Pancreatic neoplasms. In: Gore RM, Levine MS, eds. Textbook of Gastrointestinal Radiology. 2nd ed. Philadelphia: W.B. Saunders Company, 2000:1796–1811.

53. Yassa NA, Yang J, Stein S, Johnson M, Ralls P. Gray-scale and color flow sonography of pancreatic ductal adenocarcinoma. J Clin Ultrasound 1997; 25(9):473–480.

54. Oshikawa O, Tanaka S, Ioka T, Nakaizumi A, Hamada Y, Mitani T. Dynamic sonography of pancreatic tumors: comparison with dynamic CT. Am J Roentgenol 2002; 178(5):1133–1137.

55. Procacci C, Graziani R, Bicego E, et al. Serous cystadenoma of the pancreas: report of 30 cases with emphasis on the imaging findings. J Comput Assist Tomogr 1997; 21(3):373–382.

56. George DH, Murphy F, Michalski R, Ulmer BG. Serous cystadenocarcinoma of the pancreas: a new entity? Am J Surg Pathol 1989; 13(1):61–66.

57. Sarr MG, Kendrick ML, Nagorney DM, Thompson GB, Farley DR, Farnell MB. Cystic neoplasms of the pancreas: benign to malignant epithelial neoplasms. Surg Clin North Am 2001; 81(3):497–509.

58. Taouli B, Vilgrain V, O'Toole D, Vullierme MP, Terris B, Menu Y. Intraductal papillary mucinous tumors of the pancreas: features with multimodality imaging. J Comput Assist Tomogr 2002; 26(2):223–231.

59. Procacci C, Megibow AJ, Carbognin G, et al. Intraductal papillary mucinous tumor of the pancreas: a pictorial essay. Radiographics 1999; 19(6):1447–1463.

60. Choe KA. Intraductal papillary mucinous tumors and mucinous cystic tumors of the pancreas: imaging. J Hepatobiliary Pancreat Surg 2003; 10(2):137–141.

61. Procacci C, Graziani R, Bicego E, et al. Intraductal mucin-producing tumors of the pancreas: imaging findings. Radiology 1996; 198(1):249–257.

62. Anderson MA, Scheiman JM. Nonmucinous cystic pancreatic neoplasms. Gastrointest Endosc Clin N Am 2002; 12(4):769–779, viii.

63. D'Onofrio M, Malago R, Vecchiato F, et al. Contrast-enhanced ultrasonography of small solid pseudopapillary tumors of the pancreas: enhancement pattern and pathologic correlation of 2 cases. J Ultrasound Med 2005; 24(6):849–854.

64. Gupta A, Stuhlfaut JW, Fleming KW, Lucey BC, Soto JA. Blunt trauma of the pancreas and biliary tract: a multimodality imaging approach to diagnosis. Radiographics 2004; 24(5):1381–1395. Review.

65. Sato M, Yoshii H. Reevaluation of ultrasonography for solid-organ injury in blunt abdominal trauma. J Ultrasound Med 2004; 23(12):1583–1596.

66. Casadei R, Gallo C, Santini D, Zanelli M, La Donna M, Marrano D. Pancreatic foregut cyst. Eur J Surg 2000; 166(1):87–88.

67. Taouli B, Ghouadni M, Correas JM, et al. Spectrum of abdominal imaging findings in von Hippel-Lindau disease. Am J Roentgenol 2003; 181(4):1049–5104.

68. Pedersen OM, Aslaksen A, Vik-Mo H. Ultrasound measurement of the luminal diameter of the abdominal aorta and iliac arteries in patients without vascular disease. J Vasc Surg 1993; 17(3):596–601.

69. Hermsen K, Chong WK. Ultrasound evaluation of abdominal aortic and iliac aneurysms and mesenteric ischemia. Radiol Clin North Am 2004; 42(2):365–381.

70. Lumsden AB, Lin PH, Bush RL, Chen C. Chapter 22. In: Bruncardi FC, Andersen DA, Billiar TR, et al., eds. Arterial Disease in Schwartz's Principles of Surgery. 8th ed. New York, McGraw-Hill, 2005.

71. Brown LC, Powell JT. Risk factors for aneurysm rupture in patients kept under ultrasound surveillance. UK Small Aneurysm Trial Participants. Ann Surg 1999; 230(3):289–296; discussion 296–297.

72. Brown PM, Zelt DT, Sobolev B. The risk of rupture in untreated aneurysms: the impact of size, gender, and expansion rate. J Vasc Surg 2003; 37(2):280–284.

73. Lederle FA, Wilson SE, Johnson GR, et al.; Aneurysm Detection and Management Veterans Affairs Cooperative Study Group. Immediate repair compared with surveillance of small abdominal aortic aneurysms. N Engl J Med 2002; 346(19):1437–1444.

74. Brewster DC, Cronenwett JL, Hallett JW Jr, Johnston KW, Krupski WC, Matsumura JS; Joint Council of the American Association for Vascular Surgery and Society for Vascular Surgery. Guidelines for the treatment of abdominal aortic aneurysms. Report of a subcommittee of the Joint Council of the American Association for Vascular Surgery and Society for Vascular Surgery. J Vasc Surg 2003; 37(5):1106–1117. Review.

75. Brady AR, Thompson SG, Fowkes FG, Greenhalgh RM, Powell JT; UK Small Aneurysm Trial Participants. Abdominal aortic aneurysm expansion: risk factors and time intervals for surveillance. Circulation 2004; 110(1):16–21. Epub 2004.

76. Catalano O, Siani A. Ruptured abdominal aortic aneurysm: categorization of sonographic findings and report of 3 new signs. J Ultrasound Med 2005; 24(8):1077–1083.

77. Naganuma H, Ishida H, Konno K, Sato M, Ishida J, Watanabe S. Mycotic abdominal aneurysm: report of a case with emphasis on the presence of gas echoes. Abdom Imaging 2001; 26(4):420–422.

78. Cullenward MJ, Scanlan KA, Pozniak MA, Acher CA. Inflammatory aortic aneurysm (periaortic fibrosis): radiologic imaging. Radiology 1986; 159(1):75–82.

79. Auffermann W, Olofsson PA, Rabahie GN, Tavares NJ, Stoney RJ, Higgins CB. Incorporation versus infection of retroperitoneal aortic grafts: MR imaging features. Radiology 1989; 172(2):359–362.

80. Gooding GA. Ruptured abdominal aorta: postoperative ultrasound appearance. Radiology 1982; 145(3):78178–78183.

81. Mita T, Arita T, Matsunaga N, et al. Complications of endovascular repair for thoracic and abdominal aortic aneurysm: an imaging spectrum. Radiographics 2000; 20(5):1263–1278.

82. Parent FN, Meier GH, Godziachvili V, et al. The incidence and natural history of type I and II endoleak: a 5-year follow-up assessment with color duplex ultrasound scan. J Vasc Surg 2002; 35(3):474–481. Comment in: J Vasc Surg 2002; 35(3):595–597.

83. McLafferty RB, McCrary BS, Mattos MA, et al. The use of color-flow duplex scan for the detection of endoleaks. J Vasc Surg 2002; 36(1):100–104.

84. Greenfield AL, Halpern EJ, Bonn J, Wechsler RJ, Kahn MB. Application of duplex US for characterization of endoleaks in abdominal aortic stent-grafts: report of five cases. Radiology 2002; 225(3):845–851.

85. Bendick PJ, Bove PG, Long GW, Zelenock GB, Brown OW, Shanley CJ. Efficacy of ultrasound scan contrast agents in the noninvasive follow-up of aortic stent grafts. J Vasc Surg 2003; 37(2):381–385.

86. Napoli V, Bargellini I, Sardella SG, et al. Abdominal aortic aneurysm: contrast-enhanced US for missed endoleaks after endoluminal repair. Radiology 2004; 233(1):217–225.

87. Coselli JS, LeMaire SA. Chapter 21. In: Bruncardi FC, Andersen DA, Billiar TR, et al., eds. Thoracic Aortic Aneurysms and Aortic Dissection in Schwartz's Principles of Surgery. 8th ed. New York, McGraw-Hill, 2005.

88. King PS, Cooperberg PL, Madigan SM. The anechoic crescent in abdominal aortic aneurysms: not a sign of dissection. AJR Am J Roentgenol 1986; 146(2):345–348.

89. Fasouliotis SJ, Achiron R, Kivilevitch Z, Yagel S. The human fetal venous system: normal embryologic, anatomic, and physiologic characteristics and developmental abnormalities. J Ultrasound Med 2002; 21(10):1145–1158.

90. Vijayaraghavan SB, Raja V, Chitra TV. Interrupted inferior vena cava and left-sided subrenal inferior vena cava: prenatal diagnosis. J Ultrasound Med 2003; 22(7):747–752.

91. Berg C, Geipel A, Kamil D, et al. The syndrome of left isomerism: sonographic findings and outcome in prenatally diagnosed cases. J Ultrasound Med 2005; 24(7):921–931.

92. Gayer G, Zissin R, Strauss S, Hertz M. IVC anomalies and right renal aplasia detected on CT: a possible link? Abdom Imaging 2003; 28(3):395–399.

93. Yilmaz E, Gulcu A, Sal S, Obuz F. Interruption of the inferior vena cava with azygos/hemiazygos continuation accompanied by distinct renal vein anomalies: MRA and CT assessment. Abdom Imaging 2003; 28(3):392–394.

94. Gayer G, Luboshitz J, Hertz M, et al. Congenital anomalies of the inferior vena cava revealed on CT in patients with deep vein thrombosis. Am J Roentgenol 2003; 180(3):729–732.

95. Sandercoe GD, Brooke-Cowden GL. Developmental anomaly of the inferior vena cava. ANZ J Surg 2003; 73(5):356–360.

96. Obernosterer A, Aschauer M, Schnedl W, Lipp RW. Anomalies of the inferior vena cava in patients with iliac venous thrombosis. Ann Intern Med 2002; 136(1):37–41.

97. Mihmanli I, Bulakbasi N, Kantarci F, Adaletli I, Pabuscu Y. The value of ultrasonography in interrupted inferior vena cava with azygos continuation. Eur J Ultrasound 2001; 14(2–3):179–182.

98. Basile A, Certo A, Ascenti G, Lamberto S, Cannella A, Garcia Medina J. Embryologic and acquired anomalies of the inferior vena cava with recurrent deep vein thrombosis. Abdom Imaging 2003; 28(3):400–403.

99. Sakellaris G, Tilemis S, Papakonstantinou O, Bitsori M, Tsetis D, Charissis G. Deep venous thrombosis in a child associated with an abnormal inferior vena cava. Acta Paediatr 2005; 94(2):242–244.

100. Ryo E, Unno N, Nagasaka T, Taketani Y. Changes in the size of maternal inferior vena cava during pregnancy. J Perinat Med 2004; 32(4):327–331.

101. Lyon M, Blaivas M, Brannam L. Sonographic measurement of the inferior vena cava as a marker of blood loss. Am J Emerg Med 2005; 23(1):45–50.

102. Wachsberg RH. Narrowing of the upper abdominal inferior vena cava in patients with elevated intraabdominal pressure: sonographic observations. J Ultrasound Med 2000; 19(3):217–222.

103. Kitamura H, Kobayashi C. Impairment of change in diameter of the hepatic portion of the inferior vena cava: a sonographic sign of liver fibrosis or cirrhosis. J Ultrasound Med 2005; 24(3):355–359; quiz 360–361.

104. Lilova M, Velkovski IG, Velichkov NI. Budd-Chiari syndrome and inferior vena cava thrombosis in a nephrotic child. Pediatr Nephrol 2000; 14(5):412–415.

105. Savader SJ, Otero RR, Savader BL. Puerperal ovarian vein thrombosis: evaluation with CT, US, and MR imaging. Radiology 1988; 167(3):637–639.

106. Lim JH, Park JH, Auh YH. Membranous obstruction of the inferior vena cava: comparison of findings at sonography, CT, and venography. Am J Roentgenol 1992; 159(3):515–520.

107. Vijayaraghavan SB, Ramchandran P, Cherian M. Valvular-type membranous obstruction of the inferior vena cava with vertebral collaterals: color Doppler findings. J Ultrasound Med 2003; 22(2): 233–237.

108. Helmy T, Ware DL, Patterson C, Stouffer GA. Focal elastic obstruction of the inferior vena cava. Catheter Cardiovasc Interv 2000; 51(4):494–499.

109. Holland-Fischer P, Gronbaek H, Astrup L, Keiding S, Nielsen DT, Vilstrup H. Budd-Chiari and inferior caval vein syndromes due to membranous obstruction of the liver veins: successful treatment with angioplasty and transcaval transjugular intrahepatic portosystemic shunt. Scand J Gastroenterol 2004; 39(10):1025–1028.

110. Ko EY, Kim TK, Kim PN, Kim AY, Ha HK, Lee MG. Hepatic vein stenosis after living donor liver transplantation: evaluation with Doppler US. Radiology 2003; 229(3):806–810.

111. Yamagiwa K, Yokoi H, Isaji S, et al. Intrahepatic hepatic vein stenosis after living-related liver transplantation treated by insertion of an expandable metallic stent. Am J Transplant 2004; 4(6): 1006–1009.

112. Kallman DA, King BF, Hattery RR, et al. Renal vein and inferior vena cava tumor thrombus in renal cell carcinoma: CT, US, MRI and venacavography. J Comput Assist Tomogr 1992; 16(2):240–247.

113. Mehta SV, Lim-Dunham JE. Ultrasonographic appearance of pediatric abdominal neuroblastoma with inferior vena cava extension. J Ultrasound Med 2003; 22(10):1091–1095.

114. Martinez Baca-Lopez F, Ramirez-Arias E, Rayas-Gomez AL, Bernal-Ruiz EA, Saturno-Chiu G. Hepatocellular carcinoma with invasion into right cardiac cavities: report of a case and literature review. J Am Soc Echocardiogr 2004; 17(2):192–194.

115. Wang JN, Chen JS, Chuang HY, Yang YJ, Chang KC, Wu JM. Invasion of the cardiovascular system in childhood malignant hepatic tumors. J Pediatr Hematol Oncol 2002; 24(6):436–439.

116. Manavis J, Alexiadis G, Deftereos S, et al. Testicular tumors manifested as inferior vena cava thromboses. Case reports. Acta Radiol 2003; 44(1):24–27.

117. Kaszar-Seibert DJ, Gauvin GP, Rogoff PA, et al. Intracardiac extension of intravenous leiomyomatosis. Radiology 1988; 168(2):409–410.

118. Ling FT, David TE, Merchant N, Yu E, Butany JW. Intracardiac extension of intravenous leiomyomatosis in a pregnant woman: a case report and review of the literature. Can J Cardiol 2000; 16(1):73–79.

119. Kokawa K, Yamoto M, Yata C, Mabuchi Y, Umesaki N. Postmenopausal intravenous leiomyomatosis with high levels of estradiol and estrogen receptor. Obstet Gynecol 2002; 100(5 Pt 2): 1124–1126.

120. Rotter AJ, Lundell CJ. MR of intravenous leiomyomatosis of the uterus extending into the inferior vena cava. J Comput Assist Tomogr 1991; 15(4):690–693.

121. Schips L, Ratschek M, Galle G, et al. Angiomyolipoma with a caval thrombus. Urol Int 2003; 70(4):332–334.

122. Miyake H, Suzuki K, Ueda S, Yamada Y, Takeda H, Mori H. Localized fat collection adjacent to the intrahepatic portion of the inferior vena cava: a normal variant on CT. Am J Roentgenol 1992; 158(2):423–425. Comment in: Am J Roentgenol 1992; 159(6):1346. AJR Am J Roentgenol 2001; 177(1):251–252.

123. Grassi R, Di Mizio R, Barberi A, Severini S, Del Vecchio A, Cappabianca S. Case report. Ultrasound and CT findings in lipoma of the inferior vena cava. Br J Radiol 2002; 75(889):69–71.

124. Payan MJ, Xerri L, Choux R, et al. Giant leiomyoma of the inferior vena cava. Ann Pathol 1989; 9(1):44–46.

125. Dunlap HJ, Udjus K. Atypical leiomyoma arising in an hepatic vein with extension into the inferior vena cava and right atrium. Report of a case in a child. Pediatr Radiol 1990; 20(3):202–203.

126. van Rooij WJ, Martens F, Verbeeten B Jr, Dijkstra J. CT and MR imaging of leiomyosarcoma of the inferior vena cava. J Comput Assist Tomogr 1988; 12(3):415–419.

127. Hemant D, Krantikumar R, Amita J, Chawla A, Ranjeet N. Primary leiomyosarcoma of inferior vena cava, a rare entity: imaging features. Australas Radiol 2001; 45(4):448–451.

128. Abisi S, Morris-Stiff GJ, Scott–Coombes D, Williams IM, Douglas-Jones AG, Puntis MC. Leiomyosarcoma of the inferior vena cava: clinical experience with four cases. World J Surg Oncol 2006; 4:1.

129. Andonov V, Stanchev I, Cholakoval E, Nikolaeva S, Ananoshtev N, Djurkov V. A rare case of fibrosarcoma of the inferior vena cava expanding into the right atrium. Folia Med (Plovdiv) 1999; 41(4):80–82.

130. Fishman AD, Hoffman A, Volterra F, Frymus M, Gentilluci M. Intracaval and intracardiac metastatic nonseminomatous germ cell tumor: a rare cause of hemolytic anemia and thrombocytopenia. Cancer Invest 2002; 20(7–8):996–1001.

131. Sheth R, Hanchate V, Rathod K, Ahmed I, Deshmukh H, Chaubal N. Aneurysms of the inferior vena cava. Australas Radiol 2003; 47(1):94–96

The Spleen ● *Marijo A. Gillen*

EMBRYOLOGY

The spleen develops from mesenchymal cells in the dorsal mesogastrium. As the stomach rotates, the spleen moves toward the left side into its position in the left upper quadrant and there is variable fusion to the retroperitoneum. The spleen is supported by the phrenicosplenic, gastrosplenic, splenocolic, pancreatosplenic, and splenorenal ligaments. The splenorenal and gastrosplenic ligaments arise from the dorsal mesogastrium. The spleen is mostly intraperitoneal and surrounded by visceral peritoneum except for the bare area, which is a small area of variable size located between the phrenicosplenic, gastrosplenic, splenorenal, and splenocolic ligaments, in which lie the splenic vessels (1).

NORMAL ANATOMY

The spleen normally lies adjacent to the left hemidiaphragm in the left upper quadrant, lateral to the greater curvature of the stomach and cephalad to the left kidney. The tail of the pancreas is in proximity to the hilum of the spleen, which is significant in both inflammatory and neoplastic processes of the pancreas. Although a multiplicity of measurements are available for the spleen, the most common are a pole-to-pole length of 12 cm, width of 7 cm, and thickness of 4 cm as average dimensions for an adult spleen (2). The spleen consists of white pulp (lymphatic follicles) and surrounding red pulp (vascular spaces containing blood cells). The spleen is of a homogenous intermediate echotexture with smooth margins, with moderately good through transmission of sound (Fig. 1a and b); it is usually slightly more echogenic than the liver but may be isoechoic or even hypoechoic. The spleen may be lobulated. The hilar vessels are easily recognized on the medial aspect of the spleen, and both venous and arterial flows are demonstrated with color or spectral Doppler. Arterial flow is from the splenic artery and venous flow is from the splenic vein.

SCANNING TECHNIQUE

The spleen can be visualized in the supine position from a posterolateral approach or from a coronal plane with the patient's left side up. Sagittal and transverse scans are performed both subcostally and intercostally, as required. Identifying the thin echogenic arc that represents the left hemidiaphragm and the superior pole of the left kidney ensures that the splenic bed has been adequately imaged. In patients with marked splenomegaly, the inferior border is best imaged in the supine position.

Microbubble ultrasound contrast agents can be used to evaluate the spleen (Fig. 2A). The normal spleen shows immediate heterogeneity of contrast enhancement, similar to that seen on arterial phase computed tomography (CT); small arteries can be seen (Fig. 2B). After this, the spleen becomes very echogenic and homogenous (Fig. 2C) and then decreases to normal echogenicity as the contrast agent washes out (3).

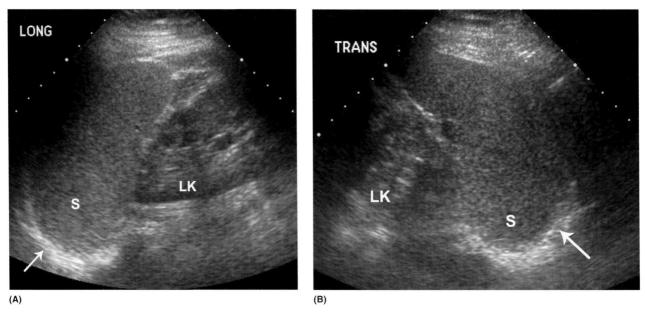

(A)　　　(B)

FIGURE 1 A AND B ■ Normal spleen. Homogeneous echotexture located between the left hemidiaphragm (*arrow*) and the left kidney. (**A**) Sagittal plane. (**B**) Transverse plane. S, spleen; LK, left kidney.

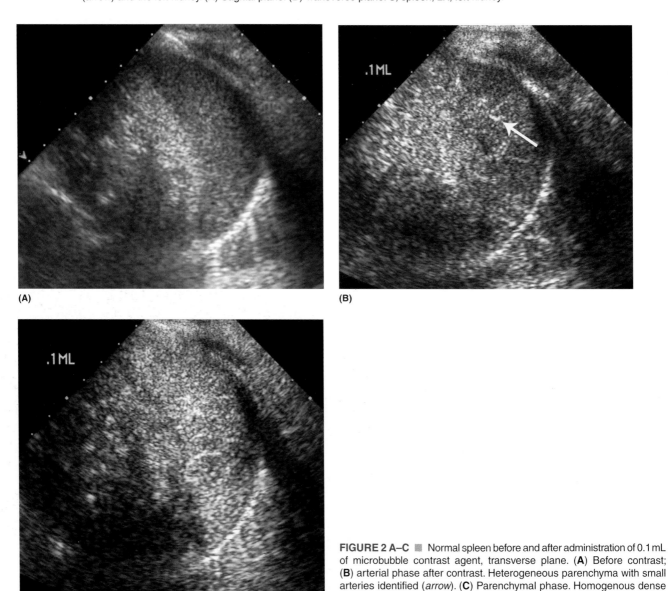

(A)　　　(B)

(C)

FIGURE 2 A–C ■ Normal spleen before and after administration of 0.1 mL of microbubble contrast agent, transverse plane. (**A**) Before contrast; (**B**) arterial phase after contrast. Heterogeneous parenchyma with small arteries identified (*arrow*). (**C**) Parenchymal phase. Homogenous dense parenchymal enhancement.

PITFALLS AND ARTIFACTS

One of the chief difficulties in complete imaging of the spleen is that substantial portions of it lie behind the ribs. For an overall length and global view of the spleen, the clinician accepts the one or two bands of near-total attenuation produced by the overlying rib and observes as the shadowed portion of the parenchyma becomes visible with variations in respiration. Oblique scans with the transducer parallel with the intercostal space also help to image the splenic texture without rib shadowing. In trauma patients, other problems include the difficulty of scanning over areas of tenderness, soft-tissue injuries in the region, and chest tubes and their bandages covering large portions of the splenic bed.

Deep clefts in the spleen that are a product of embryologic lobulation may simulate fractures. Smooth, curvilinear contours and absence of adjacent free fluid should define these lobulations as normal variants.

On occasion, the left lobe of the liver may wrap around the superolateral aspect of the spleen, creating the impression of a subcapsular hematoma of the spleen. Observing its separate motion at real time and tracing this tissue back to the liver obviates this pitfall (Fig. 3).

VARIANTS

The single or multiple aggregations of splenic tissue referred to as splenules, splenunculi, or accessory spleens can be found in 10% to 30% of the normal population (2). Their location is usually close to the splenic hilum or in the ligaments of the spleen (splenorenal and gastrosplenic) but can be in the greater omentum, in the pancreatic tail (4), or even in the pelvis (5). Accessory spleens can be identified by their smooth rounded contour, homogeneity, and echogenicity isoechoic to the spleen; they are usually less than 5 cm in diameter (Fig. 4). Their blood supply is usually from a branch of the splenic artery. They exhibit the exact same enhancement pattern as the spleen after microbubble contrast agents.

Splenogonadal fusion has been reported (6). It consists of accessory splenic tissue fused to the gonads, either in the pelvis or in the scrotum. It occurs more commonly in males, is usually on the left, and can mimic a testicular neoplasm. It can be continuous or discontinuous. In the continuous type, there is a fibrous or splenic cord connecting the spleen with the gonad and there can be associated congenital anomalies (7).

Macronodular deformity of the spleen has been reported. It has been associated with tumor, inflammatory process, or postnecrotic scar formation, but isoechoic nodules in a macronodular pattern have been reported, some seen in cases of splenic vein thrombosis (8).

The spleen can change in location with adjacent surgery such as a left nephrectomy when it can occupy the left renal fossa.

An "upside down" spleen has been reported as a variant in which the spleen is rotated on its horizontal

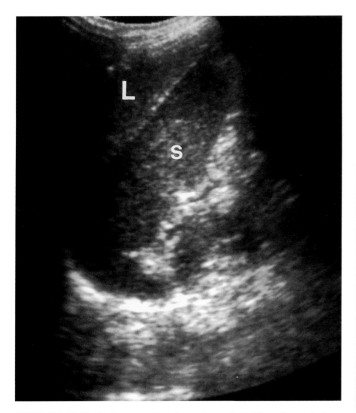

FIGURE 3 ■ Sagittal image showing enlarged slightly echogenic liver wrapping around the spleen, creating the appearance of subcapsular hematoma. S, spleen; L, liver. *Source*: Courtesy of A. Fried, University of Kentucky.

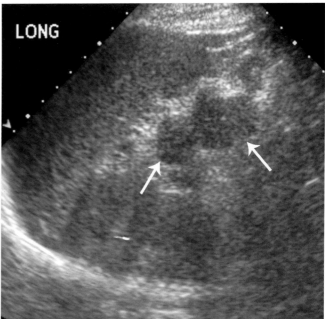

FIGURE 4 ■ Accessory spleens. Sagittal scan showing two accessory spleens (*arrows*) at the splenic hilum with echotexture identical to the splenic tissue.

anteroposterior axis; in this, the concave splenic hilus points superiorly, toward the diaphragm and the stomach fundus. This is, reportedly, of no clinical significance (9).

WANDERING SPLEEN

With severe ligamentous laxity or congenital abnormality of the peritoneal attachments, including incomplete fusion of the dorsal mesogastrium to the dorsal peritoneum, the spleen can move within the abdomen or the pelvis, called a "wandering spleen," which can be mistaken for a mass. Diagnosis can be made by detecting a mass of echotexture isoechoic to normal spleen, absence of splenic tissue in the normal location, and blood supply by vessels contiguous with the splenic artery and vein. Diagnosis can be confirmed with a heat-treated technetium (Tc)^{99m} RBC scan or sulfur colloid scan. Ligamentous laxity can also be secondary to hormonal effects of pregnancy or muscular dystrophies. A wandering spleen is most common at ages 20 to 40 (10) and in women but can be seen in children (11). In addition to being mistaken for a mass, complications of a wandering spleen include torsion, infarction, splenomegaly, and trauma to the spleen in an unprotected location. Nonsplenic complications of a wandering spleen include gastric volvulus, gastric outlet obstruction, intestinal obstruction, and pancreatitis (12). Torsion causes splenic vessel occlusion, infarction, and necrosis and can lead to abscess formation, localized peritonitis, intestinal obstruction, and necrosis of the pancreatic tail (13,14). With torsion, there is significant acute abdominal pain; with torsion and detorsion, there is chronic and intermittent abdominal pain and splenic congestion (13). Power Doppler ultrasound shows no perfusion with torsion (14). A torsed vascular pedicle at the splenic hilum may appear as a mass (15). Since the tail of the pancreas can lie within a long splenic mesentery, it can be displaced with the spleen; pancreatitis or necrosis of the pancreatic tail can occur with torsion. Treatment options include splenopexy or splenectomy (12). Accessory spleens can also be on an elongated vascular pedicle, consistent with a wandering accessory spleen; these can also torse (16).

SPLENOSIS

Splenosis occurs when small aggregates of splenic tissue are dispersed into the abdomen or thorax after splenectomy or trauma. It can occur in 26% to 67% of postsplenectomy cases after trauma (17).

These can be mistaken for abdominal masses. History is important in making this diagnosis. If the splenectomy was for an underlying hematologic disorder causing hypersplenism, areas of splenosis can hypertrophy and symptoms can reoccur. Residual accessory spleens can also hypertrophy and can become larger than 5 cm.

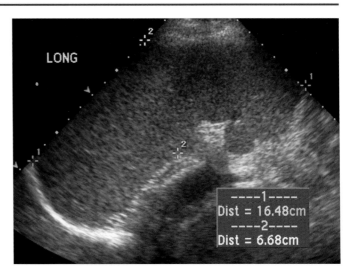

FIGURE 5 ■ Moderate splenomegaly. Sagittal measurement of 16.48 cm (*between* + *calipers*) in a patient with α thalassemia.

SPLENOMEGALY

Ultrasound provides an easy and accurate estimation of spleen size; an adult spleen measuring more than 12 cm in pole-to-pole length is considered abnormal. The enlarged spleen may be difficult to separate clinically from other causes of left upper quadrant masses, especially in children; the distinction is easily made with ultrasound, which allows confident identification of even the massively enlarged spleen extending into the iliac fossa or across the midline (Figs. 5 and 6).

Splenomegaly is seen in a variety of etiologies including infections, congestive splenomegaly, hematologic

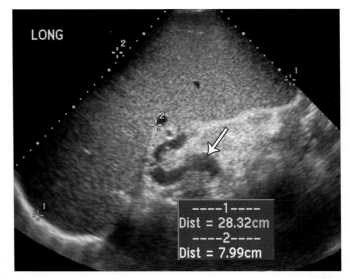

FIGURE 6 ■ Marked splenomegaly. Sagittal measurement of 28.32 cm (*between* + *calipers*) in a patient with chronic myelomonocytic leukemia with acute transformation. Prominent vessels at splenic hilum from portal hypertension (*arrow*).

TABLE 1 ■ Causes of Splenomegaly

Infection		**Collagen vascular disease**	
Bacterial	Pyogenic abscesses, bacterial endocarditis, syphilis, typhoid, tularemia, brucellosis	Systemic lupus erythematosus	
Mycobacterial	Tuberculosis	Felty syndrome (rheumatoid arthritis, splenomegaly, and neutropenia)	
Viral	Viral hepatitis, AIDS, infectious mononucleosis, CMV, herpes simplex, rubella	Juvenile rheumatoid arthritis	
		Neoplasm	
Rickettsial	Typhus, rocky mountain spotted fever	Benign	Cyst: Epidermoid, hydatid cyst, secondary or pseudocyst
Fungal	Histoplasmosis, candidiasis		Hemangioma
Parasitic	Malaria, schistosomiasis, echinococcus, leishmaniasis (Kala-azar), toxoplasmosis		Hamartoma
			Lymphangioma
		Malignant	Lymphoma
Congestive splenomegaly			Leukemia
Congestive heart failure			Angiosarcoma
Portal hypertension			Metastases: Melanoma, sarcoma
Cirrhosis	Nutritional, alcoholic, Wilson's, cystic fibrosis, α1 antitrypsin disease	**Infiltrative disease**	
		Gaucher's	
		Glycogen-storage diseases	
Splenic-vein or portal-vein obstruction	Thrombosis, pancreatic neoplasm, lymphadenopathy	Mucopolysaccharidosis	
		Mucolipidosis	
Banti's syndrome		GM1 gangliosidosis	
Acute splenic sequestration crisis in sickle-cell disease		Niemann–Pick disease	
		Hemochromatosis	
Hematologic disorders		Langerhans-cell histiocytosis	
Hemoglobinopathies	Sickle cell, thalassemia	Amyloidosis	
Elliptocytosis		Diabetes	
Hereditary spherocytosis		**Miscellaneous**	
Thrombotic thrombocytopenic purpura		Hemodialysis	
Primary neutropenia		Sarcoid	
Pyruvate kinase deficiency		Hematoma	
Autoimmune hemolytic anemia		Hemorrhagic pseudocyst	
Megaloblastic anemia		Extracorporeal membrane oxygenation in infants	
Extramedullary hematopoiesis	Myelofibrosis	Hyperthyroidism	
	Polycythemia vena	Tropical splenomegaly	
	Osteopetrosis	Drug reactions	
	Dysgammaglobulinemia		
	Myelosclerosis		

Abbreviations: CMV, cytomegalovirus; TB, tuberculosis.
Source: From Refs. 18–20.

disorders, collagen vascular disease, neoplasms, infiltrative diseases, and miscellaneous (Table 1) (18–20).

Mild splenomegaly is seen in some infections and sepsis. Moderate splenic enlargement can be seen in portal hypertension, some hematologic disorders, leukemia, and AIDS (Fig. 5). A very large spleen can be seen in lymphoma, myelofibrosis, chronic myeloid leukemia (CML), malaria, or primary splenic neoplasms (Fig. 6) (21).

THE SMALL SPLEEN

A small spleen (Fig. 7) can be seen in sickle-cell anemia and other causes of multiple splenic infarctions, occlusion of splenic vessels, post trauma, post surgery, post chemotherapy, atrophy, hereditary hypoplasia, inflammatory bowel disease, or in polysplenia and asplenia syndromes (Table 2) (18–20). Small well-functioning spleens can be seen in the elderly (Fig. 7) (22).

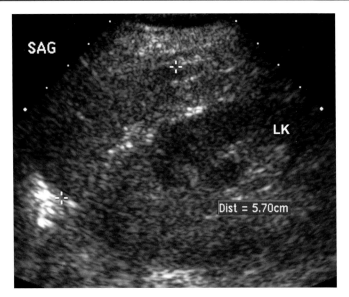

FIGURE 7 ■ Small spleen. Sagittal measurement (*between + calipers*) of 5.70 cm in an elderly female with normal splenic function. LK, left kidney.

Polysplenia and asplenia are syndromes involving situs abnormalities, congenital heart defects, and splenic abnormal number or absence.

In polysplenia, multiple small spleens are noted. It is associated with interruption of the intrahepatic portion of the inferior vena cava (IVC) with an azygous continuation, bilateral left sidedness, and congenital heart disease; it is more common in females.

With asplenia or Ivemark's syndrome, no splenic tissue is identified, the IVC and the abdominal aorta lie on the same side of the spine, there is bilateral right sidedness, and there is associated complex congenital heart disease. It is more common in males (2,19).

FUNCTIONAL ASPLENIA

Infiltrative processes may cause a functional asplenia secondary to destruction of splenic tissue in a normal-sized or enlarged spleen. Functional asplenia in the presence of splenic tissue on imaging studies is diagnosed by the presence of Howell–Jolly bodies on a peripheral blood smear or decreased activity on liver–spleen nuclear medicine scan. Functional asplenia is seen with infiltrative processes, immunologic/rheumatologic/inflammatory disorders, or in diseases that occlude splenic vessels (Table 3) (23).

TRAUMA

Although CT provides a more global view of abdominal trauma, it does have the negatives of ionizing radiation, increased cost, use of i.v. contrast, and necessity to transport the critical patient to a CT scanner. The focused abdominal sonogram for trauma (FAST) scan can be used immediately on the trauma patient during initial resuscitation efforts. It consists of limited ultrasound images of all quadrants, the pelvis (best with a full bladder), and the epigastric region (24). The presence of free fluid is used as a sign of organ injury. The presence of

TABLE 2 ■ Small or Absent Spleen

Polysplenia
Asplenia
Atrophy
Hereditary hypoplasia
Occlusion of splenic vessels
■ Auto infarction (hemoglobinopathies, especially sickle-cell disease)
■ Post infarction
■ Post pancreatitis
■ Post torsion
■ Collagen vascular disease (SLE)
■ Post radiation therapy
Post trauma
Post chemotherapy
Post surgery
Splenosis after trauma or surgery
Inflammatory bowel disease
Wandering spleen
Normal finding in elderly
Fanconi's anemia
Celiac disease
Abbreviation: SLE, systemic lupus erythematosus
Source: From Refs. 18–20.

TABLE 3 ■ Functional/Asplenia

Infiltrative processes
■ Lymphoma
■ Acute leukemia
■ Metastases
■ Metabolic disorders
■ Amyloidosis
■ Sarcoidosis
■ Chronic graft versus host disease
Immunologic/rheumatic/inflammatory disorders
■ Systemic lupus erythematosus
■ Rheumatoid arthritis
■ Systemic vasculitis
■ Ulcerative colitis
■ Celiac disease
Occlusion of splenic vessels (usually associated with a small spleen)
■ Autoinfarction (hemoglobinopathies, especially sickle cell disease)
■ Post infarction
■ Post pancreatitis
■ Post torsion
■ Post chemotherapy
■ Post radiation therapy

free fluid is not specific for injury to a particular organ, but an echogenic clot, the "sentinel clot," suggests injury to the adjacent organ (25). Depending on their hemodynamic stability and the amount of free fluid, the patient can then be taken for further evaluation with a CT scan if stable, or taken to the operating room if unstable. If the FAST scan is negative and the patient is hemodynamically stable, the patient can be monitored with further evaluation as necessary.

With a positive FAST scan, a predominance of fluid near the spleen can suggest splenic injury (26). However, with splenic injuries, free fluid can also be commonly seen in a diffuse pattern, in both upper quadrants (27), or in the pelvis, particularly in pediatric patients (28).

If evaluation of the parenchyma of the spleen is added to the FAST scan, there is improved sensitivity for detection of blunt splenic injury (24). Higher-grade injuries are more easily detected (29). Several sonographic patterns of splenic injury have been reported. The most common is a diffuse heterogeneous appearance [both hyperechoic (Fig. 8) and hypoechoic], followed by discrete hyperechoic or hypoechoic (Fig. 9) regions in the spleen. A hyperechoic (Fig. 10) or hypoechoic rim (Fig. 11), consistent with a clot or subcapsular hematoma, is often seen (29).

Microbubble contrast-enhanced ultrasound (CEUS) has been used to evaluate splenic injury and comparison made with CT and precontrast ultrasound (30). Areas of decreased echogenicity after contrast correspond to parenchymal injury (including contusion, laceration, or hematoma) or infarcts. Lacerations appear as branched or linear hypoechoic bands, usually perpendicular to the splenic capsule. Lacerocontusive areas and parenchymal hematomas correspond to inhomogeneous hypoechoic areas without vessel displacement (Fig. 12a–c) (31). Posttraumatic infarctions appear as wedge-shaped hypoechoic areas. Splenic pedicle avulsions or "shock spleen"

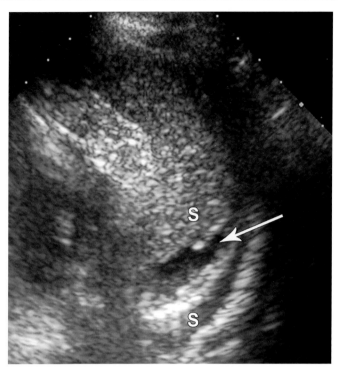

FIGURE 9 ■ Splenic laceration. FAST (focused abdominal sonogram for trauma) scan. Discrete hypoechoic region (*arrow*) within the splenic parenchyma corresponding to a laceration. S, splenic parenchyma.

(severe hypovolemia) appear as diffusely poor parenchymal enhancement, less than adjacent organs (31).

Contrast extravasation indicates ongoing bleeding. Pooling of contrast appears as a persistent round or oval

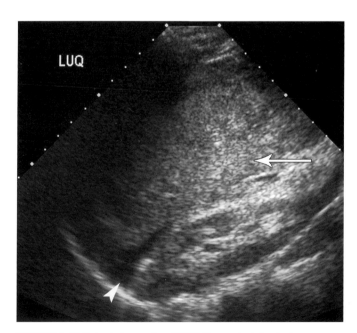

FIGURE 8 ■ Splenic laceration. FAST (focused abdominal sonogram for trauma) scan. Diffuse heterogeneous appearance of spleen. Mostly hyperechoic (*arrow*) with perisplenic free fluid (*arrowhead*).

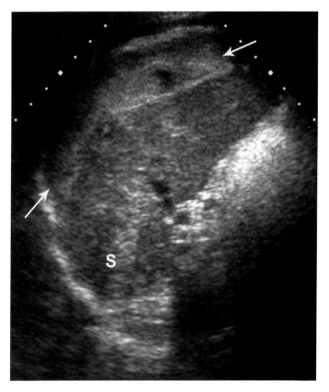

FIGURE 10 ■ Splenic laceration. FAST (focused abdominal sonogram for trauma) scan. Hyperechoic rim (*arrows*) corresponding to clot in a subcapsular hematoma anterior to the spleen. S, spleen.

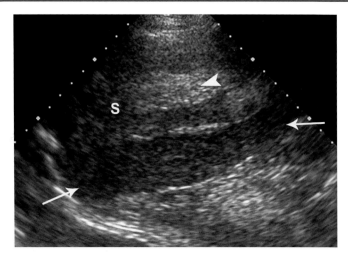

FIGURE 11 ■ Splenic laceration. FAST (focused abdominal sonogram for trauma) scan. Hypoechoic rim (*arrows*) corresponding to a subcapsular hematoma posterior to the spleen. Echogenic area within the spleen (*arrowhead*) corresponds to echogenic clot within the spleen. S, spleen.

hyperechoic area in the splenic parenchyma and is consistent with either active intraparenchymal hemorrhage or pseudoaneurysm. Hyperechoic jets of contrast, continuous or discontinuous, reaching the splenic capsule, and possibly extending around the spleen, are seen with extraparenchymal bleeding and are seen with more severe injuries (32). Subcapsular hematomas are also better seen after contrast as hypoechoic areas surrounding the enhanced splenic parenchyma (33). More splenic parenchymal lesions can be detected with CEUS than with noncontrast ultrasound and lesions are better seen, although small-to-moderate injuries can still be missed and contrast-enhanced CT is still more sensitive (34). CEUS has been used in pediatric patients with blunt abdominal trauma and has detected splenic hematomas. A greater role for CEUS in pediatric trauma patients should be considered because of the lack of ionizing radiation and lack of sedation (35). CEUS may also be useful as a follow-up modality after initial CT to evaluate for delayed pseudoaneurysms (34).

INFECTION

Pyogenic Splenic Abscesses

Pyogenic splenic abscesses can be single or multiple. Organisms include gram-positive organisms, gram-negative organisms, or anaerobic organisms; tuberculosis (TB) has also been reported (36). Abscesses are rare but are seen with high frequency in immunocompromised patients such as those with AIDS, post chemotherapy, or patients with diabetes or leukemia, or in i.v. drug users. Spread can be hematogenous (such as from bacterial endocarditis or sepsis), spread from infections of adjacent organs (such as pancreas or kidney) or can result from superinfection of a traumatic splenic hematoma or infarct (36–38).

On ultrasound, splenic abscesses appear as irregularly marginated, hypoechoic cystic collections, single or multiple, which can contain internal echoes, septa, and debris (Fig. 13A). Dirty shadowing can be seen if air is present (39). With CEUS, splenic abscesses appear as hypoechoic collections with enhancing rim and septa (3).

Abscesses can be treated with antibiotics but some may require ultrasound-guided aspiration, percutaneous drain placement (Fig. 13B), or even splenectomy.

Tuberculosis

Splenic TB occurs in micronodular or macronodular forms (40). The micronodular form is seen in miliary TB and is more common. These tiny nodules, when less than 3 mm, are too small to be seen on ultrasound; moderate splenomegaly can be seen with diffuse heterogeneity and sometimes increased echogenicity (41). If the nodules are slightly larger, the microabcesses can be seen as multiple small splenic hypoechoic lesions less than 2 cm. These can calcify, especially after treatment, and become echogenic (Fig. 14) (42).

The macronodular form of TB, also called a tuberculoma, manifests as single or multiple discrete masses greater than 2 cm with splenomegaly. On ultrasound, these are usually hypoechoic and heterogeneous but can be hyperechoic with or without calcification and can rarely be septated (41–43). Tuberculous splenic abscess have also been reported (36).

The incidence of splenic TB has increased, with an increased number of TB cases seen in AIDS patients (44).

Splenic Microabscesses

Microabscesses can be seen in the spleen and liver from disseminated infection in immunocompromised patients, especially in AIDS or postchemotherapy patients. These usually are multiple, diffuse, and size is less than 10 mm; these are usually hypoechoic but can be hyperechoic. At the usual abdominal sonographic frequency of 3.5 to 4.0 MHz, these lesions may not be seen or the spleen may appear enlarged or heterogeneous. In a study involving AIDS patients with the use of a 5.0 MHz transducer (45) and another study in HIV-infected patients using a 7.5 MHz transducer (46), more lesions were identified with the higher-frequency transducers than with the 3.5 MHz transducer. With the 5.0 MHz transducer, detection of splenic microabcesses in one study increased from 3% to 12% (45). The etiologies of splenic microabcesses in HIV patients were *Mycobacterium tuberculosis*, *Mycobacterium avium-intracellulare*, *Pneumocystis carinii*, fungal infections such as Candida (the fungal infections often show a target lesion), and less common organisms such as visceral leishmaniasis, salmonella, and *Rhodococcus equi* (45,46). In HIV patients, neoplastic causes of multiple small lesions were lymphoma (hypoechoic nodules) and Kaposi's sarcoma (hyperechoic nodules), which can mimic microabcesses (46).

Fungal

Disseminated *Candida* infection in immunocompromised patients can be separated into two main syndromes: acute disseminated candidiasis or chronic disseminated candidiasis, also known as hepatosplenic candidiasis. Although

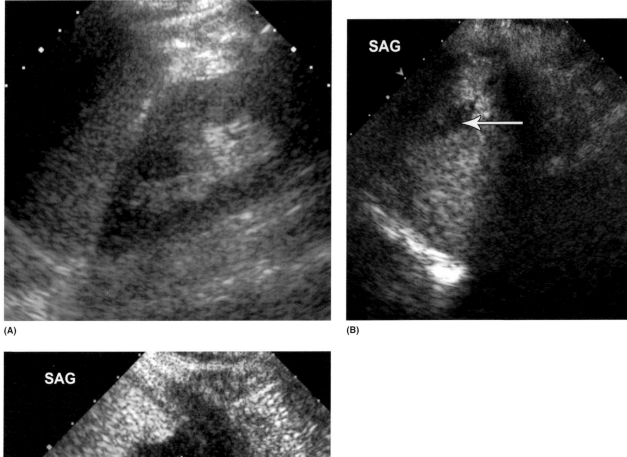

FIGURE 12 A–C ■ Splenic laceration. Scans obtained before and after 0.1 mL of microbubble ultrasound contrast agent was administered. **(A)** Sagittal precontrast ultrasound shows no parenchymal defect. **(B)** Sagittal postcontrast ultrasound showing nonenhancing laceration (*arrow*). **(C)** Transverse later postcontrast ultrasound showing nonenhancing laceration (*arrow*). S, spleen.

they may be part of the same spectrum, they have separate presentations and radiologic appearances (47). In acute disseminated candidiasis, patients have a neutropenic fever, positive *Candida* blood cultures, and no lesions seen on CT or ultrasound. In chronic disseminated candidiasis, patients have a nonneutropenic fever, negative *Candida* blood cultures, and focal lesions are seen on CT and ultrasound (47).

With chronic disseminated candidiasis, or hepatosplenic candidiasis, Pastakia et al. (48) have reported four major patterns on ultrasound. The "wheel within a wheel" type consists of a central hypoechoic area (representing necrosis), a hyperechoic wheel (consisting of inflammatory cells), and a peripheral hypoechoic wheel (representing fibrosis); this is seen early in the disease. The second type is the "bull's eye" or target pattern consisting of a central hyperechoic area surrounded by a hypoechoic rim (Fig. 15); this may evolve from the first type. The third type is a uniformly hypoechoic lesion (Fig. 15) and is most common. The fourth type is usually seen late in the disease and consists of echogenic foci (corresponding to fibrosis or calcifications) with varying degrees of shadowing.

Histoplasmosis initially presents as multiple small hypoechoic foci (Fig. 16) or target lesions, which later can calcify after healing.

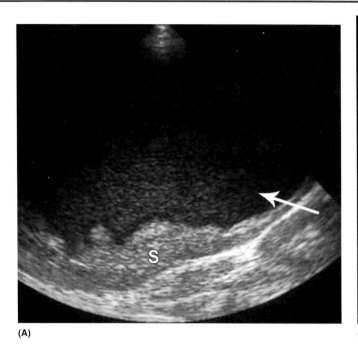

(A)

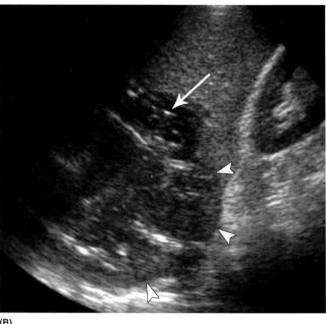

(B)

FIGURE 13 A AND B ▪ Pyogenic splenic abscess within the spleen. (**A**) Hypoechoic collection (*arrow*) with irregular margins containing internal debris. S, spleen. (**B**) Same collection (*arrowheads*) after catheter placement and drainage of the abscess. The irregular echogenic foci represent air (*arrow*). *Source*: Courtesy of A. Fried, University of Kentucky.

Parasitic Diseases

Hydatid disease from *Echinococcus* infection can involve the spleen but is rare, with a prevalence of 0.9% to 8%; it is usually seen along with other organ involvement and isolated splenic disease is rare. Echinococcal disease mani-fests as cysts that can be anechoic or can be echogenic because of parasite scolices. After microbubble contrast, there is no internal enhancement but there can be peripheral enhancement (49).

Four types of hydatid cysts have been described (50). Type I is a simple cyst but may have hydatid sand or septa; on ultrasound, turning the patient moves the sand causing a "falling snowflake" appearance. Type II is a cyst that contains daughter cysts and floating membranes;

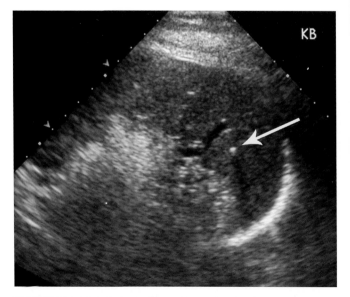

FIGURE 14 ▪ Calcified splenic granulomas, from TB. Several small echogenic foci (*arrow*) within the spleen correspond to calcified granulomas.

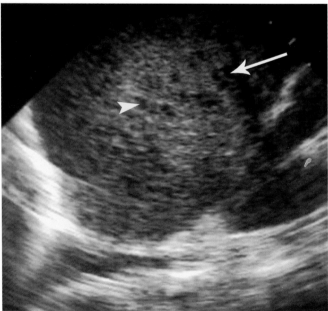

FIGURE 15 ▪ Splenic microabscesses from *Candida*. Heterogenous spleen containing multiple small hypoechoic areas of at least two types. Type II, bull's eye or target pattern with a small hyperechoic center with a hypoechoic rim (*arrow*). Type III lesions consist of a uniformly hypoechoic lesion (*arrowhead*). *Source*: Courtesy of A. Fried, University of Kentucky.

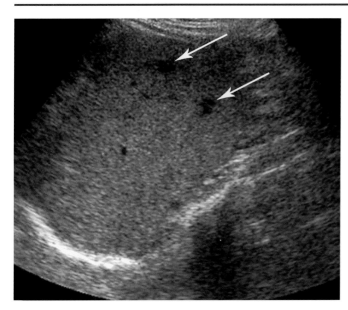

FIGURE 16 ■ Splenic histoplasmosis. Multiple small focal hypoechoic areas (*arrows*) in the spleen from disseminated histoplasmosis. *Source*: Courtesy of A. Fried, University of Kentucky.

TABLE 4 ■ Hypoechoic Splenic Lesions

Cysts	With hemorrhage or debris (including parasitic, pseudocysts, epidermoid cyst)
Abscesses	Pyogenic
Microabscesses	TB, fungal, MAI, salmonella
	Pneumocystis carinii
	Visceral leishmaniasis
	Rhodococcus equi
	Cat-scratch disease
	Septic emboli
Trauma	Laceration
	Infarction
	Hematoma
Infarcts	Usually wedge shaped
Aneurysm or pseudoaneurysm	With thrombosis or hemorrhage
Tumors—benign	Hamartomas (can also be echogenic)
	Hemangiomas (usually echogenic)
	Littoral-cell angioma (can also be iso- or hyperechoic)
Tumors—variable malignant potential	Hemangiopericytoma (can also be hyperechoic)
	Hemangioendothelioma (can also be isoechoic with a hypoechoic rim)
Tumors—malignant	Angiosarcoma (with necrosis)
	Lymphoma
	Myeloproliferative disease (can also be hyperechoic)
	Metastases (can be target lesions)
Miscellaneous	Sarcoidosis
	Peliosis (hypoechoic areas)
	Storage diseases, i.e., Gaucher's (can also be hyperechoic)
	Amyloidomas
	Inflammatory pseudotumor
	Areas of necrosis in extramedullary hematopoiesis
Acute trauma	Can also be echogenic with clot

Abbreviations: TB, tuberculosis; MAI, *Mycobacterium avium-intracellulare*.

vesicles or wall calcification can be seen. Type III is a totally calcified cyst, which is a dead cyst; on ultrasound this appears as an echogenic area with posterior shadowing. Type IV cysts are complicated hydatid cysts from either rupture or superinfection; this occurs in approximately 50% to 90% of cases. On ultrasound in a contained rupture, an undulating membrane may be identified; a "snowstorm" appearance has also been described (50).

The parasitic disease schistosomiasis often involves the spleen but most commonly presents as nonspecific splenomegaly caused by portal hypertension secondary to hepatic periportal fibrosis (51,52).

Malarial infection of the spleen commonly results in splenomegaly, but there is an increased incidence of associated complications such as splenic hematoma, subcapsular hematoma, splenic rupture, splenic torsion, or splenic cyst formation (likely from resolving hematoma). Spontaneous rupture occurs in approximately 2% of malaria cases but can be life threatening (53). Ultrasound shows an enlarged ruptured spleen and free fluid in the abdomen or pelvis. Spontaneous splenic rupture can also be seen with other diseases such as infectious mononucleosis or in splenic or hematologic malignancies (54).

Miscellaneous

Sarcoidosis, which is a granulomatous disease of unknown etiology, when present in the spleen, can present as multiple hypoechoic small nodules or can present with nonspecific splenomegaly (55).

The finding of multiple hypoechoic lesions in the spleen is nonspecific and can be seen in a variety of other etiologies (Table 4). Hypoechoic lesions have been reported with mycoplasma pneumoniae (with also some wedge-shaped lesions) (56), cat-scratch disease from *Bartonella henselae* (57), and visceral leishmaniasis (Kalaazar) from *Leishmania donovani* (58).

VASCULAR LESIONS

Infarction

Splenic infarcts can be from either arterial or venous occlusion. Arterial thrombosis occurs when the splenic artery or branches are occluded. Venous thrombosis occurs by thrombosis of the splenic sinuses or the splenic vein. Venous infarction causes massive splenomegaly, leading to congestion and thrombosis of the sinusoids. Arterial infarcts are ischemic; venous infarcts are hemorrhagic (39). Causes include post surgery (ligation of splenic artery or vein), secondary to sepsis (particularly emboli from endocarditis), arteritides, hypercoagulable states, hemolytic anemias (sickle cell and thalassemias), myeloproliferative disorders, pancreatitis, pancreatic

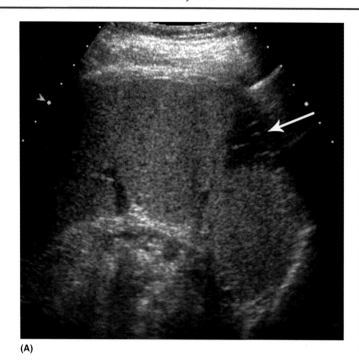

(A)

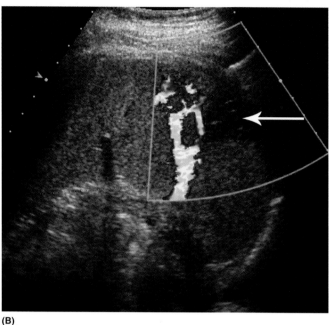

(B)

FIGURE 17 A AND B ■ Splenic infarct in a patient with acute myeloid leukemia. The spleen is enlarged. **(A)** On gray scale images, there is a wedge-shaped hypoechoic area (*arrow*) with septa, consistent with an infarct. **(B)** On color images, no flow is seen within the infarct (*arrow*).

carcinoma, or trauma (59). Infarction has been reported during acute malaria (60).

Infarcts appear as ill defined, peripheral, often wedge-shaped (but can be round or oval) hypodensities with irregular margins (Fig. 17A). No flow is seen within an infarct with color Doppler (Fig. 17B). With time, infarcts become smaller and heterogeneous, sometimes echogenic, or liquefaction may occur with pseudocyst formation (39,61).

Delayed complications of splenic infarct are intrasplenic pseudoaneurysms, splenic rupture (61), and splenic abscess (59). After splenic infarction, air seen within the splenic bed (echogenic, "dirty" shadowing) is worrisome for super infection, although cases of noninfectious air accumulation have been reported (62).

Rupture

Spontaneous, or nontraumatic, rupture of the spleen is rare, more common in males, usually associated with splenomegaly, and can be life threatening. Etiologies are infectious (infectious mononucleosis and malaria), hematologic (coagulation disorders, thrombocytopenia, infarction, and venous thrombosis), portal hypertension, vasculitis, infiltrative (Gaucher's disease), neoplastic (lymphoma, myeloproliferative diseases, and metastases), focal splenic lesions, or idiopathic (63).

Splenic rupture is graded from low grade to high grade depending on the amounts of perisplenic blood, intraparenchymal hemorrhage, free intraperitoneal hemorrhage, or the presence of flow in liquefied areas representing possible pseudoaneurysms. The presence of a pseudoaneurysm makes a rupture high grade. Low grades

may be managed conservatively but higher grades require surgical intervention. Complications of a ruptured spleen are delayed rupture and pseudocyst formation (64).

Pseudoaneurysm

Intrasplenic pseudoaneurysms are caused by injury to the wall of an intrasplenic artery; etiology may be traumatic (14% frequency with traumatic splenic rupture) or nontraumatic. Nontraumatic pseudoaneurysms occur as complications of splenic infarction or nontraumatic splenic rupture (occurs in about 12% of cases of nontraumatic splenic rupture) (65). On ultrasound, an intrasplenic pseudoaneurysm appears as an irregular hypoechoic area within the spleen on gray scale with turbulent biphasic arterial flow on color and spectral Doppler (66); a "ying-yang" pattern can be seen as well as intralesional thrombus (67).

Both traumatic and nontraumatic intrasplenic pseudoaneurysms can lead to delayed open splenic rupture into the abdomen but can rarely thrombose spontaneously (65,66). Delayed intrasplenic pseudoaneurysm has been reported after splenic conservation surgery for splenic rupture (68). The usual treatment is splenectomy or splenic artery embolization (65,66).

Splenic artery pseudoaneurysms are caused by digestion of the artery wall by pancreatic enzymes such as can be seen with pancreatitis or penetrating gastric ulcers (69).

Splenic Artery Aneurysm

Splenic artery aneurysms are the most common visceral artery aneurysms, occurring in 0.07% to 10% of autopsy series; they are multiple in 20% (69) and are more common in women. Portal hypertension, pregnancy, multiparity, mycotic aneurysm (from endocarditis), atherosclerosis, trauma, infections, fibromuscular dysplasia, Ehler–Danlos syndrome, polyarteritis nodosa, and idiopathic are suggested etiologies (70). On ultrasound, splenic artery aneurysms appear as anechoic masses, with or without mural thrombus and calcification. Most are small (<2 cm), saccular, and located at a bifurcation in the mid to distal artery. Doppler shows pulsatile flow.

A severe complication of a splenic artery aneurysm is hemorrhage and rupture; rupture can cause shock from hypovolemia and is life threatening. Incidence of rupture is from 3% to 10% with 10% to 25% mortality (69). The risk of rupture increases with aneurysm size; aneurysms greater than 2 to 2.5 cm, that are symptomatic, that are enlarging, in pregnant patients, in pre–liver transplant patients, or pseudoaneurysms should be treated. Therapy has been splenectomy or partial splenectomy but endovascular coils and Gelfoam are now being used (69) as well as percutaneous injection of thrombin and stent placement (71).

Miscellaneous

Splenic vein aneurysms are rarer and are associated with portal hypertension, pancreatitis, Osler–Weber–Render syndrome, post trauma, splenomegaly, post splenectomy, or idiopathic. Ultrasound appearance is a fusiform hypoechoic dilatation of the splenic vein with increased velocity of flow. These can rupture or cause emboli (70).

Splenic arteriovenous fistulas can be seen post trauma, post splenectomy, post rupture of a splenic artery aneurysm, post biopsy, post pancreatitis, or congenitally; they are associated with pregnancy, especially in multiparous females. Doppler ultrasound shows a dilated tortuous splenic vein with high-velocity flow in the artery and vein (70).

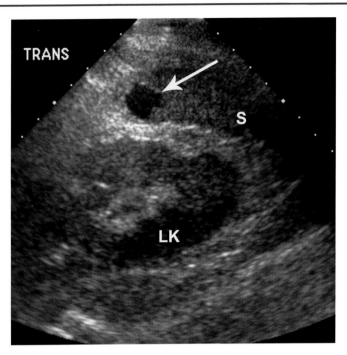

FIGURE 18 ■ Simple splenic cyst. A well-circumscribed anechoic lesion (*arrow*) with posterior enhancement. S, spleen; LK, left kidney.

polycystic kidney and liver disease. Pancreatic pseudocysts can involve the spleen (Fig. 19). The differential for splenic cysts (Table 5) includes hemangiomas, lymphangiomas, cystic neoplasms (primary or metastatic), infarcts, splenic abscesses, and parasitic cysts. Multiloculated peritoneal inclusion cysts, also known as benign multicystic mesothelioma, can involve the spleen (75).

Most splenic cysts can be treated conservatively if less than 5 cm; when symptomatic or greater than 5 cm, because

CYSTS

Nonneoplastic splenic cysts are of two types—the true (or primary) cyst with an epithelial lining and the false (or secondary cyst or pseudocyst) cyst, which has no cellular lining but may have a fibrous lining.

True cysts are congenital epidermoid cysts (21,72,73), which constitute approximately 20% of all splenic cysts (74), and parasitic cysts such as hydatid cysts, which are rare in the United States.

False splenic cysts can be secondary to trauma, infarction, infection (mononucleous, TB, or malaria), or pancreatitis, or they can be degenerative; these are approximately 80% of all splenic cysts.

Splenic cysts are usually anechoic simple cysts (Fig. 18) although they can have septa, peripheral calcification, and may contain internal echoes from debris or hemorrhage. On ultrasound, true and false cysts cannot be definitely distinguished although pseudocysts may have a thicker fibrous wall, a slightly higher incidence of debris or wall calcifications (74), and may be slightly smaller (39). Splenic cysts can be seen in autosomal-dominant

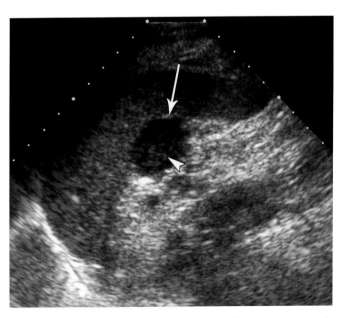

FIGURE 19 ■ Splenic pseudocyst from pancreatitis. A hypoechoic collection at the splenic margin with a slightly thick wall (*arrow*) and internal debris (*arrowhead*).

TABLE 5 ■ Cystic Masses of the Spleen

True cysts	Epidermoid cysts, parasitic cysts	
Infectious	Bacterial	Splenic abscess
	Fungal	Microabscess (multiple, small)
Posttraumatic	Pseudocysts	
	Hematoma	
	Pancreatic pseudocysts	
Vascular	Infarct	
	Peliosis	
Neoplastic	Benign	Hemangioma
		Lymphangioma
		Hamartoma (cystic areas)
		Benign multicystic mesothelioma (multiloculated peritoneal inclusion cyst)
	Malignant	Angiosarcoma (necrotic areas)
		Lymphoma (necrotic areas or can be cyst-like hypoechoic nodules)
		Metastases—(necrotic or cystic)
	Cystic metastases	Melanoma
		Breast cancer
		Ovarian cancer

of the risk of rupture, intervention such as surgery or percutaneous drainage can be performed (21). There has been a case report of malignant change with a squamous cell carcinoma nodule in a splenic cyst wall (76).

TUMORS

Benign

Benign tumors of the spleen include hemangiomas, hamartomas, lymphangiomas, littoral-cell angiomas, and angiomyolipomas.

Hemangiomas are the most common primary neoplasm of the spleen. Incidence at autopsy is 0.3% to 1.4%. On ultrasound, they appear as well-circumscribed, round, echogenic masses (Fig. 20) that may have cystic areas (77); calcifications, fibrosis, and posterior enhancement may also be seen. There may be no vascularity on color Doppler but flow has been reported on color Doppler in the solid portion of the hemangioma (39). One study reported disappearance of flow after compression of a hemangioma with reappearance of flow after pressure subsided (78). They can be less than 2cm but can be larger or multiple. Multiple hemangiomas can be seen in generalized hemangiomatosis such as Klippel–Trénaunay–Weber syndrome. After microbubble contrast, smaller lesions may enhance and larger lesions can show centripetal enhancement (49).

A splenic hamartoma, also known as a splenoma, splenadenoma, nodular hypoplasia, or fibrosplenoma, is a benign lesion consisting of an abnormal proportion and arrangement of normal splenic tissue elements. Incidence

at autopsy is 0.024% to 0.13% (79). They are usually single but can be multiple. Splenic hamartomas have been associated with tuberous sclerosis and have been associated with malignancy (79). On ultrasound, hamartomas are

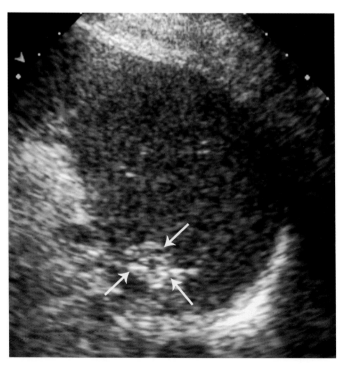

FIGURE 20 ■ Splenic hemangioma. A small (5.8 × 6.1mm) well-circumscribed, echogenic, nonshadowing mass (*arrows*) in the spleen, consistent with a hemangioma.

usually hyperechoic (79) or hypoechoic (80) solid masses that can contain cystic areas or calcifications (79,80). Increased vascularity on color Doppler ultrasound is most common (80) but there is a report of decreased vascularity on color Doppler (81). There is enhancement after microbubble contrast administration (49). Rupture of a splenic hamartoma has been described (80).

Lymphangiomas are congenital malformations of the lymphatic system, which may be single or multiple and are slow growing. Most occur in children. Lymphangioma of the spleen is a slow-growing tumor consisting of multiple thin-walled cysts of varying sizes separated by internal septations (Fig. 21); the septa consist of fibrous connective tissue with some vessels. Cysts range from a few millimeters to a few centimeters, vary in size in the same spleen, and may contain marginal calcifications. On ultrasound, the cysts are anechoic but can be hypoechoic and contain debris; the septa are hyperechoic and may show vascularity with color Doppler and echogenic calcifications. If the cysts are very small, they may not be individually seen and the area appears hyperechoic due to small reflective surfaces (82). There is no enhancement after microbubble agents (49).

Lymphangiomas can be isolated to the spleen or can be widespread, involving other areas such as the neck, mediastinum, retroperitoneum, liver, lung, extremities, and mesentery (83), as seen in the lymphangiomatosis syndrome.

Lymphangiomas usually involve the splenic capsule and trabeculae. A subcapsular location is most common but lesions can be intraparenchymal. Some lymphangiomas have the appearance of a central cyst surrounded by satellite cysts of varying sizes (79,82,84). Splenic lymphangiomas have an increased risk of splenic rupture (84). Splenic lymphangiomas are benign but there has been a reported case of malignant transformation to lymphangiosarcoma (85).

Littoral-cell angioma is a rare benign vascular tumor of the spleen. Littoral cells arise from the sinuses of the red pulp of the spleen.

On ultrasound, littoral-cell angiomas are usually multiple and are variable in appearance; cases have been reported where lesions are hyperechoic (86,87), isoechoic (88), hypoechoic (89) or even have a mottled echotexture without focal lesions (90). On CT, these lesions appear as multiple hypodensities. The lesions are often associated with splenomegaly and clinically can present with thrombocytopenia or anemia. There have been rare reported cases of a littoral-cell angiosarcoma (91), and an association with other malignancies has been suggested.

Angiomyolipomas have been reported in the spleen. They can occur in patients with tuberous sclerosis (92), in patients with renal angiomyolipomas (93), or as an isolated finding (93). These can bleed and even cause a chronic expanding hematoma of the spleen (92).

Tumors with Variable Malignant Potential

Rare tumors of the spleen include hemangiopericytoma and hemangioendothelioma. Hemangiopericytoma is a vascular lesion arising from pericytes. On ultrasound, it appears as hypoechoic (79) nodules or a heterogeneous solid mass (87); calcifications can occur (79). It has high malignant potential, with metastases common to the lungs and bone and a high incidence of local recurrence. They can be multiple. Recurrence is local but metastases to bone and lung have been reported (94).

Hemangioendothelioma usually occurs in children or young adults; it is a vascular tumor of variable malignant potential appearing on ultrasound as a hypoechoic mass that may have central areas of necrosis (79); others have been described as isoechoic with a hypoechoic rim (95). Flow is increased within the mass; flow is disordered with high arterial velocity and low resistive index (96). Calcifications may occur.

Malignant Tumors

Angiosarcoma of the spleen is the most common primary nonhematolymphoid splenic malignancy. An increased incidence with prior Thorotrast exposure was reported in a study that examined 20 cases of Thorotrast exposure; nine patients had malignancies in the liver or spleen, three of which were angiosarcomas (two with liver primaries and one in the spleen) (97). However, in a different study of 40 cases of angiosarcoma of the spleen, there were no reported cases of carcinogen exposure such as from Thorotrast, vinyl chloride, or arsenic (98).

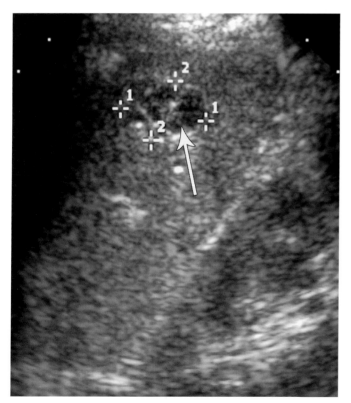

FIGURE 21 ■ Splenic lymphangioma. A 2.0 × 1.4 cm well-circumscribed mass in the spleen (+ *calipers*) that consists of multiple small cysts separated by internal septa (*arrow*).

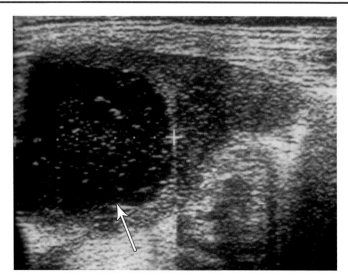

FIGURE 22 ▪ Splenic angiosarcoma. A complex heterogeneous mass (+ *calipers* and *arrow*) in the spleen. *Source*: Courtesy of B. Goldberg, Thomas Jefferson University.

For angiosarcoma, the age range is 50 to 79 years at onset. Many patients present with splenomegaly and thrombocytopenia. Spontaneous rupture can occur in up to 30% of patients (99). On ultrasound, the tumor appears as a complex heterogeneous mass with or without central hypoechoic areas of necrosis (Fig. 22); color Doppler flow is increased in the non-necrotic portions of the tumor. The tumors can be large and diffusely infiltrate the spleen. Calcifications can be present. Metastasis from angiosarcoma of the spleen can go to liver, lung, lymph nodes, omentum, bone, peritoneum, or brain (99,100); the liver is the most common site, occurring in up to 70% of cases (100).

There have been reported cases of a histiocytic sarcoma in the spleen presenting as multiple focal nodules in the spleen on ultrasound (101,102).

Lymphoma is the most common malignant tumor of the spleen. On ultrasound, lymphoma can present with homogeneous splenomegaly, as diffuse coarse echoes throughout the spleen, or as multiple focal splenic lesions (Fig. 23A). The focal lesions are hypoechoic to anechoic and can mimic cysts except for indistinct boundaries (vs. distinct boundaries in cysts) and the presence of vessels seen on color Doppler coursing through the lesions without deviation (Fig. 23B) (103). After microbubble contrast, there may be irregular peripheral enhancement (49).

Myeloproliferative diseases encompass multiple chronic hematologic diseases including CML, polycythemia vera, essential thrombocytopenia, and idiopathic myelofibrosis. Patients present with splenomegaly and can present with focal splenic nodules. These nodules have been reported as mostly hyperechoic but less commonly, hypoechoic. The appearance of these nodules may be associated with blast crises and a poor outcome (104).

Kaposi's sarcoma manifests in the spleen as small hyperechoic nodules or micronodules (45,105).

Metastases to the spleen have been described from melanoma as well as breast, ovarian, lung, gynecologic (106), colon (107), testicular (108), or gastric (109) malignancies. Melanoma metastases can be cystic (Fig. 24). The autopsy incidence is reported as 0.3% to 9% of patients with cancer (109).

Metastases can be intrasplenic or serosal. Serosal metastases are usually from ovarian or endometrial carcinoma and indent the splenic surface; intrasplenic metastases have been reported in ovarian carcinoma (110). Most splenic metastases are hypoechoic but target lesions with a hyperechoic center and hypoechoic rim

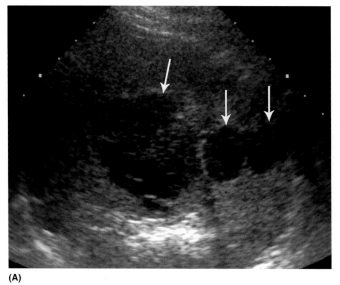

(A)

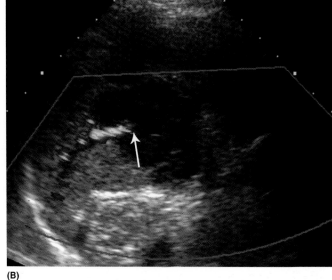

(B)

FIGURE 23 A AND B ▪ Multifocal splenic lymphoma. (**A**) Multiple hypoechoic masses in the spleen in a patient with non-Hodgkin's lymphoma (*arrows*). (**B**) Color Doppler image showing a vessel coursing without distortion through one of the lesions (*arrow*).

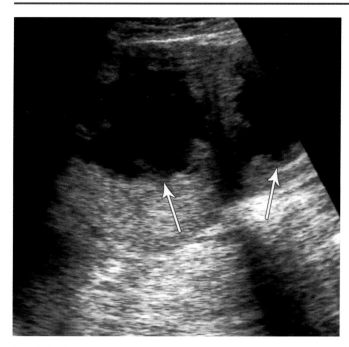

FIGURE 24 ■ Splenic metastases from melanoma. Multiple hypoechoic metastases (*arrows*) with central necrosis. *Source*: Courtesy of B. Goldberg, Thomas Jefferson University.

are also seen, especially with melanoma. Metastases generally show no flow on color Doppler. After administration of microbubble contrast, the lesions do not enhance but have a peripheral rim of enhancement; the lesions are better defined and smaller lesions can be identified in the background of normal-enhancing splenic tissue (49).

MISCELLANEOUS DISEASES

Peliosis of the spleen is characterized by multiple blood-filled spaces in the spleen, particularly in the parafollicular areas and interfollicular areas of the red pulp. It is to be distinguished from dilated splenic sinuses and from passive congestion, which are primarily in the interfollicular areas (111). Lesions may start as dilated splenic sinusoids but develop destruction of adjacent splenic tissue. Splenic peliosis is usually associated with hepatic peliosis but can be isolated (112). Splenic size is usually small. Reported associations have been with anabolic steroid use, diethylstilbestrol (113), hematologic disorders such as aplastic anemia, and chronic debilitating diseases such as AIDS, TB, and cancer. It is more common in males (111). An underlying inflammatory etiology has been suggested (114). Lesions on the surface of the spleen can rupture and lead to life-threatening hemorrhage. The ultrasound appearance is of an echogenic mass containing multiple small hypoechoic foci (79).

The spleen can be involved in storage diseases such as Gaucher's disease. Ultrasound findings include marked splenomegaly and small focal nodules in the spleen that can be hypo- or hyperechoic (115,116).

Primary amyloidosis is a disease characterized by the deposition of amyloid, an amorphous fibrillar protein, in multiple organs. Splenomegaly and calcification have been reported, as have cases of spontaneous splenic rupture. Splenic involvement often manifests with diffuse infiltration; splenomegaly is only seen in 4% to 13% of patients (117). Ultrasound shows splenomegaly with a heterogenous pattern (118); this infiltration may cause a functional hyposplenism. Calcifications can be seen. Focal amyloidomas have been reported as well-circumscribed heterogeneous masses with hypoechoic areas (119). Patients can present with splenic rupture, infarction, or functional hyposplenism.

Inflammatory pseudotumor is a benign lesion of unknown etiology made up of a heterogeneous population of inflammatory cells, acute and chronic, with areas of fibrosis and necrosis. The etiology is unknown but may be secondary to infections, autoimmune diseases, or vascular causes. It can involve the spleen, usually in middle-aged or older populations. On ultrasound, most present as hypoechoic masses that can contain calcifications (120) and are usually hypovascular (121) on color Doppler but may have increased vascularity at the margin (122).

Extramedullary hematopiesis occurs as a response to abnormal bone marrow hematopoiesis in congenital hemolytic anemias or in acquired disease with bone marrow replacement (myelofibrosis and myelodysplastic syndrome). It can occur in the spleen and usually appears as diffuse infiltration but can occur as a focal splenic mass. The focal splenic masses are well circumscribed and usually hyperechoic; hypoechoic areas of necrosis may be present (123).

DIAGNOSIS

Calcifications can be seen in multiple splenic lesions, as mentioned in Table 6. Many splenic lesions are hypoechoic (Table 4) but a smaller number are hyperechoic (Table 7).

TABLE 6 ■ Splenic Calcifications

Cysts	Epidermoid, parasitic, pseudocysts (wall calcification)
Infections	TB, histoplasmosis, treated *Candida*, abscess with wall calcification, treated *Pneumocystis carinii*
Trauma	Healed hematoma
Benign tumors	Hemangioma, hamartoma, lymphangioma
Malignant tumors	Hemangiopericytoma, hemangioendothelioma, angiosarcoma, metastases
Vascular	Arterial atherosclerosis, aneurysm, pseudoaneurysm
Infarction	Healed infarcts, sickle cell disease
Miscellaneous	Inflammatory pseudotumor
	Amyloidosis
	Sarcoid
Thorotrast	Density can mimic calcifications

Abbreviation: TB, tuberculosis.
Source: From Refs. 18–20.

TABLE 7 ■ Hyperechoic Splenic Lesions

Acute trauma	Hematoma
Infection	Abscesses with air and "dirty" shadowing
	Microabscesses (TB, histoplasmosis) (can also be hypoechoic)
	Echinococcal cysts (echogenic from scolices or hydatid sand)
Acute hemorrhagic infarct	
Treated pseudoaneurysms or aneurysms	
Tumors—benign	Hemangioma
	Hamartoma (can also have cystic areas)
	Lymphangioma (with very tiny cysts)
	Littoral-cell angioma (can also be iso- or hypoechoic)
	Angiomyolipoma
Tumors—variable malignant potential	Hemangiopericytoma (can also be hypoechoic)
Tumors—malignant	Angiosarcoma (can also be hypoechoic)
	Myeloproliferative disease (can also be hypoechoic)
	Kaposi's sarcoma
	Some metastases
Miscellaneous	Peliosis (has hypoechoic areas)
	Gaucher's (can also be hypoechoic)
	Extramedullary hematopiesis

Abbreviation: TB, tuberculosis.

Because of the numerous etiologies of splenic lesions and overlapping imaging characteristics (Tables 4–7), tissue sampling is often necessary. Percutaneous fine-needle aspiration or core biopsy, particularly with real-time ultrasound guidance or CT guidance is an effective alternative to surgical or laparoscopic biopsy for splenic lesions. Despite the spleen being a vascular organ, the risk of bleeding is small if a 22-gauge or smaller needle is used (124,125). Successful fine-needle aspiration has also been used without complications in a case of angiosarcoma of the spleen (126).

REFERENCES

1. Zhou Z, Liu S, Li Z, et al. Sectional anatomy of the peritoneal reflections of the upper abdomen in the coronal plane. J Comput Assist Tomogr 2005; 29(4):430–437.
2. Freeman JL, Jafri SZ, Roberts JL, Mezwa DG, Shirkhoda A. CT of congenital and acquired abnormalities of the spleen. Radiographics 1993; 13(3):597–610.
3. Catalano O, Sandomenico F, Matarazzo I, Siani A. Contrast-enhanced sonography of the spleen. AJR Am J Roentgenol 2005; 184(4):1150–1156.
4. Ota T, Ono S. Intrapancreatic accessory spleen: diagnosis using contrast enhanced ultrasound. Br J Radiol 2004; 77(914):148–149.
5. Nishiguchi S, Habu D, Ishizu H, et al. Accessory spleen in the pelvis diagnosed by Tc-99m phytate scintigraphy. Ann Nucl Med 2001; 15(3):263–265.
6. Nimkin K, Kleinman PK, Chappell JS. Abdominal ultrasonography of splenogonadal fusion. J Ultrasound Med 2000; 19(5): 345–347.
7. Stewart VR, Sellars ME, Somers S, Muir GH, Sidhu PS. Splenogonadal fusion: B-mode and color Doppler sonographic appearances. J Ultrasound Med 2004; 23(8):1087–1090.
8. Konno K, Ishida H, Ishida J, et al. Macronodular deformity of the spleen. Abdom Imaging 2001; 26(3):294–297.
9. Westcott JL, Krufky EL. The upside-down spleen. Radiology 1972; 105(3):517–521.
10. Bakir B, Poyanli A, Yekeler E, Acunas G. Acute torsion of a wandering spleen: imaging findings. Abdom Imaging 2004; 29(6): 707–709.
11. Romero JR, Barksdale EM Jr. Wandering spleen: a rare cause of abdominal pain. Pediatr Emerg Care 2003; 19(6):412–414.
12. Karmazyn B, Steinberg R, Gayer G, Grozovski S, Freud E, Kornreich L. Wandering spleen-the challenge of ultrasound diagnosis: report of 7 cases. J Clin Ultrasound 2005; 33(9):433–438.
13. Dalpe C, Cunningham M. Wandering spleen as an asymptomatic pelvic mass. Obstet Gynecol 2003; 101(5 Pt 2):1102–1104.
14. Danaci M, Belet Ü, Yalin T, Polat V, Nurol S, Selçuk MB. Power Doppler sonographic diagnosis of torsion in a wandering spleen. J Clin Ultrasound 2000; 28(5):246–248.
15. Kessler A, Miller E, Keidar S, et al. Mass at the splenic hilum: a clue to torsion of a wandering spleen located in a normal left upper quadrant position. J Ultrasound Med 2003; 22(5):527–530.
16. Vural M, Kacar S, Kosar U, Altin L. Symptomatic wandering accessory spleen in the pelvis: sonographic findings. J Clin Ultrasound 1999; 27(9):534–536.
17. Pumberger W, Wiesbauer P, Leitha T. Splenosis mimicking tumor recurrence in renal cell carcinoma: detection on selective spleen scintigraphy. J Pediatr Surg 2001; 36(7):1089–1091.
18. Reeder MM, Bradley WG, Merritt CR, eds. Reeder and Felson's Gamuts in Radiology Comprehensive Lists of Roentgen Differential Diagnosis. 4th ed. New York: Springer-Verlag, 2003:715–718.
19. Paterson A, Frush DP, Donnelly LF, Foss JN, O'Hara SM, Bisset GS III. A pattern-oriented approach to splenic imaging in infants and children. Radiographics 1999; 19(6):1465–1485.

20. Gore RM. Spleen: differential diagnosis. In: Gore RM, Levine MS, eds. Textbook of Gastrointestinal Radiology. WB Saunders Co, 2000:1925–1928.

21. Hansen MB, Moller AC. Splenic cysts. Surg Laparosc Endosc Percutan Tech 2004; 14(6):316–322.

22. Ravaglia G, Forti P, Biagi F, Maioli F, Boschi F, Corazza GR. Splenic function in old age. Gerontology 1998; 44(2):91–94.

23. Görg C, Eichkorn M, Zugmaier G. The small spleen: sonographic patterns of functional hyposplenia or asplenia. J Clin Ultrasound 2003; 31(3):152–155.

24. McGahan JP, Richards J, Gillen M. The focused abdominal sonography for trauma scan: pearls and pitfalls. J Ultrasound Med 2002; 21(7):789–800.

25. McGahan JP, Wang L, Richards JR. From the RSNA refresher courses: focused abdominal US for trauma. Radiographics 2001; 21(Spec No):S191–S199.

26. Richards JR, McGahan PJ, Jewell MG, Fukushima LC, McGahan JP. Sonographic patterns of intraperitoneal hemorrhage associated with blunt splenic injury. J Ultrasound Med 2004; 23(3):387–394.

27. Sirlin CB, Casola G, Brown MA, Patel N, Bendavid EJ, Hoyt DB. Patterns of fluid accumulation on screening ultrasonography for blunt abdominal trauma: comparison with site of injury. J Ultrasound Med 2001; 20(4):351–357.

28. Nance ML, Mahboubi S, Wickstrom M, Prendergast F, Stafford PW. Pattern of abdominal free fluid following isolated blunt spleen or liver injury in the pediatric patient. J Trauma 2002; 52(1):85–87.

29. Richards JR, McGahan JP, Jones CD, Zhan S, Gerscovich EO. Ultrasound detection of blunt splenic injury. Injury 2001; 32(2): 95–103.

30. Catalano O, Lobianco R, Sandomenico F, Siani A. Splenic trauma: evaluation with contrast-specific sonography and a second-generation contrast medium: preliminary experience. J Ultrasound Med 2003; 22(5):467–477.

31. Catalano O, Cusati B, Nunziata A, Siani A. Real-time, contrast-specific sonography imaging of acute splenic disorders: a pictorial review. Emerg Radiol 2004; 11(1):15–21.

32. Catalano O, Cusati B, Nunziata A, Siani A. Active abdominal bleeding: contrast-enhanced sonography. Abdom Imaging 2006; 31(1):9–16.

33. Thorelius L. Contrast-enhanced ultrasound in trauma. Eur Radiol 2004; 14(suppl 8):P43–P52.

34. Poletti PA, Platon A, Becker CD, et al. Blunt abdominal trauma: does the use of a second-generation sonographic contrast agent help to detect solid organ injuries? AJR Am J Roentgenol 2004; 183(5):1293–1301.

35. Oldenburg A, Hohmann J, Skrok J, Albrecht T. Imaging of paediatric splenic injury with contrast-enhanced ultrasonography. Pediatr Radiol 2004; 34(4):351–354.

36. Sangchan A, Mootsikapun P, Mairiang P. Splenic abscess: clinical features, microbiologic finding, treatment and outcome. J Med Assoc Thai 2003; 86(5):436–441.

37. Aessopos A, Politou M, Farmakis D, et al. Staphylococcus aureus abscess of the spleen in a β-thalassemia patient. Scand J Infect Dis 2002; 34(6):466–468.

38. Ng KK, Lee TY, Wan YL, et al. Splenic abscess: diagnosis and management. Hepatogastroenterology 2002; 49(44):567–571.

39. Urrutia M, Mergo PJ, Ros LH, Torres GM, Ros PR. Cystic masses of the spleen: radiologic-pathologic correlation. Radiographics 1996; 16(1):107–129.

40. Pereira JM, Madureira AJ, Vieira A, Ramos I. Abdominal tuberculosis: imaging features. Eur J Radiol 2005; 55(2):173–180.

41. Akhan O, Pringot J. Imaging of abdominal tuberculosis. Eur Radiol 2002; 12(2):312–323.

42. Chandra S, Srivastava DN, Gandhi D. Splenic tuberculosis: an unusual sonographic presentation. Int J Clin Pract 1999; 53(4):318–319.

43. Topal U, Savci G, Sadikoğlu MY, Parlak M, Tuncel E. Splenic involvement of tuberculosis: US and CT findings. Eur Radiol 1994; 4:577–579.

44. Porcel-Martin A, Rendon-Unceta P, Bascunana-Quirell A, et al. Focal splenic lesions in patients with AIDS: sonographic findings. Abdom Imaging 1998; 23(2):196–200.

45. Murray JG, Patel MD, Lee S, Sandhu JS, Feldstein VA. Microabscesses of the liver and spleen in AIDS: detection with 5-MHz sonography. Radiology 1995; 197(3):723–727.

46. Bernabeu-Wittel M, Villanueva JL, Pachon J, et al. Etiology, clinical features and outcome of splenic microabscesses in HIV-infected patients with prolonged fever. Eur J Clin Microbiol Infect Dis 1999; 18(5):324–329.

47. Kontoyiannis DP, Luna MA, Samuels BI, Bodey GP. Hepatosplenic candidiasis: a manifestation of chronic disseminated candidiasis. Infect Dis Clin North Am 2000; 14(3):721–739.

48. Pastakia B, Shawker TH, Thaler M, O'Leary T, Pizzo PA. Hepatosplenic candidiasis: wheels within wheels. Radiology 1988; 166(2):417–421.

49. Peddu P, Shah M, Sidhu PS. Splenic abnormalities: a comparative review of ultrasound, microbubble-enhanced ultrasound and computed tomography. Clin Radiol 2004; 59(9):777–792.

50. Polat P, Kantarci M, Alper F, Suma S, Koruyucu MB, Okur A. Hydatid disease from head to toe. Radiographics 2003; 23(2):475–494.

51. De Jesus AR, Miranda DG, Miranda RG, et al. Morbidity associated with Schistosoma mansoni infection determined by ultrasound in an endemic area of Brazil, Caatinga do Moura. Am J Trop Med Hyg 2000; 63(1–2):1–4.

52. Barata CH, Pinto-Silva RA, Lambertucci JR. Abdominal ultrasound in acute schistosomiasis mansoni. Br J Radiol 1999; 72(862):949–952.

53. Ozsoy MF, Oncul O, Pekkafali Z, Pahsa A, Yenen OS. Splenic complications in malaria: report of two cases from Turkey. J Med Microbiol 2004; 53(Pt 12):1255–1258.

54. Yagmur Y, Kara IH, Aldemir M, Buyukbayram H, Tacyildiz IH, Keles C. Spontaneous rupture of malarial spleen: two case reports and review of literature. Crit Care 2000; 4(5):309–313.

55. Kessler A, Mitchell DG, Israel HL, Goldberg BB. Hepatic and splenic sarcoidosis: ultrasound and MR imaging. Abdom Imaging 1993; 18(2):159–163.

56. Zou CC, Liang L. Multiple hypoechoic lesions in spleen and *Mycoplasma pneumoniae* infection. Indian Pediatr 2005; 42(4):379–382.

57. Danon O, Duval-Arnould M, Osman Z, et al. Hepatic and splenic involvement in cat-scratch disease: imaging features. Abdom Imaging 2000; 25(2):182–183.

58. Bükte Y, Nazaroglu H, Mete A, Yilmaz F. Visceral leishmaniasis with multiple nodular lesions of the liver and spleen: CT and sonographic findings. Abdom Imaging 2004; 29(1):82–84.

59. Miller LA, Mirvis SE, Shanmuganathan K, Ohson AS. CT diagnosis of splenic infarction in blunt trauma: imaging features, clinical significance and complications. Clin Radiol 2004; 59(4):342–348.

60. Bonnard P, Guiard-Schmid JB, Develoux M, Rozenbaum W, Pialoux G. Splenic infarction during acute malaria. Trans R Soc Trop Med Hyg 2005; 99(1):82–86.

61. Goerg C, Schwerk WB. Splenic infarction: sonographic patterns, diagnosis, follow-up, and complications. Radiology 1990; 174(3 Pt 1):803–807.

62. Barzilai M, Schlag-Eisenberg D, Peled N, Bitterman A. Noninfectious gas accumulation in an infarcted spleen. Dig Surg 2000; 17(4):402–404.

63. Gorg C, Colle J, Gorg K, Prinz H, Zugmaier G. Spontaneous rupture of the spleen: ultrasound patterns, diagnosis and follow-up. Br J Radiol 2003; 76(910):704–711.

64. Sinha PS, Stoker TA, Aston NO. Traumatic pseudocyst of the spleen. J R Soc Med 1999; 92(9):450–452.

65. Gorg C, Colle J, Wied M, Schwerk WB, Zugmaier G. Spontaneous nontraumatic intrasplenic pseudoaneurysm: causes, sonographic diagnosis, and prognosis. J Clin Ultrasound 2003; 31(3):129–134.

66. Fitoz S, Atasoy C, Dusunceli E, Yagmurlu A, Erden A, Akyar S. Post-traumatic intrasplenic pseudoaneurysms with delayed rupture: color

Doppler sonographic and CT findings. J Clin Ultrasound 2001; 29(2):102–104.

67. Saad NE, Saad WE, Davies MG, Waldman DL, Fultz PJ, Rubens DJ. Pseudoaneurysms and the role of minimally invasive techniques in their management. Radiographics 2005; 25(suppl 1):S173–S189.

68. Paya K, Wurm J, Graf M, et al. Intrasplenic posttraumatic pseudoaneurysm secondary to spleen-salvaging surgery. J Trauma 2002; 52(4):783–785.

69. Guillon R, Garcier JM, Abergel A, et al. Management of splenic artery aneurysms and false aneurysms with endovascular treatment in 12 patients. Cardiovasc Intervent Radiol 2003; 26(3):256–260.

70. De Schepper AM, Vanhoenacker F, Op de Beeck B, Gielen J, Parizel P. Vascular pathology of the spleen, part I. Abdom Imaging 2005; 30(1):96–104.

71. Madoff DC, Denys A, Wallace MJ, et al. Splenic arterial interventions: anatomy, indications, technical considerations, and potential complications. Radiographics 2005; 25(suppl 1):S191–S211.

72. Kabra NS, Bowen JR. Congenital splenic cyst: a case report and review of the literature. J Paediatr Child Health 2001; 37(4):400–402.

73. Lopes MA, Ruano R, Bunduki V, Miyadahira S, Zugaib M. Prenatal diagnosis and follow up of congenital splenic cyst: a case report. Ultrasound Obstet Gynecol 2001; 17(5):439–441.

74. Van Dyck P, Vanhoenacker F, Corthouts B, De Schepper AM. Epidermoid cyst of the spleen. JBR-BTR 2002; 85(3):166–167.

75. Guzzo MH, Davis CA, Belzer GE, Virata RL. Multiloculated peritoneal inclusion cysts with splenic involvement: a case report. Am Surg 2001; 67(7):619–621.

76. Elit L, Aylward B. Splenic cyst carcinoma presenting in pregnancy. Am J Hematol 1989; 32(1):57–60.

77. Willcox TM, Speer RW, Schlinkert RT, Sarr MG. Hemangioma of the spleen: presentation, diagnosis, and management. J Gastrointest Surg 2000; 4(6):611–613.

78. Niizawa M, Ishida H, Morikawa P, Naganuma H, Masamune O. Color Doppler sonography in a case of splenic hemangioma: value of compressing the tumor. AJR Am J Roentgenol 1991; 157(5):965–966.

79. Abbott RM, Levy AD, Aguilera NS, Gorospe L, Thompson WM. From the archives of the AFIP: primary vascular neoplasms of the spleen: radiologic-pathologic correlation. Radiographics 2004; 24(4):1137–1163.

80. Tang S, Shimizu T, Kikuchi Y, et al. Color Doppler sonographic findings in splenic hamartoma. J Clin Ultrasound 2000; 28(5):249–253.

81. Chou YH, Chiou HJ, Tiu CM, Chiou SY, Hsia CY, Tsay SH. Splenic hamartoma: presentation on contrast-enhanced sonography. J Clin Ultrasound 2004; 32(8):425–428.

82. Bezzi M, Spinelli A, Pierleoni M, Andreoli G. Cystic lymphangioma of the spleen: US-CT-MRI correlation. Eur Radiol 2001; 11(7):1187–1190.

83. Komatsuda T, Ishida H, Konno K, et al. Splenic lymphangioma: US and CT diagnosis and clinical manifestations. Abdom Imaging 1999; 24(4):414–417.

84. Solomou EG, Patriarheas GV, Mpadra FA, Karamouzis MV, Dimopoulos I. Asymptomatic adult cystic lymphangioma of the spleen: case report and review of the literature. Magn Reson Imaging 2003; 21(1):81–84.

85. Feigenberg Z, Wysenbeek A, Avidor E, Dintsman M. Malignant lymphangioma of the spleen. Isr J Med Sci 1983; 19(2):202–204.

86. Espanol I, Lerma E, Fumanal V, et al. Littoral cell angioma with severe thrombocytopenia. Ann Hematol 2000; 79(1):46–49.

87. Goldfeld M, Cohen I, Loberant N, et al. Littoral cell angioma of the spleen: appearance on sonography and CT. J Clin Ultrasound 2002; 30(8):510–513.

88. Oliver-Goldaracena JM, Blanco A, Miralles M, Martin-Gonzalez MA. Littoral cell angioma of the spleen: US and MR imaging findings. Abdom Imaging 1998; 23(6):636–639.

89. Anton-Pacheco J, Ayuso RM, Cano I, Martinez MA, Cuadros J, Berchi FJ. Splenic littoral cell angioma in an infant. J Pediatr Surg 2000; 35(3):508–509.

90. Kinoshita LL, Yee J, Nash SR. Littoral cell angioma of the spleen: imaging features. AJR Am J Roentgenol 2000; 174(2):467–469.

91. Meybehm M, Fischer HP. Littoral cell angiosarcoma of the spleen. Morphologic, immunohistochemical findings and consideration of histogenesis of a rare splenic tumor. Pathologe 1997; 18(5):401–405.

92. Asayama Y, Fukuya T, Honda H, et al. Chronic expanding hematoma of the spleen caused by angiomyolipoma in a patient with tuberous sclerosis. Abdom Imaging 1998; 23(5):527–530.

93. Tang P, Alhindawi R, Farmer P. Case report: primary isolated angiomyolipoma of the spleen. Ann Clin Lab Sci 2001; 31(4):405–410.

94. Hosotani R, Momoi H, Uchida H, et al. Multiple hemangiopericytomas of the spleen. Am J Gastroenterol 1992; 87(12):1863–1865. Review.

95. Ng WH, Ching AS, Chan KF, Fung WT. Clinics in diagnostic imaging (89). Infantile hepatosplenic haemangioendotheliomas. Singapore Med J 2003; 44(9):491–495.

96. Ferrozzi F, Bova D, De Chiara F. Hemangioendothelioma of the spleen: imaging findings at color Doppler, US, and CT. Clin Imaging 1999; 23(2):111–114.

97. Levy DW, Rindsberg S, Friedman AC, et al. Thorotrast-induced hepatosplenic neoplasia: CT identification. AJR Am J Roentgenol 1986; 146(5):997–1004.

98. Falk S, Krishnan J, Meis JM. Primary angiosarcoma of the spleen. A clinicopathologic study of 40 cases. Am J Surg Pathol 1993; 17(10):959–970.

99. Vrachliotis TG, Bennett WF, Vaswani KK, Niemann TH, Bova JG. Primary angiosarcoma of the spleen—CT, MR, and sonographic characteristics: report of two cases. Abdom Imaging 2000; 25(3):283–285.

100. Thompson WM, Levy AD, Aguilera NS, Gorospe L, Abbott RM. Angiosarcoma of the spleen: imaging characteristics in 12 patients. Radiology 2005; 235(1):106–115.

101. Audouin J, Vercelli-Retta J, Le Tourneau A, et al. Primary histiocytic sarcoma of the spleen associated with erythrophagocytic histiocytosis. Pathol Res Pract 2003; 199(2):107–112.

102. Kimura H, Nasu K, Sakai C, et al. Histiocytic sarcoma of the spleen associated with hypoalbuminemia, hypo γ-globulinemia and thrombocytopenia as a possibly unique clinical entity—report of three cases. Leuk Lymphoma 1998; 31(1–2):217–224.

103. Ishida H, Konno K, Ishida J, et al. Splenic lymphoma: differentiation from splenic cyst with ultrasonography. Abdom Imaging 2001; 26(5):529–532.

104. Görg C, Riera-Knorrenschild J, Görg K, Zugmaier G. Focal splenic lesions in myeloproliferative disease: association with fatal outcome. Ann Hematol 2004; 83(1):14–17.

105. Valls C, Canas C, Turell LG, Pruna X. Hepatosplenic AIDS-related Kaposi's sarcoma. Gastrointest Radiol 1991; 16(4):342–344.

106. Chen LW, Chien RN, Yen CL, Chang LC. Splenic tumour: a clinicopathological study. Int J Clin Pract 2004; 58(10):924–927.

107. Okuyama T, Oya M, Ishikawa H. Isolated splenic metastasis of sigmoid colon cancer: a case report. Jpn J Clin Oncol 2001; 31(7):341–345.

108. Nguyen MM, Corr AS, Evans CP. Testicular cancer metastatic exclusively to the brain and spleen. Urology 2004; 63(1):176–178.

109. Natarajan P, Varshney S. Spontaneous splenic rupture secondary to metastatic gastric carcinoma. Trop Gastroenterol 2000; 21(1):28.

110. Carrington BM, Thomas NB, Johnson RJ. Intrasplenic metastases from carcinoma of the ovary. Clin Radiol 1990; 41(6):418–420.

111. Tada T, Wakabayashi T, Kishimoto H. Peliosis of the spleen. Am J Clin Pathol 1983; 79(6):708–713.

112. Tsokos M, Püschel K. Isolated peliosis of the spleen: report of 2 autopsy cases. Am J Forensic Med Pathol 2004; 25(3):251–254.

113. Supe A, Desai C, Rao PP, Madiwale C, Joshi A. Isolated massive splenic peliosis. Indian J Gastroenterol 2000; 19(2):87–88.

114. Gugger M, Gebbers JO. Peliosis of the spleen: an immune-complex disease? Histopathology 1998; 33(4):387–389.

115. Poll LW, Koch JA, vom Dahl S, Sarbia M, Haussinger D, Modder U. Gaucher disease of the spleen: CT and MR findings. Abdom Imaging 2000; 25(3):286–289.

116. Patlas M, Hadas-Halpern I, Abrahamov A, Elstein D, Zimran A. Spectrum of abdominal sonographic findings in 103 pediatric patients with Gaucher disease. Eur Radiol 2002; 12(2):397–400.

117. Kim SH, Han JK, Lee KH, et al. Abdominal amyloidosis: spectrum of radiological findings. Clin Radiol 2003; 58(8):610–620.

118. Monzawa S, Tsukamoto T, Omata K, Hosoda K, Araki T, Sugimura K. A case with primary amyloidosis of the liver and spleen: radiologic findings. Eur J Radiol 2002; 41(3):237–241.

119. Maffe GC, Ruga A, Nava A. Splenic amyloidoma. Haematologica 2002; 87(1):EIM02.

120. Noguchi H, Kondo H, Kondo M, Shiraiwa M, Monobe Y. Inflammatory pseudotumor of the spleen: a case report. Jpn J Clin Oncol 2000; 30(4):196–203.

121. Moriyama S, Inayoshi A, Kurano R. Inflammatory pseudotumor of the spleen: report of a case. Surg Today 2000; 30(10):942–946.

122. Yesildag E, Sarimurat N, Ince U, Numan F, Buyukunal C. Nonsurgical diagnosis and management of an inflammatory pseudotumor of the spleen in a child. J Clin Ultrasound 2003; 31(6):335–338.

123. Singer A, Maldjian P, Simmons MZ. Extramedullary hematopoiesis presenting as a focal splenic mass: a case report. Abdom Imaging 2004; 29(6):710–712.

124. Lal A, Ariga R, Gattuso P, Nemcek AA, Nayar R. Splenic fine needle aspiration and core biopsy. A review of 49 cases. Acta Cytol 2003; 47(6):951–959.

125. Venkataramu NK, Gupta S, Sood BP, et al. Ultrasound guided fine needle aspiration biopsy of splenic lesions. Br J Radiol 1999; 72(862):953–956.

126. Delacruz V, Jorda M, Gomez-Fernandez C, Benedetto P, Ganjei P. Fine-needle aspiration diagnosis of angiosarcoma of the spleen: a case report and review of the literature. Arch Pathol Lab Med 2005; 129(8):1054–1056.

Urinary Tract • *Dennis L. Cochlin*

ANATOMY

The Kidneys

The kidneys lie on the posterior abdominal wall, angled in the sagittal and axial planes (Fig. 1). This angulation has important implications for choosing the best ultrasonic scan plane, which must match the anatomic planes to achieve true longitudinal and transverse images of the kidneys. This plane also displays the proximal ureter and displays the blood vessels with good Doppler studies. Anterior to the right kidney lie the liver and the hepatic flexure. The upper pole and sometimes the whole kidney may be imaged through the liver on an anterior plane. The lower pole, however, usually is obscured in this plane by the hepatic flexure. An oblique approach is then necessary. Anterosuperior to the left kidney lies the spleen, which offers a poor sonic window unless enlarged. The colon lies anterior to the rest of the left kidney, so that the only possible ultrasound plane usually is a posterior oblique one (Fig. 1).

The kidneys (Fig. 2) consist of a collecting system (calyces, infundibula, and renal pelvis), surrounded by a variable thickness of fat, and surrounding this, the renal parenchyma, which consists of the medullary pyramids and the cortex. The cortex can be divided into the peripheral portion and the columns of Bertin, which extend between the medullary pyramids. The whole is surrounded by a renal capsule, and the kidney is in turn surrounded by perinephric fat.

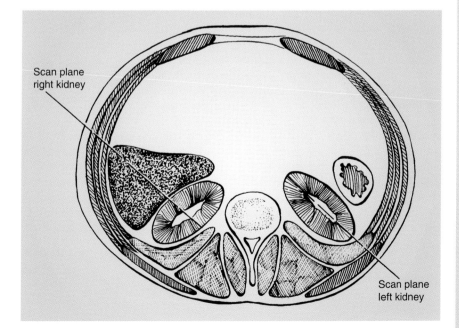

FIGURE 1 ■ Renal anatomy. The diagram shows the obliquity of the kidneys in the axial plane, which should be recognized when choosing appropriate scan planes.

The interface between the uroepithelium of the collecting system and the urine contained within it is seen as a dense white line. The cavity of the collecting system is variably seen, depending on the degree of distension.

In children and in adults with little sinus fat, the uroepithelium itself appears as a narrow echogenic band. In those with more fat, the uroepithelium has an echodensity similar to the sinus fat and merges with it to produce an irregular renal sinus complex.

The renal pyramids (medulla) contain the renal tubules, supporting tissue, and blood vessels. These tissues are tightly packed, with few reflecting interfaces. The pyramids are anisotropic. They are least echogenic when the ultrasound beam runs along the line of the tubules and become increasingly more echogenic as the angle changes, until they become iso-echoic with the renal cortex. The pyramids are therefore commonly seen as triangular structures with an echodensity lower than the cortex, but only at the mid pole of the kidney. Toward the poles, because of the changing scan angle, they become less prominent, or isoechoic, and thus not distinguishable from the cortex (Fig. 2). The cortex contains the glomeruli, which are moderately powerful reflectors. Because of this, the renal cortex has higher echogenicity than the medulla. The renal capsule and the interfaces between the perinephric tissue, the capsule, and the cortex produce an echogenic line around the kidney, having a crisp outline. The perinephric fat is variable both in its extent and in its echodensity. Usually of medium-high echodensity, it occasionally may be of low echogenicity, in which case it may simulate a perinephric fluid collection.

The normal ultrasonic image in the adult kidney, therefore, has the following features. The renal cortex is traditionally described as having an echodensity slightly lower than or equal to that of the liver and spleen. Newer ultrasound machines, however, have improved tissue differentiation and show the renal cortex as significantly less echoic than liver and spleen. The renal pyramids are of lower echodensity compared with the cortex, but they may be seen only as separate structures when the ultrasound beam is at a near right angle to the renal surface and in slim patients. (In large patients and particularly when scanning through the muscles of the back, corticomedullary differentiation may be poor or absent.) The renal sinus complex has the highest echodensity. The normal collecting system has a narrow urine-filled space, which is usually invisible but may be seen as a narrow anechoic space in well-hydrated patients. The renal pelvis also is variable in appearance, ranging from a hardly discernible, small intrarenal structure to a large, anechoic extrarenal structure. Because of the shape of the kidney, the renal outline in the longitudinal plane varies, depending on the angle of the scan. An anterior approach produces a fairly narrow outline, with the sinus complex lying centrally, whereas an oblique posterolateral plane produces a wider outline, with the renal pelvis shown at the lower end of the image, similar to the image on an intravenous urogram (IVU). Most sonologists scan the right kidney from an anterior oblique approach using the liver as a sonic window, whereas the left kidney often is shown only by a posterolateral oblique approach. This results in the two kidneys appearing different on the scan. In addition, the more posterior the scan plane, the greater the muscle bulk between the kidney and the transducer. This degrades the ultrasound image, resulting in less well-defined tissue planes within the kidney and in particular loss of differentiation of cortex and medulla (1–3).

The Neonatal and Infant Kidney

The infant kidney differs from the adult kidney in four ways (Fig. 3) (Table 1) (4–10):

1. The infant kidney has a greater concentration of glomeruli in the cortex, resulting in a higher cortical echodensity than in the adult.

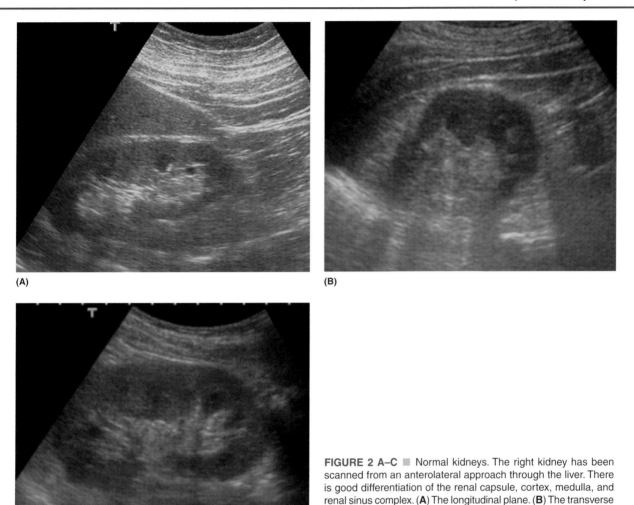

(A)

(B)

(C)

FIGURE 2 A–C ■ Normal kidneys. The right kidney has been scanned from an anterolateral approach through the liver. There is good differentiation of the renal capsule, cortex, medulla, and renal sinus complex. (**A**) The longitudinal plane. (**B**) The transverse plane. (**C**) The left kidney has been scanned from a posterolateral approach through the lumbar muscles.

2. The renal pyramids of the infant kidney are larger in relation to the cortex than in the adult and may be relatively hypoechoic. In the infant kidney, the proximity

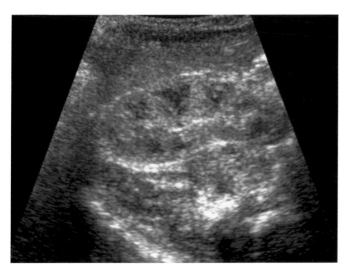

FIGURE 3 ■ The infant kidney showing the hyperechoic cortex, large pyramids, and lack of renal sinus fat, which is typical of the infant kidney.

of the kidney to the skin surface and the ability to use a higher frequency transducer also increase the corticomedullary differentiation, so that, compared to the adult, the renal pyramids appear to be prominent.
3. The infant kidney has little or no renal sinus fat, so that the sinus complex consists solely of the narrow structures of the calyceal system.
4. The calyceal system is relatively distended in about 75% of infants, so that the calyces and infundibula are seen fairly distinctly as fluid-filled structures.

The cortical changes persist until 6 to 24 months of age, at which time the kidney changes to the adult pattern. The amount of renal pelvic fat increases gradually during adolescence. Infants and young children continue to have better differentiation of cortex from the medulla on the ultrasound image, but this is because they usually are slim and higher frequency transducers often are used. Similar appearances may be found in slim adults.

The Ureters

The ureters are tubular retroperitoneal structures connecting the renal pelvis with the bladder. The abdominal portions lie

TABLE 1 ■ Neonatal and Infant Kidneys: Differences from the Adult Pattern

Differences	Comment
More echodense cortex	Equal to or slightly less than the liver. May be greater than the liver in premature infants. Changes to the adult pattern at 6–24 mo
Prominent pyramids	The pyramids are large in relation to the cortex and may be hypoechoic. They change to the adult pattern at 6 mo
Less echodense renal sinus	The sinus complex lacks fat. This changes to the adult pattern at adolescence
Distended calyceal system	Most infants (75%) have slightly distended calyceal systems, whereas in older children and adults, only a few show this pattern

on the medial edge of the psoas muscles, and the pelvic portions lie on the lateral walls of the pelvis anterior to the iliac arteries to about the level of the ischial spines, at which point they turn anteriorly and medially to enter the bladder. In the male anatomy, these portions lie above the seminal vesicles; in the female anatomy, they lie close to the lateral fornices of the vagina. The intramural portions then pass obliquely through the bladder wall for a length of about 2 cm in the adult to enter the bladder lumen at the trigone.

The Bladder

The bladder is an ovoid structure lying in the pelvic cavity. The exact shape varies with the degree of distension. The ureters enter the bladder and the urethra leaves the bladder at the three corners of the trigone. The trigone itself is a triangular area of bladder wall that is smoother than the surrounding muscle on cystoscopy but has no distinguishing features on the ultrasound image. The ureteric orifices occasionally may be identified if they pout slightly into the bladder (Fig. 4). In most cases, their position may be identified by the ureteric jets (Fig. 5). The

position of the urethra sometimes is seen as a small depression at the bladder base (Fig. 6).

The full bladder has the shape of a rounded triangle in the sagittal plane and a rounded oblong in the transverse

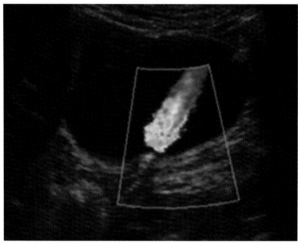

(A)

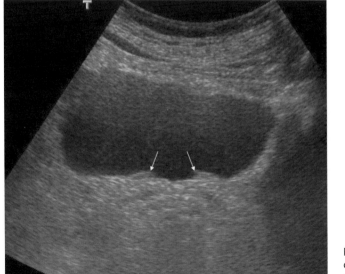

FIGURE 4 ■ Ureteric orifices. The positions of the ureteric orifices may be seen as small protuberances at the bladder base (*arrows*).

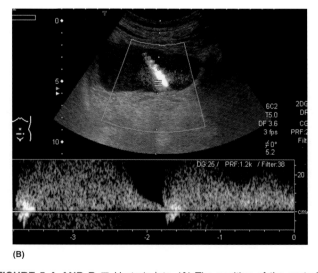

(B)

FIGURE 5 A AND B ■ Ureteric jets. (**A**) The position of the ureteric orifices is more easily seen by observing the ureteric jets, seen here on a color Doppler image. The position and angle have a correlation with the intramural ureteric angle and length, which in turn correlate (although poorly) with vesicoureteric reflux. (**B**) Spectral Doppler shows a normal biphasic flow pattern.

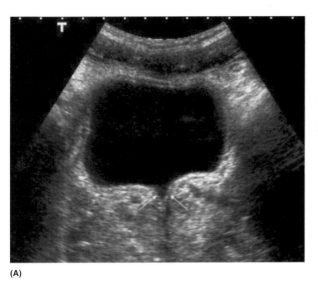 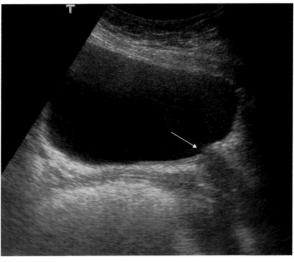

(A)   (B)

FIGURE 6 A AND B ■ Urethral orifice is shown by a shallow depression at the bladder base in the female transverse view (**A**) and in the male sagittal view (**B**).

plane, although when full, it becomes more spherical. In female patients, the uterus bulges into the posterior wall of the bladder; in male patients, the prostate causes an impression at the bladder base. In either sex, bowel loops may cause impressions on the bladder outline.

The bladder wall is of even thickness of 4 to 6 mm. These measurements apply at any age (Table 2) (11,12).

The normal bladder empties completely on micturition. Urine, however, starts to refill the bladder immediately at a rate of up to 2 mL/min. Even a short delay in taking a postmicturition measurement therefore may result in a small bladder residue. Also, some normal patients do not empty their bladder completely. Whether this is truly normal is debatable, but in practice, a postmicturition residue of less than 10 mL in a child and less than 20 mL in an adult is regarded as normal (Table 2).

The Urethra

The male urethra measures 7.5 to 20 cm in length and is divided into prostatic, membranous, and spongy (penile) segments. The urethral orifice often is seen as a small depression in the bladder base on transabdominal scans (Fig. 6), whereas the normal prostatic urethra is not seen transabdominally, although the surgical defect after a transurethral resection of the prostate often is clearly seen. The prostatic urethra is seen on transrectal scans as a V- or C-shaped structure that distends on micturition. The membranous and spongy urethra are seen on transperineal and penile scans as an echogenic ovoid structure in the transverse plane and as parallel lines in the longitudinal plane that distend on micturition, especially against a pinched penile tip or otherwise occluded distal urethra (13–15).

The female urethra is about 4 cm long and has a membranous portion only. The urethral orifice may be seen as a shallow depression in the bladder base.

Vascular Anatomy and Normal Doppler Pattern

The renal arteries originate from the lateral sides of the aorta, directed slightly anteriorly, about 1.5 cm below the superior mesenteric artery origin. The right usually lies slightly lower than the left (Figs. 7 and 8). The right renal artery runs posterior to the inferior vena cava (Fig. 9). The left renal artery runs posterior to the left renal vein and into the renal hilum (Fig. 10). About 10% of kidneys have multiple renal arteries, with one or more accessory renal arteries usually supplying a portion of the lower pole. Their anatomy is variable. They may arise near to or from the main renal trunk, or they may arise far distally. They enter the kidney at variable sites. Because of this variation in anatomy, accessory renal arteries are difficult to detect on Doppler studies, and most are missed (Fig. 8). The main artery branches at the hilum, either within or outside of the kidney, into anterior and posterior branches that further divide into segmental arteries, and then interlobar arteries. Small branches supply the renal sinus and columns of Bertin. The interlobar arteries further divide into a network of arcuate arteries that run across the cortico–medullary junction and give off cortical branches, which run radially to the renal periphery and medullary branches, and then pass back to supply the renal pyramids (Fig. 11). About 90% of the normal renal blood flow supplies the cortex; only 10% supplies the medulla.

The renal veins approximately follow the arteries and join at the hilum to form the main renal vein. The right

TABLE 2 ■ Normal Bladder Measurements

■ Wall thickness (any age)	2–4 mm
■ Postmicturition volume—adult	<20 mL
■ Postmicturition volume—child	<10 mL
■ Female vesicoureteric junction movement on straining or micturition	<10 mm

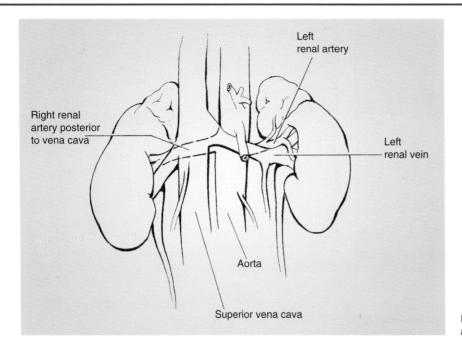

FIGURE 7 ▨ Anatomic diagram of the renal arteries and veins.

renal vein runs a relatively short course to enter the vena cava. The left crosses anterior to the aorta and posterior to the superior mesenteric artery to enter the vena cava (Figs. 7, 9, and 10).

The Doppler signal in the renal arteries is a low-resistance signal, similar to that found in all the solid organs of the body (Fig. 12). The important features of this signal are the rapid systolic rise and the continuing high-velocity flow throughout diastole. It is important to identify the small spike that occurs at the end of the systolic rise when measuring the systolic acceleration.

This feature is seen only in the main renal artery and its major branches.

The systolic velocity in the main renal artery and its major branches is 0.8 to 1.4 m/sec. The velocity slowly decreases in the intrarenal arteries as they branch into the kidney. The diastolic velocity is a little less than half of the systolic velocity. This value normally is expressed as a ratio of end diastole to peak systolic flow, the most commonly used ratio being the resistance index (RI), which measures 0.56 to 0.7 in the normal kidney (Table 3).

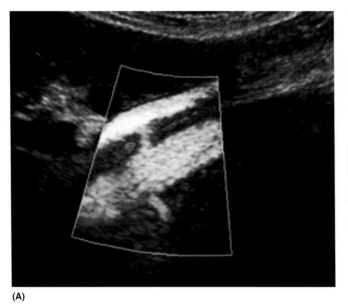

(A)

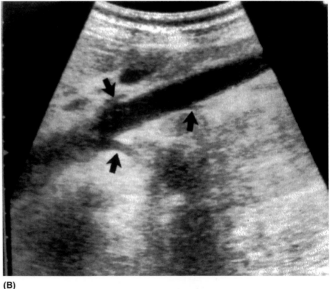

(B)

FIGURE 8 A AND B ▨ Renal artery origins. (A) In this oblique right lateral view of the aorta, the renal artery origins are shown as small sections of the trunk as they leave the aorta. (B) In this case, an accessory right renal artery is shown, although most of the accessory renal arteries are missed on ultrasound.

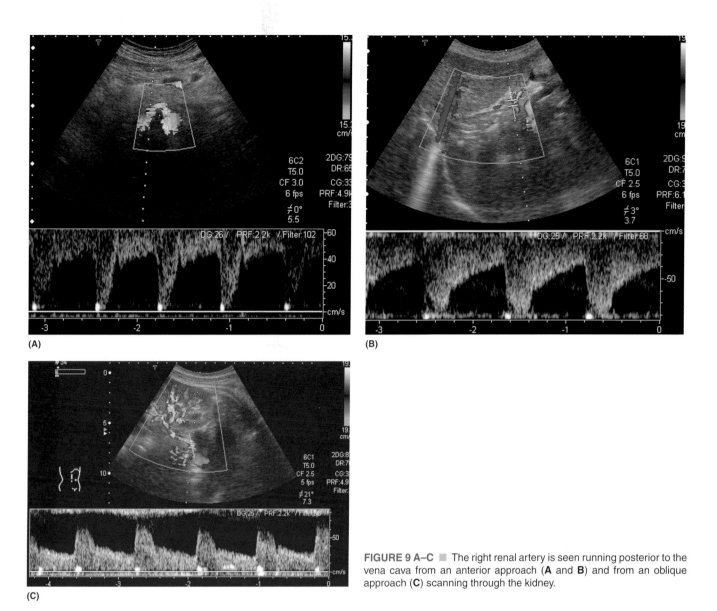

(A)

(B)

(C)

FIGURE 9 A–C ■ The right renal artery is seen running posterior to the vena cava from an anterior approach (**A** and **B**) and from an oblique approach (**C**) scanning through the kidney.

(A)

(B)

FIGURE 10 A AND B ■ The left renal artery is seen (**A**) from an anterior approach and (**B**) from an oblique longitudinal approach from the right side.

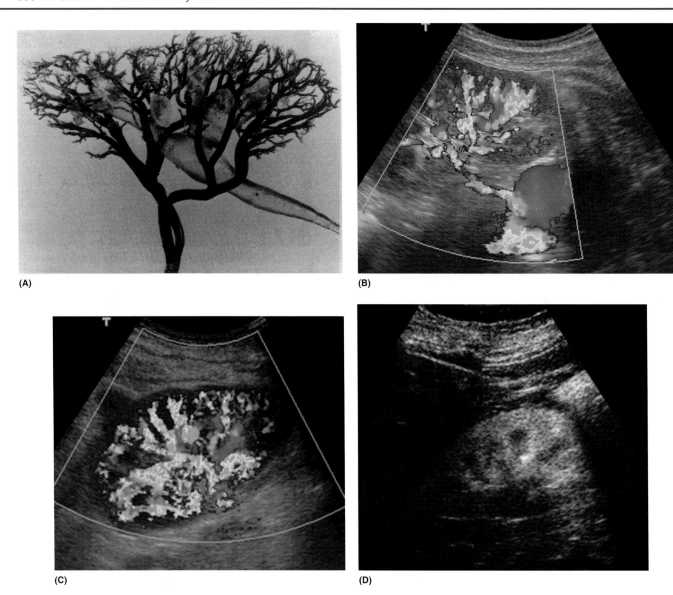

(A)

(B)

(C)

(D)

FIGURE 11 A–D ■ Intrarenal arteries. (**A**) Injected anatomic specimen showing the renal arteries. (**B**) The renal trunk and larger renal vessels are shown on a color Doppler image. (**C**) The cortical vessels are shown on a color flow image. (**D**) Cortical perfusion is shown on a contrast ultrasound image using a low MI technique and Sonovue®. The image is taken 20 seconds after injection and shows cortical perfusion. The medullary pyramids have not yet filled. *Source*: (**A**) From Ref. 16.

The renal vein signal is continuous in the smaller veins and slightly undulates with respiration in the main veins. The left renal vein shows little or no phasic swing within the cardiac cycle, whereas the right shows a variable amount of pulsatility, reflecting changes in right atrial pressure (Fig. 13) (17,18).

SCANNING TECHNIQUE

The Kidneys

Both kidneys are scanned in multiple longitudinal and transverse planes to ensure that the whole volume of renal tissue has been studied. Carefully obliqued planes are necessary to show the pelviureteric junctions.

The right kidney initially is scanned from an antero-lateral approach using the liver as a sonic window. A more posterior approach may be needed to image the lower pole. Respiration can be used to move the kidney relative to the ribs and any overlying bowel gas. A more oblique posterior approach is however often advantageous.

The left kidney requires a more posterior approach. The upper pole may be scanned through the spleen, but most of the kidney usually must be scanned through the lumbar muscles. This degrades the image, but usually there is no choice. The patient must be turned into varying degrees of obliquity to get complete images of both kidneys. Scanning with the patient prone is rarely advantageous, although this position must be used for ultrasonic guidance of renal biopsy or antegrade pyelography.

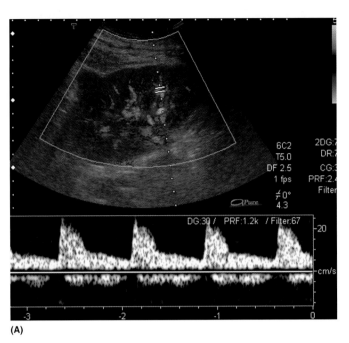

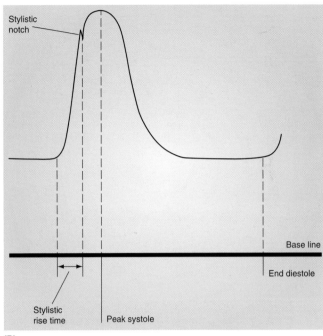

FIGURE 12 A AND B ■ Normal renal artery spectral signal. (**A**) Notice the rapid systolic rise and gradual descent into diastole, with end diastolic flow velocity a little less than half of the peak systolic velocity. (**B**) Diagrammatic representation of the important features of the spectral waveform.

The Ureters

Unless dilated, only the proximal and distal ends of the ureters are seen ultrasonically (Figs. 14 and 15). Usually the central portions comprising most of the abdominal and pelvic ureters are obscured by bowel gas. In slim patients, however, bowel can be displaced by graded compression, but even then it is not usually possible to distinguish the normal ureter from other retroperitoneal and pelvic tissues except at the point where they cross the iliac vessels. The graded compression technique does, however, enable a proportion of dilated ureters to be seen, and in some cases, the level and cause of obstruction may be established. In most cases, however, the upper and lower ureters only can be seen.

The upper ureters at and just distal to the pelviureteric junction are best shown by scanning in a lateral oblique longitudinal plane using the kidney itself as a sonic window. The ureter is identified by its continuity with the renal pelvis (Fig. 14).

The lower ureters are scanned through a full bladder (Fig. 15). Their approximate positions are chosen from their anatomic landmarks. They often are identified when a peristaltic wave is seen passing along them.

The intramural portions of the ureters occasionally are just visible but are not seen in most patients. The ureteric jets into the bladder may be seen as slightly hyperechoic intermittent jets directed obliquely into the bladder lumen on real time but are better demonstrated with color Doppler imaging (Fig. 5). The presence of a strong jet excludes ureteric obstruction. The position of the jets may be used to assess the position and obliquity of the intramural ureters, this having a correlation (although not a good one) with vesicoureteric reflux. The spectral pattern of the jets is also changed in refluxing ureters (19–21).

The Bladder

A curved linear transducer is usually used though in some cases, the small footprint of a sector transducer facilitates angulation behind the symphysis pubis for better visualization of the bladder base.

Transverse (axial) images are obtained in the true axial plane and angled caudad to show the bladder base. Sagittal and oblique sagittal images complete the examination. In both planes, moving the transducer

TABLE 3 ■ Normal Renal Doppler Indices

Index	Formula	Normal value
Peak systolic velocity: main renal artery and branches	–	0.6–1.4 m/sec (<1.8 m/sec)
Resistance index	$S - D/S$	0.56–0.7
Pulsatility index	$S - D$/mean	0.7–0.14
Renal/aortic ratio	Renal systolic velocity/aortic systolic velocity	<3.5
Systolic rise time	Time to early systolic peak	0.11 ± 0.06
Systolic acceleration	–	11 ± 8 m/sec^2

Abbreviations: S, peak systolic velocity; D, end diastolic velocity.

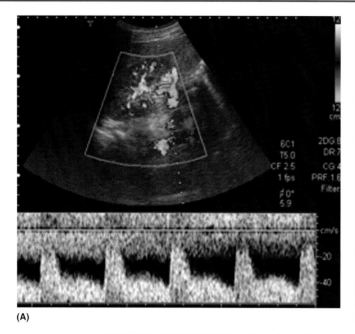 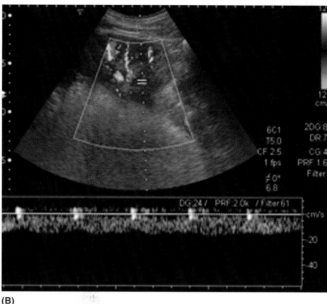

(A)   (B)

FIGURE 13 A AND B ▧ Normal renal vein flow patterns. **(A)** Left renal vein. (The artery is also included in the spectral gate.) **(B)** Right renal vein.

cephalad and then steeply angling caudad are necessary to show the bladder base (Fig. 16).

The relatively "blind" areas of the bladder are as follows: the lateral walls, where, in conventional scan planes, the beam is nearly parallel to the wall; the base, which lies behind the symphysis pubis; and the anterior bladder wall, the image of which is degraded by reverberation. Angulation of the transducer helps to show lateral walls and bladder base. Careful manipulation of gain settings and the use of a higher frequency transducer may reduce reverberation in the region of the anterior wall (Fig. 16). The lower anterior wall of the bladder, which lies behind the symphysis, remains a problem.

Transrectal scanning shows this area well but is regarded by many as too invasive for routine use in this area. Transperineal scanning also may show this area and the bladder base but is less effective than the transrectal approach. Nevertheless, it is a useful and underused scan plane. Intravesical scanning with small endoprobes is possible but still experimental (11,22–24).

The Urethra

In male patients, the prostatic urethra may be scanned transrectally using the standard prostatic scanning technique, and the membranous urethra may be imaged by

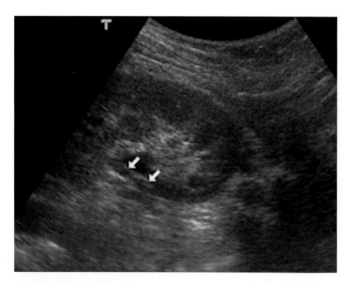 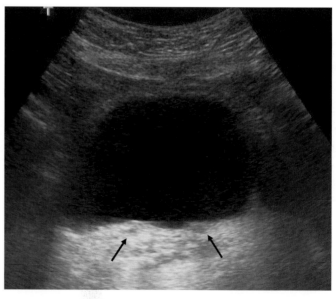

FIGURE 14 ▧ Upper ureter. The upper end of the ureter (*arrows*) is shown by scanning through the kidney. On the real-time image, peristalsis aids its recognition.

FIGURE 15 ▧ Lower ureters (*arrows*) viewed through the bladder.

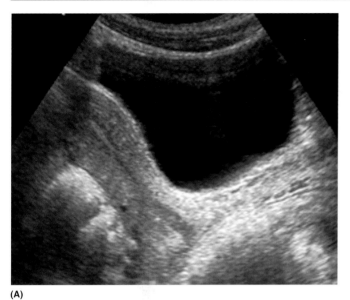

(A)

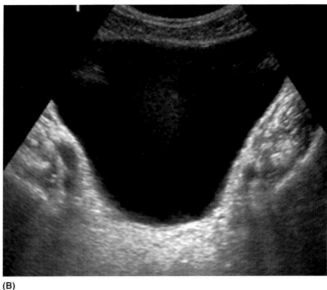

(B)

FIGURE 16 A AND B ■ The normal full bladder is shown. (**A**) A sagittal view. The uterus is seen posterior to the bladder. (**B**) Transverse view. The psoas muscles and iliac vessels are seen lying posterolateral to the bladder.

the transperineal plane. The pendulous or penile urethra is visualized using a high-frequency linear transducer from the ventral or dorsal aspect of the penis. The ventral approach may require the use of standoff. The urethra may be seen in its collapsed state, but for most diagnostic purposes, visualization of the distended urethra is necessary; this may be achieved either by the instillation of sterile water through the urethral orifice, as in a contrast urethrogram, or by micturition while pinching or otherwise occluding the penile tip. This is done near the end of micturition to minimize discomfort (Fig. 17).

The female urethra may be seen transvaginally, transrectally, or, less satisfactorily, transperineally, but it is

difficult to distend. The main use of ultrasound in female patients is to show movement of the vesicourethral junction during straining and micturition in cases of suspected pelvic floor weakness. For these studies, a catheter usually is placed with the balloon against the vesicourethral junction to aid visualization (25–28).

Renal Doppler Studies

Renal Doppler studies may be performed in the investigation of renal artery stenosis; this technique is discussed at the end of the chapter. Doppler studies of the intrarenal vessels are performed as an adjunct to the gray scale

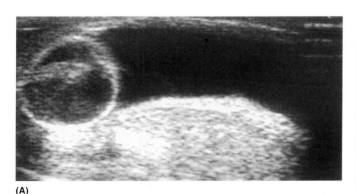

(A)

FIGURE 17 A AND B ■ Male pendulous (penile) urethra. The urethra has been scanned while distended with saline. (**A**) The anterior urethra. (**B**) The bulbar urethra.

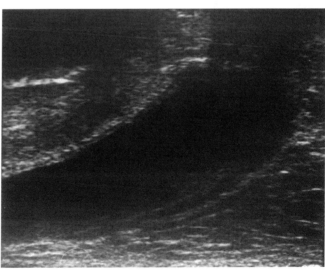

(B)

study in appropriate cases. Whereas intrarenal Doppler spectral signals may be obtained without the use of color flow mapping, the use of color is a major advantage in the kidney. Doppler studies of the kidneys are not easy. The kidneys move considerably during respiration, and patients can hold their breath only for a limited time. The kidneys also lie relatively deep to the skin surface, and Doppler loses sensitivity with depth.

The first requirement is to choose a good scan plane. The larger intrarenal arteries run from the renal hilum toward the renal periphery, mainly in a posterolateral plane. Scanning must be done in or near this plane to identify renal vessels for the Doppler study. Power Doppler is non–angle dependent, but the appropriate plane is still required to identify a sufficient length of artery. The longitudinal plane of the kidney usually is best used, although occasionally a transverse plane works better.

After the appropriate Doppler plane is chosen, a medium pulse repetition frequency is selected. Further adjustments to the scan plane are made with the patient breathing quietly until the ideal vascular plane is achieved. Even with a good technique, in large patients, only a few vessels may be identified. The vessel for study is chosen, and the patient is instructed to hold the breath, usually in mid-inspiration. The Doppler gate must be moved quickly into the desired vessel. Rapid adjustments must be made at this stage to obtain a Doppler spectral signal within the time of a breath hold. Some ill patients cannot hold their breath. In these cases, a Doppler spectral signal may be snatched during respiration, usually at the point of end expiration or inspiration. Usually, only one cardiac cycle is obtained, but this is sufficient for a spectral study.

The choice of vessel for study depends on the purpose of the Doppler study. If the purpose is to seek the tardus parvus waveform of renal artery stenosis, then the main renal trunk at the hilum or one of the major segmental arteries is required. If the investigation is the assessment of renal parenchymal disease, however, an artery well within the kidney is required to minimize central effects. Interlobar vessels are best for this study. Some workers have advocated the use of arcuate vessels, but these are small and their velocity is relatively low, making their study difficult.

Doppler studies of the main renal trunks require a different technique. This involves imaging the renal arteries from an anterior approach in the axial plane, angling toward the side of interest. The right renal artery usually is identified as it crosses posterior to the vena cava, and the left as it runs posterior to the renal vein (Figs. 9 and 10). An alternative method of imaging the origins is an oblique longitudinal approach, with the patient in a 45° right anterior oblique position. This shows the renal arteries as they leave the aorta. The disadvantage of this approach is that only the origins are shown (Fig. 8). With the axial approach, the arteries often may be followed to the renal hilum. In other cases, the arteries at the hilum are best shown by a posterior oblique longitudinal scan through the kidney (Fig. 11B). In practice, all of these techniques often are necessary, and even

after prolonged scanning, the technique often does not show the whole of both the arteries.

Studies of cortical perfusion are possible using relatively high-frequency (at least 5 MHz), high-resolution transducers and preferably using power Doppler. The use of Doppler contrast agents not only facilitates this study but also enables perfusion studies—similar to those created by isotope studies—to be performed (Figs. 11D, 19B, 27C, 60D, 93). Study of cortical perfusion is new and is under evaluation.

Doppler measurements are discussed later and are listed in Table 3.

MEASUREMENTS

Various measurements may be derived from the ultrasound scan (Table 4).

Renal Length

The most widely used measurement of renal size is the pole-to-pole length. This is a quick, easily obtained measurement, but accurate reproducibility requires careful technique. The main problem is underestimation of the size by misinterpreting an oblique plane as the true length. The normal adult renal length as measured by ultrasound is quoted as a normal range for male and female patients (29). However, as shown by Hodgson and Edwards (30), on IVU measurements, normal measurements are more properly related to height, weight, and age. Surprisingly, little use of such data has been made in ultrasonic measurements. Ultrasound-derived measurements are 10% to 15% smaller than IVU measurements because of the magnification factor present on IVUs. Numerous tables of renal length have been produced for children (31), all having their own relative merits.

TABLE 4 ◼ Normal Renal Measurements in Adults

◼ *Length—male*	
Right kidney	11.3 ± 0.8 cm
Left kidney	11.5 ± 0.9 cm
◼ *Length—female*	
Right kidney	10.8 ± 0.8 cm
Left kidney	10.9 ± 1.0 cm
Difference in renal sizes	Right < 2 cm smaller than left
	Left < 1.5 cm smaller than right
◼ *Renal volume—male*	
Right kidney	147 ± 38 mL
Left kidney	154 ± 37 mL
◼ *Renal volume—female*	
Right kidney	118 ± 27 mL
Left kidney	125 ± 26 mL
Cross-sectional area	16–30 cm²
◼ *Parenchymal thickness*	
Male	14.8 ± 3.7 mm (range 11–18 mm)
Female	13.6 ± 3.6 mm [range 11–16 mm (practically, more than 10 mm)]

Measurements of children's kidneys may be related to age, height, and weight, and many suitable tables are available.

Cross-Sectional Area

The cross-sectional area of the kidney at the level of the hilum is another easy, reproducible measurement. The measurement should include the renal hilum itself, assuming a regular contour, but excluding an extrarenal pelvis. The measurement is made by identifying the longitudinal axis of the kidney and scanning at 90° to this axis at hilar level. Depending on the software facilities available, the renal cross-sectional area may be measured by tracing around the outline, from which the area may be directly calculated, or by constructing an ellipse at the best fit around the outline. This is less satisfactory since the outline of many kidneys is a rounded triangle. Another method is to measure two diameters at 90° to each other, although this method also assumes an elliptical shape in calculating the area. Although the trace method is most accurate, all three methods are sufficiently accurate for clinical use. The main source of error is in choosing a scan plane that is not at 90° to the longitudinal axis. Normal cross-sectional areas in adults vary between 18 and 30 cm^2.

Volume and Surface Area

Renal volume and surface area may be calculated by two methods. Multiple cross-sectional areas may be measured at set distances along the renal length and calculations made from these measurements (32,33). A far simpler method may also be employed—measuring the pole-to-pole length and the hilar cross-sectional area. The volume and surface area calculation assumes an ellipsoid shape. For most clinical uses, the second, simpler method is preferable, because it is quick, reproducible, and sufficiently accurate. It loses accuracy when the kidneys have an irregular shape. The more complicated method of multiple cross-sectional areas is mainly reserved for research, but when extreme accuracy is necessary, computed tomography (CT) is preferable. Whenever two or more measurements are multiplied, errors also are multiplied, and even with great care, neither method is reproducible to greater than ±10% accuracy. A careless measurement technique makes the results so inaccurate as to be meaningless.

Cortical Size

True cortical volume is impossible to estimate ultrasonically. The cortical width from the renal pyramids to the renal surface may be measured when the corticomedullary boundary is seen sufficiently well. With irregular cortical size, it may be necessary to take an average of several measurements. In cases of marked hydronephrosis and some cases of altered sonodensity, the corticomedullary junction may not be well seen, and in these cases, the distance between the calyces and the renal surface or from the edge of the sinus complex to the surface may be substituted (34).

Renal Pelvis Measurements

The anteroposterior diameter of the renal pelvis is used in the fetus and the neonate to assess obstruction. The measurement normally is not used, however, in adults in whom hydronephroses usually are described as mild, moderate, or severe, with or without cortical loss.

The Ureters

A dilated ureter may be described in terms of its diameter, but reports usually are descriptive only.

The Bladder

The normal full bladder has a wall thickness of 4 to 6 mm at any age (Table 2). Wall measurements are used in cases of hypertrophy. Bladder volume measurements are discussed in the section entitled Incomplete Bladder Emptying.

The Urethra

The position of the urethrovesical junction may be assessed in female patients by introducing a urethral catheter and scanning transvaginally or transrectally. The normal junction moves less than 1 cm on straining or micturition, with greater movement suggesting pelvic floor weakness.

NORMAL VARIANTS AND ARTIFACTS

Variations in Renal Shape

Table 5 provides a list of normal variants.

Splenic or Dromedary Hump
A splenic hump is a bulge in the lateral border of the midpole of the left kidney (Table 5). The feature that establishes normality is that the calyces underlying the hump extend further laterally into the hump than the other calyces, and the echotexture of the hump is similar to the rest of the kidney (35). If in doubt, an isotope scan, preferably using dimercaptosuccinic acid (DMSA), will show normal uptake in a splenic hump, whereas a tumor will cause a photon-deficient area, with normal perfusion indicating normal renal tissue (Fig. 18).

Fetal Lobulation
Fetal lobulation consists of indentations in the renal outline. These lie between the renal pyramids or calyces, unlike scars that lie directly over the calyces. Isotope and possibly contrast ultrasound studies may show poor perfusion beneath scars (2).

Hypertrophied Column of Bertin
A hypertrophied column of Bertin is a rounded enlargement of a column of Bertin displacing the adjacent infundibula (Fig. 19) (36). It is discussed more fully under the section entitled Renal Masses and Cysts. Isotope and ultrasound contrast studies may be used in a similar way to that discussed for splenic humps.

TABLE 5 ■ Normal Variants in Renal Anatomy

Cause	Comment	Confirmatory test
Splenic hump (dromedary hump; may simulate a tumor)	Hump on the midpole of the left kidney; calyces extend into it	Isotope (DMSA) scan ? Power Doppler or CEUS
Fetal lobulation (may simulate scarring)	Indentation of the renal cortex between pyramids and calyces	Isotope (DMSA) scan ? Power Doppler or CEUS
Hypertrophied column of Bertin	Enlarged, rounded column of Bertin that displaces the infundibula and simulates a tumor	Isotope (DMSA) scan ? Power Doppler or CEUS
Duplex kidney	Long thin kidney that varies from duplication of the collecting system only to complete separation. May be accompanied by disease	IVU or CT
Congenitally small kidney; hypotrophic kidney; (may simulate pathologically small kidney)	Small but otherwise normally appearing and functioning kidney	Isotope study, IVU
Malrotated kidney	Renal pelvis and ureter lies anteriorly	IVU or CT
Ptotic kidney	Low lying	
Ectopic kidney	Pelvic or crossed renal ectopia	
Horseshoe kidney	Low-lying kidneys fused in the midline	
Congenital absence	One kidney may be absent; the ureter also is absent	CT, cystoscopy

Abbreviations: DMSA, dimercaptosuccinic acid; IVU, intravenous urogram; CT, computed tomography; CEUS, contrast enhanced ultrasound.

Duplex Kidney

The duplex kidney is a complex subject, and it is debatable whether a duplex kidney is truly a normal variant or a pathologic condition. It is mentioned here because most are long, thin kidneys with double collecting systems but no pathologic features (Fig. 51). An IVU confirms the diagnosis.

Horseshoe Kidney

In a horseshoe kidney, the lower poles of the kidneys are joined across the midline. The tissue that joins them, called the isthmus, may be a thin band of fibrous tissue or a thicker band of renal tissue. The lower poles of the kidneys are pulled medially so that the kidneys lie with their long axes in an oblique plane. The ureters exit the kidneys anteriorly. It is the abnormal lie of the kidneys that is the first feature to be usually seen. If the isthmus is thick, it may initially be confused with a retroperitoneal mass (Fig. 20) (37).

Congenitally Small (Hypotrophic) Kidney

A congenitally small (hypotrophic) kidney is a small (less than 5 cm) kidney but of otherwise normal appearance, with reduced total renal function but normal function for its size. An IVU shows normal excretion for the renal size, as does an isotope study. Small kidneys from other causes have disproportionately reduced function.

Malrotated Kidney

There is a spectrum of malrotation, varying from minor changes in the normal renal angulation to kidneys in which the renal pelvis and ureter lie anterior to the kidney (see also the section entitled Horseshoe Kidney).

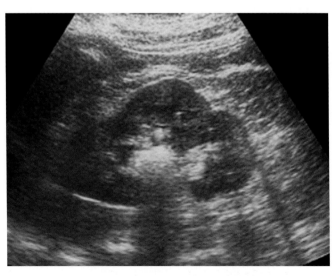

FIGURE 18 ■ Dromedary (splenic) hump.

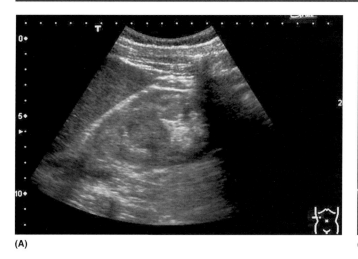
(A)

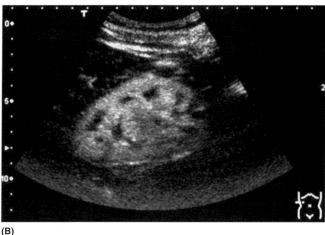
(B)

FIGURE 19 A AND B ▦ Hypertrophied column of Bertin. (**A**) An isoechoic mass is seen displacing adjacent structures. (**B**) A contrasted ultrasound scan (Sonovue® with low MI technique) shows that the perfusion pattern is identical to the rest of the kidney. A tumor would have a different perfusion pattern.

Ptotic Kidney

More often affecting the right kidney, ptotic kidneys lie lower than usual in the abdomen, with their pelviureteric junctions angled cephalad. Once thought to be symptomatic, they are regarded as innocent normal variants.

Ectopic Kidney

Ectopic kidneys usually are pelvic in position. Rarely, both kidneys lie on the same side (crossed renal ectopia) (38). Horseshoe kidneys (already discussed) may be regarded as ectopic. They lie low in the abdomen, with their lower poles joined by an isthmus of normal renal tissue or fibrous tissue. The ureters pass anterior to this (37).

Congenitally Absent Kidney

In congenital absence, both the kidney and the ureter are absent. Confirmation of the diagnosis is made by establishing the absence of a ureteric orifice at cystoscopy.

Medially Placed or Retrocaval Ureters

Medially placed or retrocaval ureters are anomalies seen on the IVU, but these show no diagnostic features on the ultrasound image.

Duplex Ureters

Duplex renal pelves and upper ureters sometimes are seen, although they often are difficult to recognize on the ultrasound image. The kidney is usually long and thin, and this shape suggests a duplex kidney. Only if there is a waist or if two renal pelves or ureters are identified is duplication definite. The insertion of the ureter into the bladder sometimes is demonstrated by observing the ureteric jet (Fig. 5A), although ectopic insertions rarely are demonstrated.

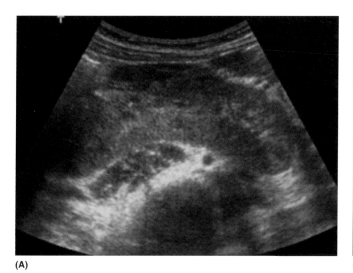
(A)

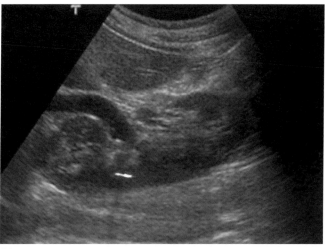
(B)

FIGURE 20 A AND B ▦ Horseshoe kidneys. (**A**) In this case, the isthmus joining the two halves is wide and easily identified crossing the midline. (**B**) In this case, the isthmus was narrow, but the malrotation with the anteromedial hilum is easily appreciated.

Variants in Bladder Anatomy

The bladder is variable in shape, particularly in female patients, where it may be relatively hypotonic when half full, sometimes with floppy lateral extremities called bladder ears. Major bladder anomalies such as exstrophy are clinically obvious, and ultrasound plays no part except in checking for associated renal and other anomalies.

A patent urachus results from failure of closure of the fetal structure, resulting in a fistula between the bladder and the umbilicus when the whole structure is patent, a sinus at the umbilicus or the bladder if only the cephalad or caudal portion is patent, or a cyst between the bladder and the umbilicus if only the mid-portion is patent. Cysts occasionally are found incidentally on ultrasound studies (Fig. 81d). Malignant change produces a complex, mostly solid tumor between the dome of the bladder and the umbilicus (39–42). A connection with the bladder or umbilicus may be demonstrated, but is often more clearly seen on a magnetic resonance imaging (MRI) study.

Variants in Urethral Anatomy

Ultrasound has a minimal role in examining variants in urethral anatomy apart from seeking associated anomalies.

Artifacts and Pitfalls

Asymmetry of the Renal Image

As discussed in the section entitled Anatomy, the right kidney usually is scanned through an oblique anterior approach and the left through an oblique posterior approach. Because of the shape of the kidneys, these different planes result in the right kidney appearing narrower than the left. Because of the different tissues between the kidneys and the transducer, the echo pattern of the two kidneys also appears different, the right showing better corticomedullary differentiation than the left (Fig. 2). This should be appreciated as the normal pattern.

Hyperechoic Areas of Renal Sinus Fat

In some patients, parts of the renal sinus complex fat are hyperechoic and may cast weak shadows. It may be difficult to distinguish these from calculi. Calculi normally cast a strong shadow but, in cases of doubt, a plain kidney–ureter–bladder (KUB) radiograph should be performed, and if doubt persists, a CT study should be performed.

Hyperechoic Cortical Foci

Small hyperechoic foci are often seen in the renal cortex. They may usually be distinguished from calculi by their peripheral position, though such distinction is sometimes difficult. Their nature is uncertain. They are often loosely termed granulomas. Whatever they are, they are known to be innocent.

Hypoechoic Perinephric Fat

Perinephric fat usually has a medium echodensity with a speckled pattern. In a few cases, it may be hypoechoic, in which case it may simulate a perinephric collection. The distribution of the fat, the similar appearance on both sides, and the lack of supportive clinical and ultrasonic evidence for a perinephric collection suggest the correct diagnosis. But in cases of doubt, a CT scan differentiates between these entities.

Prominent Renal Pyramids

Either pathologically prominent pyramids or normal pyramids that are well seen in slim patients and children have been mistaken in the past for hydronephrosis. With the good resolution of current machines, this should not be a problem. The pyramids lie outside of the renal sinus complex echoes; hydronephrotic calyces lie inside.

Cysts Simulating Hydronephrosis

Cysts simulating hydronephrosis is a perennial problem. Both pathologic conditions produce fluid-filled spaces within the kidneys. Scanning in the anatomic plane that shows the infundibula connecting at the renal hilum usually solves the problem. In a few cases of coexisting cysts and possible hydronephrosis, the diagnosis still may be difficult. In such cases, an IVU should be performed, or, if the patient is in renal failure, a retrograde study should be obtained. An antegrade study is less useful since cysts may be entered and outlined with contrast, but this does not exclude a coexisting hydronephrosis.

Normally Prominent Calyces Simulating Hydronephrosis

Some texts state that if the sinus complex is "split" (i.e., the calyces and infundibula are visible), this constitutes hydronephrosis. Modern ultrasound machines, however, may show normal calyces in some slim patients. In well-hydrated patients and children, these may be more obvious. Differentiation between normal calyces and hydronephrosis is made on the same criteria as those used in the IVU, that is, preservation of the normal pattern of the fornices.

A full bladder may cause actual distension of the calyces. This reverts to normal when the bladder is emptied.

Normal (Nondistended) Calyces in an Obstructed System

In cases of acute obstruction, the physiologic response of the kidney is to reduce its excretion. This response may be sufficient to prevent calyceal dilatation, so that absence of calyceal dilatation does not exclude acute obstruction. In cases of chronic obstruction, dilatation usually does occur, with the exception of cases of retroperitoneal fibrosis in which calyceal dilatation occurs late or occasionally not at all in the disease.

Apparently Absent Kidney

Absence of the kidney in the normal position should initiate a search for a pelvic or crossed ectopic kidney. A small kidney—particularly if it has increased echodensity—may blend with the perinephric fat and be difficult to see. In cases of doubt, CT or MRI studies readily distinguish between renal tissue and surrounding fat (Fig. 21).

Problems with Renal Measurement

Renal length measurement is reasonably accurate, although a few millimeters' error is usual. If the kidney is not visualized in the true longitudinal plane, however, serious

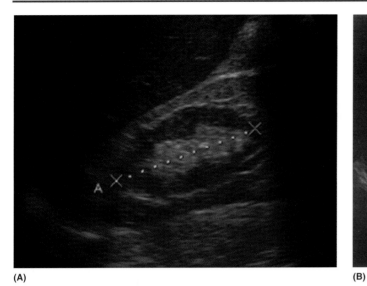

(A)

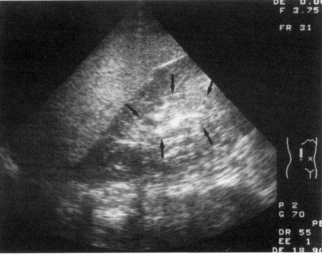

(B)

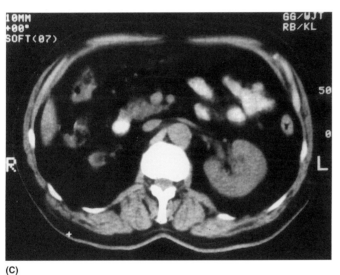

(C)

FIGURE 21 A–C ■ Small end-stage kidney. (**A**) A small 6.6 cm kidney. (**B**) In this case, the kidney is seen indistinctly (*arrows*) within the perinephric fat. (**C**) The findings were confirmed in this case by CT scan.

underestimation of length may occur. Careful technique solves this problem. Cross-sectional areas may be overestimated if the true transverse cross-section is not obtained.

Measurement of small, echodense kidneys also is a problem since differentiating the kidney from the perinephric fat may be difficult, and overestimations of size are common (Fig. 21). In cases of doubt, CT or MRI may be used.

Renal Cyst Simulating Suprarenal, Hepatic, or Splenic Cyst
Cysts in the upper pole of the kidney may be difficult to differentiate from suprarenal, hepatic, or splenic cysts. Persistence with imaging in multiple planes may solve the problem. In any case, differentiation usually is academic since treatment in all cases is conservative.

Postnephrectomy Pseudokidney
After a nephrectomy, organizing tissue and bowel loops fill the old renal bed and produce a reniform complex that may superficially look like a kidney. This should be appreciated since it is embarrassing, to say the least, to report a kidney as being present after a nephrectomy. Tumor

recurrence is another possibility with these appearances. Tumor vascularity may be shown on Doppler studies in such cases. If doubt remains, CT should be performed.

Large Renal Pelvis Simulating Hydronephrosis
An extrarenal pelvis may be large. This appearance suggests a pelviureteric junction obstruction, but a large renal pelvis may be a normal but prominent renal pelvis. In such cases, the calyces must be carefully examined for dilation. When in doubt, a diuretic renogram is necessary.

Iliac Blood Vessels Simulating Dilated Ureters
When seeking the lower ureters posterior to the bladder, it is easy to mistake the iliac vessels for dilated ureters. The plane of the vessels is different to the ureters, the arteries pulsate, and a Doppler study readily confirms their vascular nature.

Bladder Reverberation Artifact
A band of reverberation artifact across the anterior portion of the bladder is inevitable, and although it may be

reduced by gain manipulation, it can never be truly eradicated. The main problem is partial obscuring of lesions in the anterior wall. Reverberation also sometimes occurs in the posterior part of the bladder. In these cases, reverberation must be distinguished from layering caused by blood, pus, or debris. Gain manipulation or turning the patient distinguishes between the two entities.

One or several narrow lines of reverberation apparently originating from the posterior bladder and extending anteriorly are more difficult to explain, but they are some form of artifact.

Doppler Artifacts

The subject of Doppler artifacts is long and complex. Space does not permit discussion here. The reader is referred to texts specializing in this subject (43–45).

PATHOLOGY

Renal Masses: General Considerations

Renal masses may be detected clinically if large, may be found on an IVU examination or a plain abdominal radiograph, or may be primarily detected with ultrasound study (Fig. 22). The most important role of ultrasound is to determine whether these masses are simple cortical cysts, the most common masses, or solid lesions. Large solid lesions commonly are hypernephromas, and if a large solid tumor is detected in a patient with hematuria, it usually is assumed to be a hypernephroma and treated accordingly. Small, smooth, hypoechoic or isoechoic lesions raise the possibility of a benign condition, and further tests are necessary to establish this (Table 6).

Solid Renal Masses in Adults

Isoechoic Renal Lesions

Some renal-cell carcinomas are isoechoic with the renal cortex, although most show some areas of mixed echo pattern caused by variable interfaces, within them (Table 7). They also destroy the normal architecture of that part of the kidney in which they develop. Isoechoic lesions lying centrally, however, may be hypertrophied columns of Bertin. These typically displace the renal pyramids and parainfundibular fat on either side of them. The pattern is fairly typical (Fig. 19) (36). If, however, there was any doubt on the ultrasound interpretation or on clinical grounds, a renal isotope scan, preferably using DMSA, should be performed. A hypertrophied column of Bertin contains normal renal tissue and takes up the isotope, whereas a renal tumor gives a "cold" area. It is likely, although not proven, that a normal perfusion pattern on Doppler study may be helpful. An alternative that has become available recently is a contrast ultrasound study. This appears to be a useful tool to characterize equivocal masses (46,47), though no large studies have been performed.

Isoechoic protuberances from the renal outline, particularly on the left, may be innocent bulges or splenic (dromedary) humps. With these also, their shape and position usually are characteristic and calyces extend partly into them (Fig. 18), whereas tumors destroy or displace calyces medially (35). Again, any doubt should be investigated with an isotope scan or possibly a contrast ultrasound study.

Hypoechoic Lesions

Renal cell carcinomas also may be predominantly hypoechoic (Fig. 23) (Table 8) (48–50), but a relatively small, smooth, usually hypoechoic lesion should raise the suspicion of an

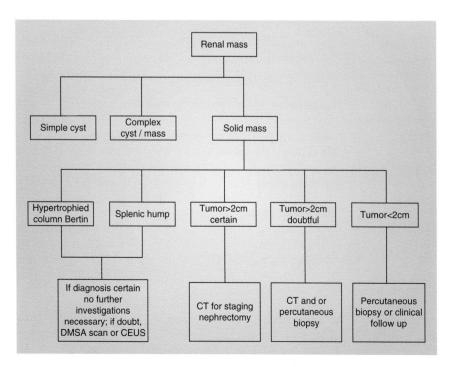

FIGURE 22 ■ Flow chart for the investigation of renal masses.

TABLE 6 ■ Solid Renal Tumors

Low	Isoechoic	Mixed with hyperechoic elements	Areas of calcific density
Echodensity			
May be an oncocytoma	Probably a carcinoma	May be an angiomyolipoma	If central, probably a renal-cell carcinoma If peripheral may be benign
? Biopsy	May be a hypertrophied column of Bertin or a splenic hump ? DMSA scan	? CT	? CT
Size			
<3 cm	>3 cm	Invading vessels or perinephric tissues	
Hamartoma, oncocytoma, granuloma	Probably carcinoma or angiomyolipoma	Carcinoma	
Multiple			
Lymphoma			
Secondary deposits			

Abbreviations: DMSA, dimercaptosuccinic acid; CT, computed tomography.

oncocytoma. Typically, oncocytomas are 3 to 6 cm, containing a central stellate scar (Fig. 24) (51,52). The central scar often is seen on CT but rarely on ultrasound. If this feature is seen, then percutaneous biopsy may be obtained to confirm the diagnosis, though histology is not always straightforward. However, oncocytoma often is indistinguishable from carcinoma on imaging, the diagnosis being made only on the postnephrectomy specimen.

Cysts are anechoic or hypoechoic, but their nature is obvious. A more detailed description of cysts is found later in this chapter. Xanthogranulomatous pyelonephritis may produce an enlarged kidney but also may give hypoechoic areas. The condition usually is associated with calculi. The picture often is confusing but usually is not confused with a tumor (53–56).

Focal pyelonephritis can cause an echo-poor or hyperechoic area in the kidney that may bulge outside the renal outline. Abscesses may cause identical appearances. These often may not be distinguished on ultrasound from tumors, but the history and the confirmation of infection from urinalysis usually establish the diagnosis (57–59). CT may often be helpful particularly for demonstration of inflammatory stranding in the perinephric fat. If doubts persist, percutaneous biopsy may be performed, although

TABLE 7 ■ Predominantly Isoechoic Renal Masses

Cause	Comment	Confirmatory test
Renal-cell carcinoma (hypernephroma)	Often predominantly isoechoic with some variation in pattern; there are often areas of calcification	Biopsy
Hypertrophied column of Bertin	Displaces infundibula; normal uptake of isotopes and contrast US	Isotope (DMSA) scan. ? contrast US
Splenic hump (dromedary hump)	Calyces extend partly into the area; normal isotope uptake and contrast US	Isotope (DMSA) scan. ? contrast US

Abbreviations: DMSA, dimercaptosuccinic acid; US, ultrasound.

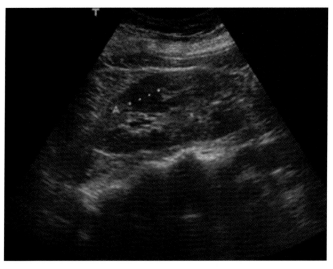

FIGURE 23 ■ Hypoechoic renal-cell carcinoma.

TABLE 8 ▨ Hypoechoic Renal Lesions

Cause	Comment	Confirmatory test
Common lesions		
Cysts	Typical features of cyst	
Oncocytoma	Usually hypoechoic rounded lesion	CT to show central scar, biopsy (though histological interpretation is difficult)
Renal cell carcinoma	Often slightly hypoechoic	
Rare lesions		
Xanthogranulomatous pyelonephritis	Usually associated with calculi	
Pyelonephritis or abscess	Diagnosis implied from the history	? Aspiration, biopsy

Abbreviation: CT, computed tomography.

usually it is sufficient to repeat the examination after appropriate antibiotic treatment.

Malakoplakia occurs in patients with chronic renal infections, who are often immunocompromised patients. It typically causes an enlarged kidney with ill-defined hypoechoic areas (60–62).

Hyperechoic and Mixed Hyperechoic Lesions

Renal cell carcinomas also may display a mixed pattern, predominantly hyperechoic (Fig. 25) (Table 9) (49,50), but a predominance of hyperechoic elements suggests the high fat content and multiple vessel–tissue interfaces of an angiomyolipoma (Fig. 26). Small angiomyolipomas often are of even, high echodensity (Fig. 27), and this pattern does not occur in renal cell carcinomas. Although hyperechoic renal cell carcinomas do occur, they are less echoic than angiomyolipomas. A confident diagnosis therefore may be made on ultrasound alone (63–69). Larger lesions of mixed but predominantly high echodensity should be further studied by CT. The high fat content of angiomyolipomas is readily evident on CT (69). Contrasted ultrasound studies have shown early even enhancement greater than the normal renal cortex. This has however only been reported in case reports and there is no large series to validate this finding.

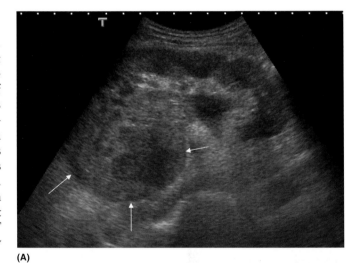

(A)

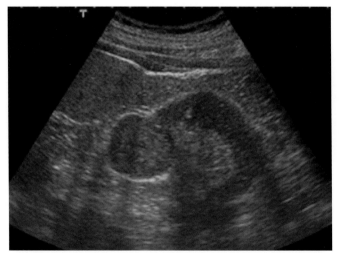

FIGURE 24 ▨ Oncocytoma. A typically smooth though not hypoechoic tumor is shown. A stellate scar is just visible at its center.

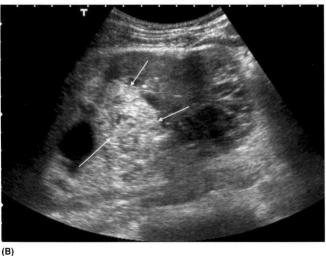

(B)

FIGURE 25 A AND B ▨ Renal cell carcinoma. (**A**) This tumor shows a mixed, predominantly hyperechoic pattern. (**B**) A more hyperechoic renal cell cancer.

TABLE 9 ■ Hyperechoic and Mixed Hyperechoic Lesions

Cause	Comment	Confirmatory test
Angiomyolipoma	Small lesions of even high echodensity; larger lesions mixed	CT to demonstrate fat content
Renal cell carcinoma	Large lesions commonly have a mixed hyperechoic pattern	

Abbreviation: CT, computed tomography.

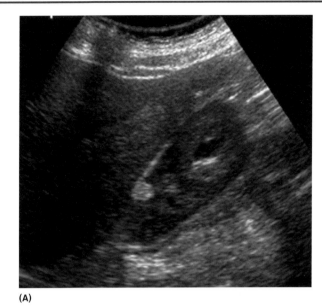

(A)

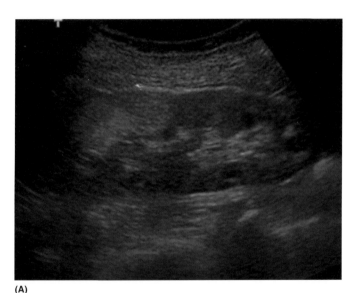

(A)

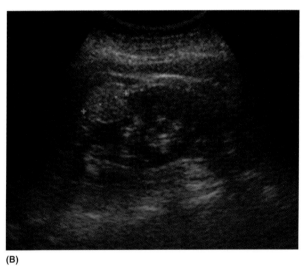

(B)

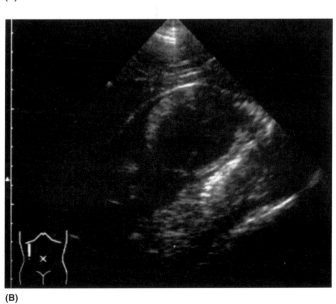

(B)

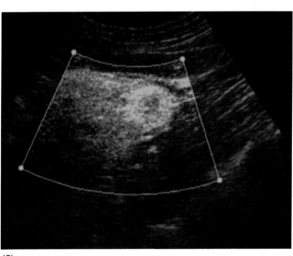

(C)

FIGURE 26 A AND B ■ Angiomyolipoma. Patchy high echodensity (**A**) and a rim of higher echodensity (**B**) both suggest the fat content of an angiomyolipoma. This was confirmed by computed tomography.

FIGURE 27 A–C ■ Small angiomyolipoma. Small angiomyolipomas are often of an even, high echodensity. (**A**) A typical small rounded hyperechoic lesion. (**B**) A slightly larger, less hyperechoic lesion. In this case, a hyperechoic renal cell cancer is a differential diagnosis. (**C**) A contrast ultrasound study in another case (Sonovue® low MI technique) shows increased perfusion of the angiomyolipoma in the arterial phase compared with the normal renal cortex. The less perfused center is probably an area of fat, but this is speculative.

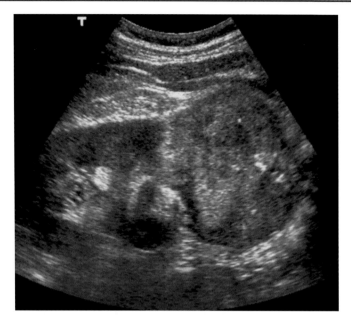

FIGURE 28 ■ Renal cell carcinoma with calcification. Dense hyperechoic areas of calcification are seen within the tumor.

Calcification in Renal Masses

Calcific areas occurring within a tumor may be identified on ultrasound as dense shadowing areas (Fig. 28) (Table 10) (48,49). Such lesions are characteristic of renal-cell carcinomas, although calcification is shown more often on CT images than on ultrasound. Peripheral or rim calcification may occur in renal cell carcinomas or benign conditions (such as simple cysts or hydatid cysts). There may be differential features, however, in the nature of the calcification. A smooth, thin calcific rim typically occurs in benign conditions; a rim with irregular thick areas suggests a malignant lesion (70). Because of shadowing, this differentiation is difficult on ultrasound and better made on plain radiographs or CT.

Multiple Renal Masses

Secondary deposits are found in 2% to 20% of cases of malignancy at autopsy, with colon, lung, breast, and melanoma being the most common primaries (Table 11). However, they are only rarely found on renal imaging. One reason is that they tend to occur late, in advanced disease, when aggressive treatment and imaging may not be justified. Most are small, but larger ones may be seen.

TABLE 10 ■ Calcification in Renal Masses

Cause	Comment	Confirmatory test
Renal cell carcinoma	Rim or intratumoral calcifications occur in about 50% of cases	CT
Hydatid cyst	Usually rim calcification but variable	CT
Simple cortical cyst	Rarely thin rim calcification	CT

Abbreviation: CT, computed tomography.

TABLE 11 ■ Multiple Renal Masses

Cause	Comment
Secondary deposits	Occur late in disease, so rarely found on ultrasound imaging
Lymphoma	May produce multifocal hypoechoic lesions or an infiltrative pattern
Angiomyolipoma	Multiple angiomyolipomas occur in tuberose sclerosis

Ultrasonically, they are indistinguishable from primary lesions, although multiple lesions clearly suggest secondary deposits (71,72). Lymphoma sometimes infiltrates the kidney, but multifocal hypoechoic lymphoma deposits are more common (Fig. 29) (73,74). The kidney also may be involved by spread from adjacent lymph nodes. Papillary renal cancers are uncommon. They are indistinguishable on imaging from renal cell cancers. They have a tendency to recur, and a proportion are multifocal or bilateral at the initial diagnosis. They tend to be only slightly hyperechoic or hypoechoic to the renal cortex (Fig. 30). These features may suggest the diagnosis but are not pathognomonic. Multiple angiomyolipomas occur in the kidneys of patients with tuberose sclerosis (Fig. 35) (95) (see also the section entitled Renal Masses in Children).

Infiltrative Renal Masses

Infiltrative lesions of the kidney typically occur in lymphoma and amyloidosis (Table 12). However, renal-cell carcinomas and transitional cell carcinomas also may infiltrate, and the patterns are similar in all cases. The kidney is enlarged, with loss of the normal architecture: the corticomedullary differentiation is lost, and the sinus fat echo pattern is ill defined or lost. The infiltrative tissue itself may be of low or mixed echodensity but not of increased echodensity (Fig. 30). A definitive diagnosis requires percutaneous biopsy (75).

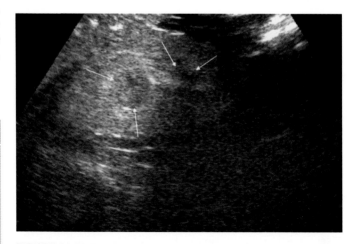

FIGURE 29 ■ Renal lymphoma. A large hypoechoic tumor deposit is seen in the upper pole with a smaller one in the midpole. Further deposits were seen on other scan planes.

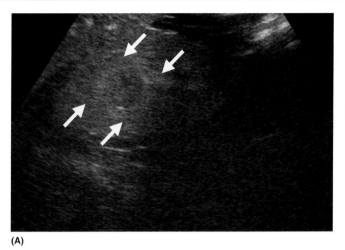

(A)

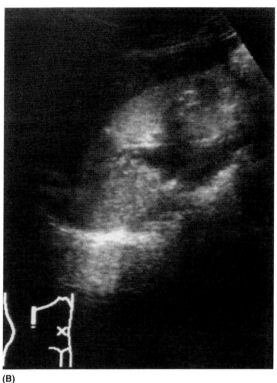

(B)

FIGURE 30 A AND B ■ ■ (**A**) Papillary renal cancer. There are two hypoechoic tumors. The patient had undergone a partial nephrectomy on the other side for papillary cancer. These were found on follow-up. (**B**) Infiltrated kidney (lymphoma). The kidney is enlarged and the internal architecture is destroyed.

Solid Renal Masses in Children

General Considerations

Determining the nature of pediatric renal masses depends as much on the age of the patient as the appearance (Table 13) (76–79). It is also useful to distinguish between common and uncommon masses.

Common Masses Considered by Age

First Year of Life: Mesoblastic Nephroma ■ In the first year of life, the most common renal tumor is the mesoblastic nephroma (also termed fetal renal hamartoma, congenital Wilms' tumor, mesenchymal hamartoma, and congenital fibrosarcoma). They appear as well-circumscribed, homogeneous, hypoechoic masses, rarely with an irregular area of hypoechoic or anechoic necrosis at the center (Fig. 31). They occasionally contain concentric hyperechoic and hypoechoic rings. They may be locally invasive, although they do not invade the hilar vessels and do not metastasize (80,81). They are often found on a prenatal scan (82,83).

Older Than One Year of Age: Wilms' Tumor (Nephroblasoma) ■ Wilms' tumor is the most common tumor in children older than one year of age, with most presenting before five years of age. They usually are large by the time they present and appear ultrasonically as well-circumscribed masses with a well-defined hyperechoic or hypoechoic rim of compressed renal tissue (Fig. 32). They may be homogeneous or heterogeneous because of areas of necrosis, hemorrhage, fat, and calcification (81,84–86). They may invade locally through the renal capsule, spread along the renal vein and vena cava, and metastasize to local lymph nodes, liver, and lung.

Older Children: Renal Cell Carcinoma ■ Renal-cell carcinoma is generally rare in children, except those with Von Hippel Lindau disease. In other children, it rarely occurs, with a peak at nine years of age, so that a tumor

TABLE 12 ■ Infiltrative Lesions

Cause	Comment	Confirmatory test
Lymphoma; amyloidosis; transitional cell carcinoma	All give enlarged homogeneous kidney; similar pattern in infiltrations from any cause	Biopsy

TABLE 13 ■ Common Pediatric Renal Masses by Age

Age	Most common tumor	Appearances
0–1 yr	Mesoblastic nephroma	Well-circumscribed homogeneous, sometimes necrotic, center; occasional concentric rings
1–5 yr	Wilms' tumor	Well-defined; capsule of compressed renal tissue; homogeneous or heterogeneous
>5 yr	Renal cell carcinoma	Poorly defined; hyperechoic, isoechoic, hypoechoic, or mixed

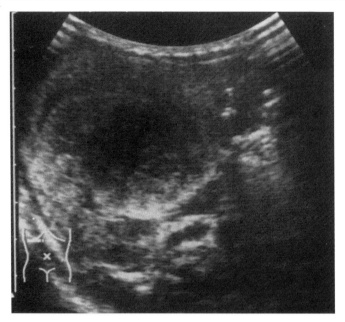

FIGURE 31 ■ Mesoblastic nephroma. An eight-week-old infant presented with a palpable renal mass. The lesion is typically well circumscribed with a homogeneous rim and a stellate hypoechoic necrotic center.

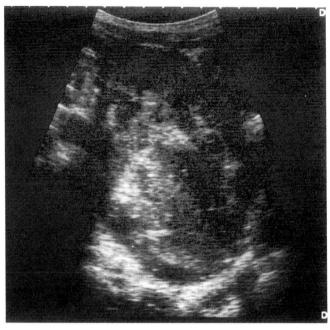

FIGURE 33 ■ Renal cell carcinoma. This tumor in a 14-year-old boy is typically less well defined than a Wilms' tumor.

occurring in children older than five years of age should suggest the diagnosis. Ultrasound appearances are similar to those in adults. Ultrasound patterns are variable, with a hyperechoic, isoechoic, hypoechoic, or mixed echoic mass that is less well defined than a Wilms' tumor. The tumor may invade locally, spread along the renal veins, and metastasize to local lymph nodes, lung, or liver (Fig. 33) (87,88).

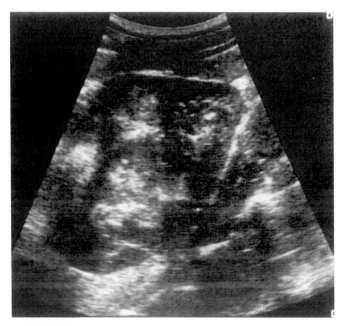

FIGURE 32 ■ Wilms' tumor. The tumor is of a mixed echodensity, well circumscribed, with a hypoechoic rim of compressed renal tissue.

Less Common Pediatric Renal Masses

Secondary Deposits ■ Secondary deposits usually result from undifferentiated sarcomas and cause multiple lesions, usually in patients with a known primary.

Lymphoma ■ Renal involvement occurs late in the disease, by which time a diagnosis invariably has been made. As in adults, there are four patterns of renal involvement: (*i*) multiple hypoechoic or, rarely, hyperechoic lesions; (*ii*) solitary lesions; (*iii*) infiltration; and (*iv*) local invasion from adjacent nodes (89).

Leukemia ■ Hyperechoic or hypoechoic masses rarely occur with leukemia, the usual pattern being infiltration, which causes enlarged kidneys with loss of corticomedullary differentiation (90).

Clear-Cell Sarcoma ■ Clear-cell sarcoma is a rare tumor. The appearances are similar to Wilms' tumor and most are misdiagnosed as Wilms' tumor prenephrectomy (91).

Malignant Rhabdoid Tumor ■ Malignant rhabdoid tumor also is rare. Some tumors have a characteristic subcortical fluid collection containing tumor nodules, which provides the diagnosis. If this feature is not present, differentiation from a Wilms' tumor is not possible. Peak incidence is at 13 months of age (Fig. 34) (92–94).

Angiomyolipoma ■ Angiomyolipoma is a rare pediatric tumor except in cases of tuberose sclerosis, 80% of whom have one or often multiple tumors, sometimes replacing most of the renal tissue. In the general pediatric population, the lesions usually are found incidentally when

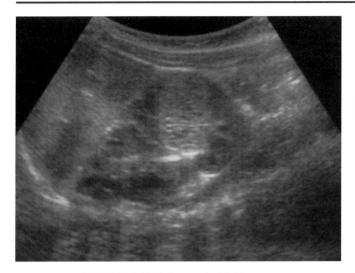

FIGURE 34 ■ Malignant rhabdoid tumor.

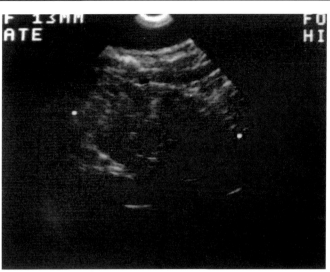

FIGURE 36 ■ Nephroblastomatosis. Hypoechoic areas are seen displacing the renal sinus complex.

scanning for other reasons and appear, as in the adult, as small echogenic lesions, although they rarely cause larger complex masses (Fig. 35) (95,96).

Nephroblastomatosis ■ Nephroblastomatosis is a persistence of fetal renal tissue into childhood and is a precursor of Wilms' tumor. The deposits sometimes are microscopic, but otherwise they are visible ultrasonically, with the appearances depending on the distribution, which has three distinct patterns: pancortical, in which the whole cortex is hypoechoic; superficial, in which a hypoechoic rim is seen in the subcapsular region; and multifocal, in which multiple hypoechoic areas are seen. Rarely, the lesions in any of the patterns may be hyperechoic or isoechoic (Fig. 36).

XanthogranulomatousPyelonephritis ■ Xanthogranulomatous pyelonephritis may cause hypoechoic areas in the renal parenchyma that mimic tumors (97).

Malakoplakia ■ Malakoplakia is rare in children. It occurs in cases of chronic infection. The few reported cases had enlarged kidneys with multifocal hypoechoic areas in the cortex (98).

Renal Cysts: General Considerations

The etiology and classification of renal cystic disease is complex. Some conditions are relevant only in the neonatal or childhood period, and these are discussed separately. The classification of cystic disease has been

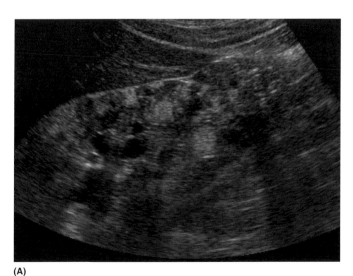

(A)

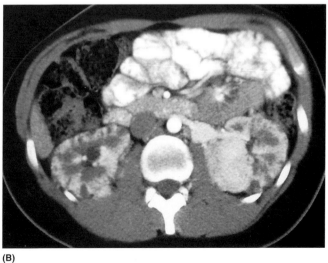

(B)

FIGURE 35 A AND B ■ Multiple angiomyolipomas. In this patient with tuberose sclerosis, multiple angiomyolipomas are seen as small echogenic lesions throughout the kidney. (**A**) Ultrasound scan. (**B**) Computed tomography scan of the same case.

attempted on histologic and clinical grounds. Neither classification is particularly helpful to a practicing sonologist. I therefore first describe the more common cystic conditions and then the less common ones, with differentiating features when possible.

Solitary or Few Renal Cysts in Adults

Simple Cysts

Simple Cortical Cysts ■ Simple cortical cysts have the ultrasound features of any simple cyst (Table 14). They are thin-walled, smoothly outlined structures with anechoic contents (Fig. 37). They are extremely common, the frequency increasing with age. They occasionally reach a considerable size of more than 10 cm, although they are usually 4 cm or less (99,100). Although cortical, they may be peripheral, extend from the surface of the kidney, or lie centrally, originating in the columns of Bertin. They often are multiple, particularly in the elderly, and when they are numerous, it is difficult to distinguish multiple cortical cysts from autosomal dominant polycystic kidney disease (ADPKD).

Parapelvic Cysts ■ Parapelvic cysts lie adjacent to the renal pelvis at the hilum (Fig. 38). They are histologically

TABLE 14 ■ Renal Cystic Disease in Adults

Cause	Comment
Solitary or few cysts	
Simple cortical cyst	Increases in frequency and number with age; thin walled, with no solid elements
Parapelvic cyst	Appears identical to cortical cysts, though their histology differs. They occur in the parapelvic area
Complex cysts	
Hydatid disease	Complex septate cysts typically with solid areas representing daughter cysts, although this feature is not always present
Malignant change in a cortical cyst	Solid elements; thickened areas of wall
Malakoplakia	Hypoechoic areas; complex cysts; calculi
Cystic tumor	Significant solid elements
Multiple bilateral cysts	
Autosomal dominant polycystic kidney disease	Multiple cysts in enlarged kidneys; may be coexisting cysts in other organs
Dialysis (renal failure) cysts	Small cysts with malignant potential in patients with chronic renal failure
Other pathologic conditions simulating cysts	
Renal artery aneurysm	Appearances can be similar to a cyst; the lesion is pulsatile, and flow is shown with Doppler
Hydronephrosis	Dilated calyces may simulate cysts, but the infundibula join at the renal pelvis

different from cortical cysts. Their nature may be inferred from their position, but since cortical cysts also may lie centrally, the distinction cannot be made with certainty. Such distinction is academic, since both entities are innocent and require no treatment.

Complex Cysts

Simple cortical and parapelvic cysts are thin-walled spherical structures with anechoic contents. Anything other than these features makes them a complex cyst, which may be caused by a number of pathologic conditions.

Malignant Change in a Cortical Cyst ■ Considering the prevalence of cortical cysts, malignant change is rare but does occur (101). There are varying degrees of complexity that suggest malignancy. The probability of malignant change being present or developing increases with the complexity. The risk has been studied by Bosniak (102–105). His classification was based on CT appearances (Table 15) and is not strictly applicable to ultrasound appearances. It is nevertheless widely used when describing the ultrasound appearances and the prognosis of cysts and determining treatment (Fig. 37).

Cystic Hypernephroma ■ Cystic hypernephroma also are rare, but some hypernephromas contain large cystic elements. However, there is always a coexisting large solid element to the tumor (48–50,106).

Hydatid Cysts ■ Hydatid cysts typically are multiloculated or septated cysts, with solid elements representing daughter cysts (Fig. 39) (107).

Malakoplakia ■ Malakoplakia causes renal enlargement, with usually hypoechoic areas. Some may appear cystic but there may also be variably loculated multicystic areas. The diagnosis is suggested in an immunocompromised patient, and particularly if there are coexisting renal calculi (Fig. 40).

Multiple Bilateral Renal Cysts in Adults

Autosomal-Dominant Polycystic Kidney Disease

Apart from multiple cortical cysts in the elderly, ADPKD is the most common cause of multiple cysts in adults. Typically, the kidneys are enlarged and full of cysts of varying sizes (Fig. 41), often with coexisting liver cysts. Cysts often occur in the pancreas, spleen, and most other organs of the body (108,109). Difficulties in diagnosis arise in young patients in whom only a few cysts are visible. Although simple cortical cysts may occur in the young, multiple cysts—perhaps three or more in each kidney before 40 years of age—suggest polycystic disease. CT may help by showing multiple smaller cysts that are not visible on ultrasound. In the elderly, the distinction is more difficult since multiple cortical cysts are common in this age group. A family history of polycystic disease changes the probability. Gene markers for ADPKD may be available soon. The coexistence of cysts in other organs strongly suggests ADPKD.

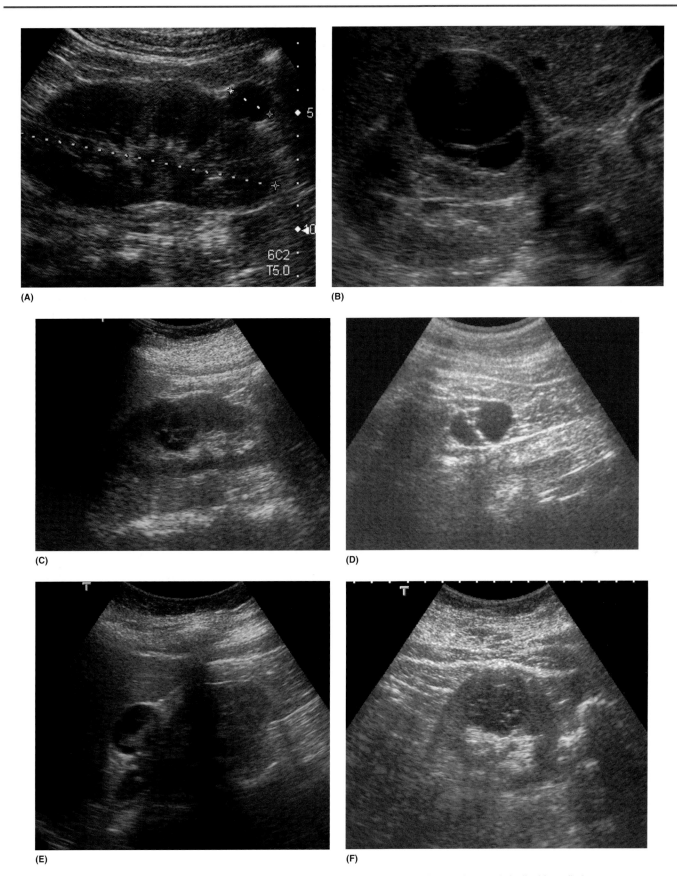

FIGURE 37 A–F ■ Cortical cysts. (**A**) A simple (Bosniak 1) cortical cyst. This is characteristically thin walled with an even shape and anechoic contents. There are no associated solid masses. (**B**) A Bosniak II cyst with a thin septum. (**C**) Bosniak II cysts with closely packed multiple cysts. (**D**) A Bosniak III cyst with a thick septum. (**E**) Bosniak III with a solid inclusion. (**F**) A clearly malignant tumor with cystic elements (Bosniak IV).

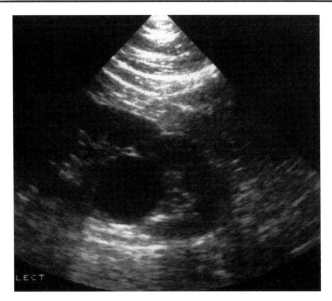

FIGURE 38 ■ Parapelvic cyst. This is similar in appearance to a cortical cyst. The diagnosis is suggested only by the position.

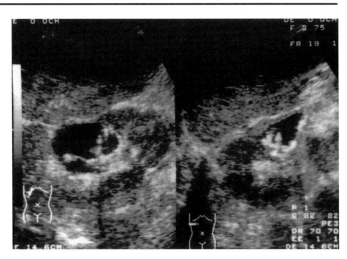

FIGURE 39 ■ Hydatid cyst. The cyst is typically multiloculated, with echogenic daughter cysts and areas of fine calcification in the walls.

The main complications of ADPKD are renal failure, hypertension, bleeds into cysts, and, less often, infection in cysts. Bleeds and infection both present with pain because of increased pressure in the infected cyst. Ultrasound may show a cyst that has increased echogenicity of its contents (Fig. 42). In these cases, percutaneous aspiration confirms the diagnosis and relieves symptoms. MRI or CT of polycystic kidneys, however, shows old hemorrhage in more cysts than is seen on ultrasound, indicating that this is a more common occurrence than previously thought and not always symptomatic.

Acquired Renal Cystic Disease (Dialysis Cysts)

Patients who have been on long-term renal dialysis have a high incidence of renal cysts, the incidence rate being about 70% (53). The cysts are of varying size but are relatively small (Fig. 43). They are often clearly visible ultrasonically, although CT detects cysts in patients who have no cysts visible on ultrasound. They may undergo malignant change. The incidence of malignant change, once thought to be high, is in fact quite low (110–112).

Primary Polycystic Liver Disease

In primary polycystic liver disease, there are multiple hepatic cysts and there also may be renal cysts. It is a different disease from ADPKD, although it is sometimes found in families with ADPKD. The ultrasound images are similar to those found in autosomal recessive polycystic kidney disease (ARPKD) except for the predominance of hepatic cysts (113).

TABLE 15 ■ Bosniak Classification of Renal Cysts

Class I: benign cysts requiring no follow-up	Well-defined, rounded, homogeneous, lucent mass with thin imperceptible wall
Class II: minimally complex but benign, requiring no follow-up	Minimal irregularity, clusters of cysts, high-attenuation cysts, infected cysts, minimally calcified cysts, minimally septated cysts (septae < 1 mm, smooth, attached to walls of cyst with no associated soft tissue mass or enhancement)
Class IIF: require follow-up at 3, 6, and 12 mo	Hyperdense cysts, more wall calcification, slightly more complicated lesions
Class III: may be malignant, require surgical intervention	Thickened irregular septae ± contrast enhancement, thickened or irregular calcifications. Irregular margination, a multilocular mass, uniform wall thickening, small nonenhancing nodular mass
Class IV: malignant lesions, require surgical intervention	Clearly malignant lesions with a cystic or necrotic component, irregular wall thickening, solid elements with contrast enhancement

Source: From Refs. 101, 102.

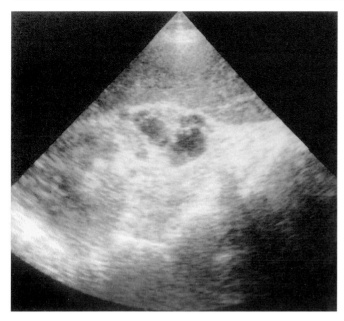

FIGURE 40 ▓ Renal malakoplakia. Multiple hypoechoic areas are seen in an enlarged kidney.

Bilateral Renal Cystic Disease in Neonates and Infants

Autosomal-Recessive Polycystic Kidney Disease

Formally termed infantile polycystic kidney disease, ARPKD presents as renal failure (Table 16). The kidneys are enlarged and of increased sonodensity, with loss of corticomedullary differentiation (Fig. 44) (114–116). In about 50% of cases, a rim of lower echodensity is seen around the periphery of the kidney. Care must be taken in the interpretation of these appearances since neonatal kidneys normally have more sonodense cortices than those of older children, but in normal infants, the renal pyramids are of low echodensity and are clearly seen (Fig. 3).

The increased sonodensity in ARPKD is caused by the interfaces between the cysts, which are really cystic dilations of the tubules. In most cases, they are too small to appear as cysts, although in some patients, a few of the larger ones may be just visible as cysts.

The liver also is affected in this condition, with hepatic fibrosis causing increased sonodensity, enlarged ducts, and signs of portal hypertension. In patients presenting in the neonatal period, however, the renal changes tend to

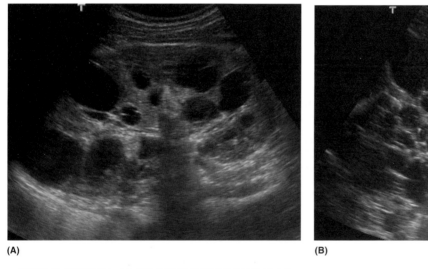

(A)

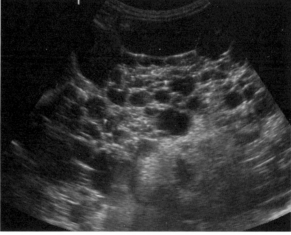

(B)

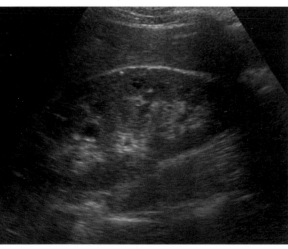

(C)

FIGURE 41 A–C ▓ (**A**) Autosomal-dominant polycystic kidney disease. The kidney is enlarged and full of cysts of varying sizes. (**B**) A more typical example in which the kidney is enlarged to a size that obscures the renal outline. (**C**) An early case with no renal enlargement but multiple small cysts. Such early changes are better shown by computed tomography.

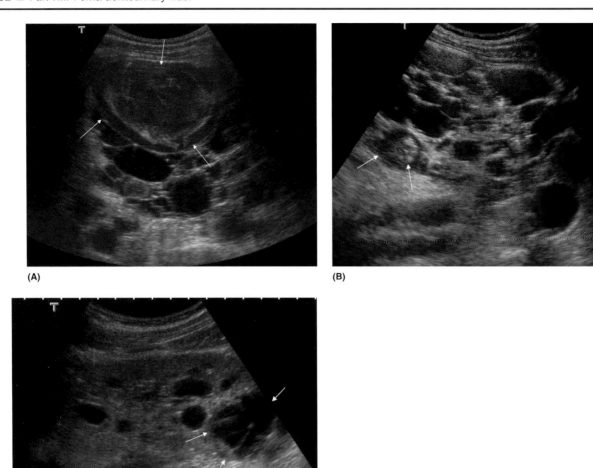

(A)

(B)

(C)

FIGURE 42 A–C ■ Complicated autosomal-dominant polycystic kidney disease. (**A**) There are echogenic hemorrhagic cysts. (**B**) A similar echogenic cyst, but the patient was pyrexial. Aspiration revealed pus. (**C**) A more worrisome case with a complex cyst that could have been malignant. Aspiration biopsy was negative, but the lesion progressed and was malignant.

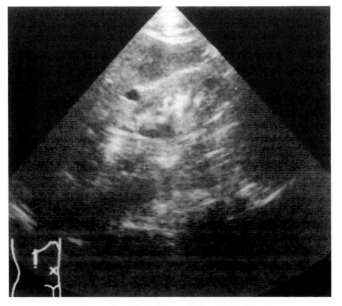

FIGURE 43 ■ Acquired cystic disease (dialysis cysts). In this end-stage kidney, small cysts are seen near the periphery.

predominate and the hepatic changes are less marked, whereas in those patients presenting in later childhood, the liver changes predominate. Rarely, the renal enlargement may be predominantly unilateral (117). If there is any doubt about the ultrasonic diagnosis, an IVU shows a characteristic pattern of radiating streaks of contrast representing the dilated tubules.

Autosomal-Dominant Polycystic Kidney Disease

ADPKD rarely presents in the neonate. When it does occur, it causes enlarged kidneys with increased sonodensity, with cysts visible in about 50% of cases. The presence of several ultrasonically visible cysts suggests ADPKD rather than ARPKD, but the diagnosis usually is made from the family history (Fig. 45) (118). Genetic markers for the disease may be available soon.

Glomerulocystic Disease

Glomerulocystic disease is a rare condition that also causes enlarged sonodense kidneys similar to ADPKD

TABLE 16 ■ Bilateral Multiple Renal Cysts in Neonates and Infants

Cause	Comment	Confirmatory tests
Autosomal recessive (infantile) polycystic kidney disease	Appearances are of sonodense kidneys. Cysts may be seen in a few cases only	IVU shows streaks of contrast in dilated tubules
ADPKD	Rarely presents in neonates. It causes sonodense, enlarged kidneys. Small cysts are visible in about 50% of cases	Positive family history. Gene markers may soon be available
Glomerulocystic disease	A rare condition. Appearances are similar to ADPKD but visible cysts may be larger, up to 1 cm	There may be associated syndromes
Medullary cystic disease:		
Medullary sponge kidney (renal collecting tubular ectasia)	Sonogram findings usually are normal. Sometimes the pyramids are enlarged	
Juvenile nephronophthisis (uremic medullary cystic disease)	Small kidneys with cysts in the medulla and at the corticomedullary junction. Cortex is thin	

Abbreviations: ADPKD, autosomal dominant polycystic kidney disease; IVU, intravenous urogram.

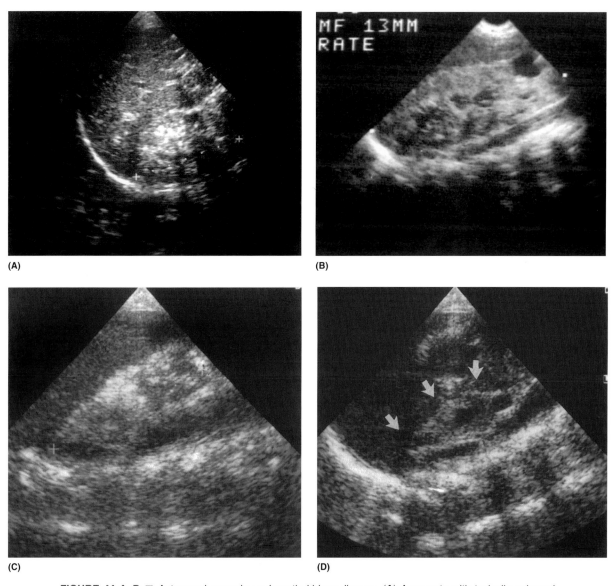

(A)

(B)

(C)

(D)

FIGURE 44 A–D ■ Autosomal-recessive polycystic kidney disease. (**A**) A neonate with typically enlarged hyperechoic kidneys. (**B**) In this six-week-old infant, a few of the cysts are large enough to be ultrasonically visible as cysts. (**C**) A six-month-old infant. (**D**) In this neonate, a rim of lower echodensity is seen around the periphery of the kidney.

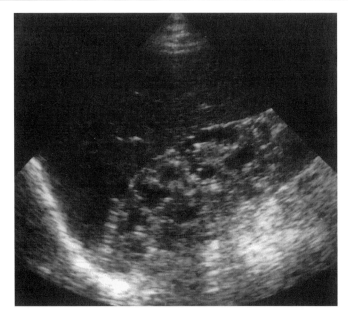

FIGURE 45 ■ Autosomal-dominant polycystic kidney disease in a child. The kidneys are hyperechoic, but multiple cysts of varying sizes also are visible.

(119–122), but in this condition, larger cysts (up to 1 cm) also may be seen (Fig. 46). It has no familial pattern but may be associated with Zellweger's syndrome, orofaciodigital syndrome, or renal retinal dysplasia. There also may be associated hepatic adenomas and cysts.

Medullary Cystic Disease

Medullary cystic disease includes medullary sponge kidney and juvenile nephronophthisis. Medullary sponge

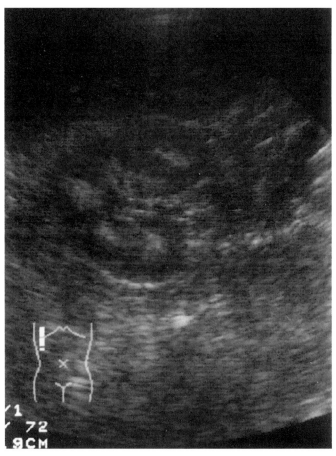

FIGURE 47 ■ Medullary sponge kidney. In this nine-year-old patient, increased echodensity is seen in the medullary pyramids from multiple small cysts.

kidney may cause enlarged pyramids (Fig. 47), but more often, the ultrasound images are normal (123). Juvenile nephronophthisis (uremic medullary cystic disease) may cause kidneys with visible cysts in the medulla and corticomedullary junction (Fig. 48) (124,125).

Bilateral Renal Cystic Disease in Older Children

Children past the neonatal and infant stage may present with a different picture from infants with the same diseases (Table 17). It is relevant, therefore, to consider them separately.

Autosomal-Recessive Polycystic Kidney Disease

In older children, although ARPKD may give the same ultrasound appearance as in neonates with enlarged homogeneous sonodense kidneys, some cases have prominent hyperechoic pyramids with a hypoechoic cortex (116,126). The hepatic changes are more pronounced in this age group, with generalized increase in hepatic sonodensity and particularly increased sonodensity in the periportal region caused by fibrosis. There may be duct ectasia and signs of portal hypertension.

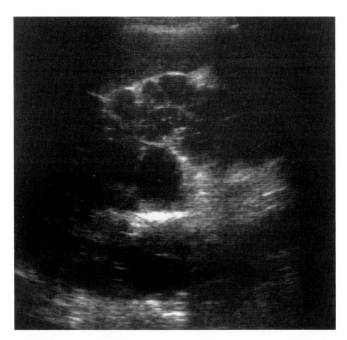

FIGURE 46 ■ Glomerulocystic disease. The kidneys are enlarged with multiple cysts of varying size.

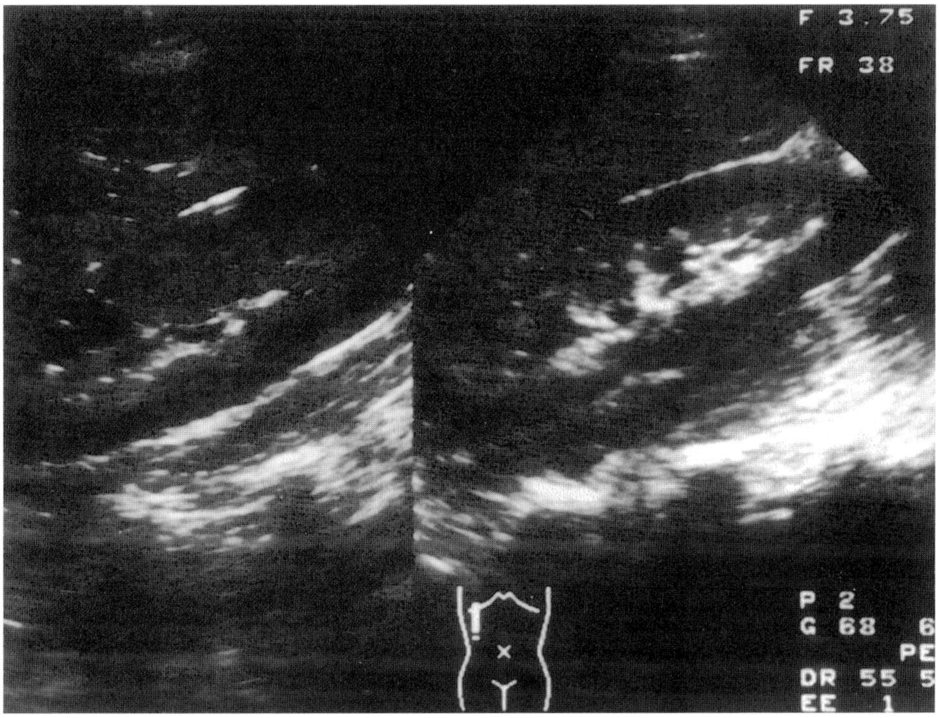

FIGURE 48 ■ Juvenile nephronophthisis. Several cysts are visible at the corticomedullary junction.

Autosomal-Dominant Polycystic Kidney Disease

As affected children get older, the pattern of ADPKD resembles that seen in the adult (Fig. 41), with enlarged kidneys full of multiple cysts, and often cysts in other organs (108,109). However, manifestations of the disease in infancy and childhood are unusual, and most affected patients do not develop ultrasonically visible cysts until at least the third or fourth decade.

Glomerulocystic Disease and Medullary Cystic Disease

The pattern in glomerulocystic disease and medullary cystic disease is similar to that seen in neonates.

Acquired Cystic Disease (Dialysis Cysts)

Older children on long-term dialysis may develop small renal cysts that have a low malignant potential. The ultrasound appearances are similar to those seen in the adult (66).

Unilateral Renal Cysts in Neonates, Infants, and Children

Unilateral cysts represent a different spectrum of disease from bilateral cystic disease, so it is useful to consider them separately (Table 18). Whereas bilateral diseases such as ARPKD rarely affect one kidney more severely than the other, cysts are always actually bilateral.

Simple Cortical Cysts

Simple cortical cysts are rare in childhood, affecting less than 1% of children, but they are seen occasionally. When seen, they have an appearance similar to that in adults (127). The detection of more than one, or at most, two cysts should raise the strong possibility of one of the other cystic diseases.

TABLE 17 ■ Bilateral Cystic Disease in Older Children

Cause	Comment
Autosomal recessive polycystic kidney disease	May show the neonatal pattern or prominent hyperechoic pyramids and hypoechoic cortex
	Hepatic changes are more marked, with increased hepatic sonodensity, periportal fibrosis, and duct ectasia
Autosomal dominant polycystic kidney disease	In older children, the pattern is similar to the adult form, with enlarged kidneys and multiple cysts
Glomerulocystic disease	Similar to the neonatal pattern
Medullary cystic disease	Similar to the neonatal pattern
Dialysis cysts	Similar to the adult pattern

TABLE 18 ■ Unilateral Renal Cysts in Children

Cause	Comment
Simple cortical cyst	Rare in children but seen occasionally
MDK	Multiple cysts of varying size, with no renal pelvis or multiple cysts surrounding a larger cyst
Multilocular cystic nephroma	Affects boys younger than 4 yr and women older than 40 yr. Well-circumscribed lesion containing multiple cysts separated by septa. When the cysts contain mucin, they appear solid

Abbreviation: MDK, multicystic dysplastic kidney.

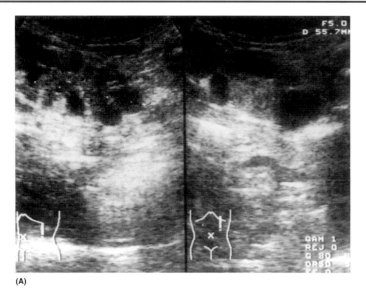
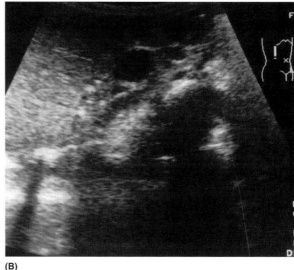

(A) (B)

FIGURE 49 A AND B ■ Multicystic dysplastic kidney. (**A**) The kidney contains multiple cysts and no renal pelvis. (**B**) In this rarer form, multiple cysts surround a larger central cyst. There is no ureter.

Multicystic Dysplastic Kidney

Multicystic dysplastic kidney (MDK) is caused by obstruction in the first 10 weeks of intrauterine life, resulting in a dysplastic kidney full of cysts of varying sizes and with no renal pelvis (Fig. 49) (128,129). The rare bilateral form is not compatible with life. A less common pattern is the hydronephrotic form caused by obstruction occurring after the 10th intrauterine week, in which cysts surround a larger central cyst, representing calyces and pelvis. There is no ureter. Atresia of the renal vasculature occurs in both forms, and a Doppler study reveals either no demonstrable renal blood flow or low-velocity systolic peaks with absent diastolic flow (70).

Abnormality of the contralateral kidney—usually vesicoureteric reflux or pelviureteric junction obstruction—occurs in up to 20% of cases (130).

The usual natural history of an MDK is that the kidneys shrink to a small size in later childhood, often making them invisible on ultrasound. A small proportion, however, develop Wilms' tumor, so they should be carefully monitored by repeat ultrasound studies unless they are excised, usually because they cause hypertension or infection (131).

Multilocular Cystic Nephroma

Multilocular cystic nephroma is unusual in that it has two sex-related age distributions, occurring in boys younger than five years of age, and in women older than 40 years of age. It causes a well-circumscribed lesion containing multiple cysts separated by thin fibrous septa (Fig. 50) (78). Occasionally, the cysts contain mucin, in which case, the

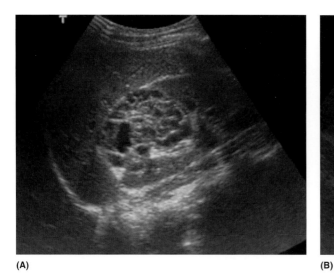
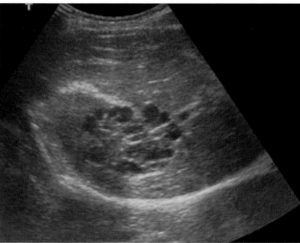

(A) (B)

FIGURE 50 A AND B ■ Multilocular cystic nephroma. (**A**) Longitudinal view. (**B**) Transverse view. There is a well-circumscribed lesion containing multiple cysts and septa.

TABLE 19 ■ Syndromes Associated with Childhood Renal Cysts

- Tuberosa sclerosis
- Turner's syndrome
- Meckel's syndrome
- Jeune's asphyxiating thoracic dystrophy
- Zellweger's syndrome
- Orofaciodigital syndrome

lesion appears to be solid. The terminology of the lesion is confused since it has several synonyms: benign cystic nephroma, cystic hamartoma, cystic Wilms' tumor, and partially polycystic kidney.

Syndromes Associated with Renal Cysts

Renal cysts may be associated with several syndromes (Table 19). There are few features to differentiate the cysts in the different syndromes, and it is sufficient to list the associations.

The Enlarged Kidney: General Considerations

Although many pathologic conditions cause renal enlargement, most cause only moderate enlargement, so that unless baseline measurements are available, such enlargement cannot be appreciated on an ultrasound image.

The cause of the renal enlargement often is obvious, for example, with cysts, tumors, or hydronephrosis. Otherwise, the cause of the enlargement may be ascertained from the patient's history and other tests.

When analyzing cases of renal enlargement, it is useful to divide them into those with unilateral (Table 20) enlargement and bilateral (Table 21) enlargement, and those with intrarenal masses and those without. However,

some of the causes of unilateral enlargement may affect both kidneys in some patients. Therefore, some overlap occurs between the groups discussed.

Unilateral Renal Enlargement

Compensatory Hypertrophy

Compensatory hypertrophy occurs when the opposite kidney is absent, nonfunctioning, or poorly functioning. It occurs within a few months of the reduction of contralateral function. Increase in length may be up to 30%, but there is also an increase in cross-sectional area of up to 30%, so that the increase in volume is as much as 80%. The increase in size is sufficient to be subjectively obvious and to produce measurements that are well above the normal values for the patient's age, sex, and build. The echo pattern of the kidney remains normal.

Duplex Kidney

In a duplex kidney, the renal length is increased by up to 30%, but the renal volume is normal because the cross-sectional area is decreased. The kidney thus appears as a long thin kidney (Fig. 51). A narrowing or waist sometimes is visible between the two moieties; the sinus complex may be double and two renal hila may be visible, but some or all of these signs often are absent, and the only clue to a duplex kidney may be the long narrow shape (132,133). In such cases, if clinically important, confirmation requires an IVU.

Pathologic features associated with a duplex kidney also should be sought. The main ones are dilation of the upper moiety from obstruction of the lower end of its ureter, calyceal dilation, and scarring of the lower pole moiety from reflux, ureterocele, or ectopic ureteric implantation, and other less common ureteric anomalies (134).

TABLE 20 ■ Unilateral Renal Enlargement

Cause	Comment
Compensatory hypertrophy	Physiologic response in a single functioning kidney; kidney appears large but otherwise normal
Duplex kidney	Kidney is long but with decreased cross-sectional area and normal volume; other features such as a double calyceal system and a waist may be seen
Acute pyelonephritis	Enlarged only in severe cases; the cross-sectional area is enlarged most
Renal vein thrombosis	Other associated ultrasonic and Doppler features
Hydronephrosis	Obvious calyceal dilation
Acute arterial infarct	Uncommon; no distinctive gray scale features
Any space-occupying lesion	Cysts are the most common cause; tumors usually are obvious
Multicystic dysplastic kidney	Enlarged in early childhood but often shrinks by later childhood or adulthood
Xanthogranulomatous pyelonephritis	Multiple areas of altered echodensity; associated with calculi
Malakoplakia	Multiple hypoechoic masses

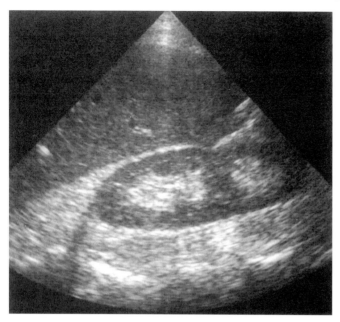

FIGURE 51 ■ Duplex kidney. The kidney is long and thin with a small waist between the two collecting systems.

Acute Pyelonephritis

Acute pyelonephritis may cause marked enlargement of the kidney both in length and in cross-sectional area. Whereas the increase in size may be large, many cases of acute pyelonephritis show little or no demonstrable increase in renal size. In uncomplicated cases, the renal echo pattern remains normal, although in others, there may be decreased corticomedullary echodensity, resulting in an apparently prominent renal sinus complex (135,136). In severe cases, a complicating pyonephrosis may cause calyceal dilation with echogenic contents, focal nephronia may give areas of altered echodensity (see the section entitled Increased Cortical Echodensity with Normal Medulla), and perinephric abscesses may occur. Study of renal size in urinary tract infection is valuable in children, particularly young children, in whom an increase in renal volume to more than 140% gives a high probability that a urinary tract infection is affecting the upper urinary tract (Fig. 52) (137).

Renal Vein Thrombosis

Renal vein thrombosis causes renal enlargement. The echogenicity of the kidney may be altered, with areas of increased and decreased echodensity from hemorrhage and edema, and there may be a collection of serous perinephric fluid (Fig. 53). However, there may be only mild enlargement, with no other gray scale features. The Doppler study is the most useful diagnostic test. Typically, reduced or absent venous flow is accompanied by a characteristic pattern of arterial flow consisting of a narrow systolic peak and sharp reversal of diastolic flow, often with a biphasic reversed M pattern (138–142). Collateral venous pathways may, however, occur rapidly, particularly in the left kidney in male patients, so that the Doppler pattern may not be so characteristic, and in some cases, may be almost normal.

Hydronephrosis

Hydronephrosis causes renal enlargement, but the cause is obvious on the scan and needs no further discussion.

Acute Arterial Infarct

Acute arterial infarct is an uncommon event that may cause increase in renal size, although some reports deny

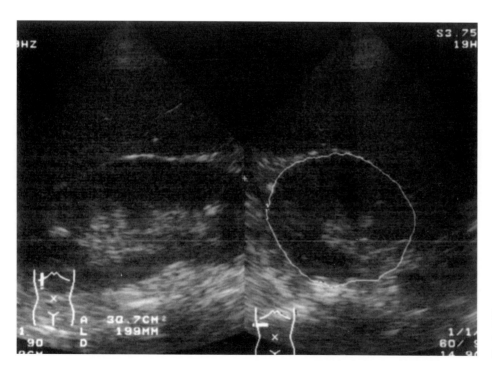

FIGURE 52 ■ Acute pyelonephritis. This 14-year-old girl has a swollen kidney at 13 cm in length and more than 30 cm² in cross-sectional area.

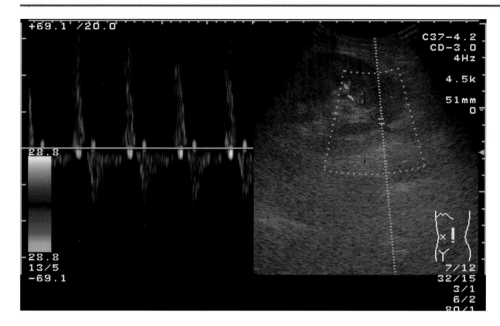

FIGURE 53 ▦ Renal vein thrombosis. The kidney is enlarged, with areas of increased and decreased echodensity. The Doppler flow pattern shows the typical reversed M.

that renal swelling occurs. There are hyperechoic and hypoechoic areas of hemorrhage and edema similar to those found in renal vein thrombosis. Doppler studies may show absent arterial flow in the segment affected or a few vessels with low systolic and low diastolic flow. However, a normal finding on Doppler study probably does not exclude the diagnosis (143). Contrast ultrasound studies may be useful in the diagnosis. Personal experience suggests that in most of infarcted kidneys or in total renal artery occlusion, but the kidney may show no perfusion, there are small irregular patches of perfusion in many cases, perhaps from capsular vessels.

Xanthogranulomatous Pyelonephritis

Xanthogranulomatous pyelonephritis is an unusual reaction to an infection that usually occurs in association with renal calculi and in diabetics or otherwise immunocompromised patients. There are disorganized areas of mixed echodensity within the kidney with moderate renal enlargement. Calculi often are seen ultrasonically (60–62).

Renal Malakoplakia

Renal malakoplakia also is an unusual reaction to chronic infection in diabetic or otherwise immunocompromised patients, resulting in an enlarged kidney with irregular hypoechoic areas and sometimes multilocular cystic areas throughout the kidney (Fig. 40).

Multicystic Dysplastic Kidney

MDK, where the whole kidney is replaced by multiple, often irregular cysts, causes renal enlargement in infants (Fig. 49), although, by later childhood, the kidney shrinks to a small size (see the earlier discussion on MDK) (128,129).

Any Space-Occupying Lesion

Any space-occupying lesion within the kidney such as a tumor, cyst, or hematoma causes renal enlargement. The

primary disease usually is the obvious cause for the enlargement.

Bilateral Renal Enlargement

Numerous pathologic conditions cause bilateral renal enlargement (Table 21). Most cause only mild-to-moderate enlargement with no differentiating features. These are listed but not discussed.

"Unilateral" Causes

Many of the causes listed under "unilateral enlargement" occasionally occur in both kidneys.

Infiltrations

Amyloid infiltrations, lymphomas, and other infiltrations cause a diffuse bilateral renal enlargement with loss of corticomedullary differentiation and loss of definition of

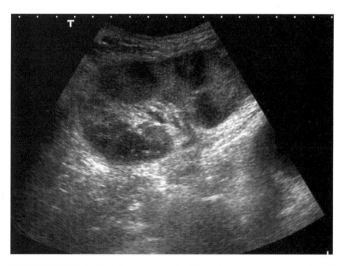

FIGURE 54 ▦ Acute tubular necrosis. There is renal enlargement and marked enlargement of the medullary pyramids.

TABLE 21 ■ Bilateral Renal Enlargement

Cause	Comment
Causes listed under unilateral	Any of these (except compensatory hypertrophy) may occur bilaterally
Infiltrations	Loss of differentiation of internal renal structure
Autosomal dominant polycystic kidney disease	Multiple cysts in kidneys and possibly other organs
Autosomal recessive polycystic kidney disease	Large hyperechoic kidneys in young children; shrink in those that survive
Glomerulonephritis	No differentiating features
Acute tubular necrosis	Enlargement in severe cases only; pattern depends on cause
Diabetic nephropathy	No differentiating features
Uncommon causes	
Acute interstitial nephritis	Lupus erythematosus
Acute urate nephropathy	Polyarteritis nodosa
Beckwith–Weidemann syndrome	Membranous glomerulonephritis
Acute cortical necrosis	IgA glomerulosclerosis
Diabetic glomerulosclerosis	Thrombocytopenic purpura
Goodpasture's syndrome	Amyloidosis
Henoch–Schonlein purpura	Multiple myeloma
Wegner's granulomatosis	Leukemia
	Preeclampsia

the renal sinus complex (75). There are no differentiating features between the various causes of infiltration.

Autosomal-Dominant Polycystic Kidney Disease

ADPKD causes renal enlargement with multiple cysts in both kidneys (Fig. 41), often with coexisting cysts in the liver, spleen, and many other organs. When advanced sufficiently to cause renal enlargement, the diagnosis is obvious (108,109).

Autosomal-Recessive Polycystic Kidney Disease

In ARPKD, a cause for renal enlargement in childhood, the kidneys have increased echodensity from the multiple interfaces of the small cyst walls. Most of the cysts are too small to see on the ultrasound image, although a few may be seen. The kidneys are moderately enlarged in infancy, but in the infants who survive, reduction of size occurs with age (Fig. 44) (116,126).

Acute Glomerulonephritis

Acute glomerulonephritis is one of the more common causes of renal enlargement, although there are no differentiating ultrasonic features.

Acute Tubular Necrosis

Acute tubular necrosis (ATN) causes renal enlargement in severe cases, although less severely affected cases

may have no appreciable enlargement. Increase in cross-sectional area is more marked than increase in length. The kidneys otherwise appear normal when the cause is ischemia, but have increased cortical echodensity in cases of nephrotoxicity and enlarged renal pyramids when there is production of Tamm–Horsfall protein (143,144). The Doppler pattern of reduced or, in severe cases, diastolic flow strengthens the diagnosis (Fig. 54).

Preeclampsia

Preeclampsia causes renal enlargement with significant increase in cortical echodensity. The cause is clinically obvious (145).

Diabetic Nephropathy

Type 1 diabetes may cause a series of changes in renal size, depending on the stage of the disease. Study of these changes may correlate with prognosis (146).

Other Causes

Other causes are numerous and are listed in Table 21. Because they are uncommon or have no particular differentiating features, they are not further discussed here.

Unilateral Small Kidneys

Congenitally Small Kidneys

Congenitally small or hypotrophic kidneys are small, often less than 5 cm in pole-to-pole length, but otherwise appear entirely normal (Table 22). The opposite kidney shows compensatory hypertrophy. The main differential diagnosis is ischemia or severe global scarring. Normal function for the renal size on IVU or isotope study suggests the diagnosis.

Ischemia: Renal Artery Stenosis

A hemodynamically significant renal artery stenosis may rapidly lead to a decrease in renal size, although, conversely, a normal renal size does not totally exclude significant renal ischemia. The ischemic kidney is small but with a smooth outline and normal echo pattern (147). A history of hypertension suggests the diagnosis, which is confirmed by Doppler studies, MR, CT, or contrast angiography.

Reflux Nephropathy: Cortical Scarring

Reflux nephropathy with or without recurrent infection may lead to cortical scarring and decrease in renal size. There may be scarring in a normal-sized kidney, the scars appearing as echogenic depressions in the renal outline above the calyces, often with deformity of those calyces (Fig. 55). More severe cases have scarring with generalized loss of cortex and decrease in renal size. In so-called global scarring, there is marked cortical loss and a decrease in renal size, but the outline may be relatively smooth (Fig. 56) (148,149). Coexisting calyceal deformity suggests the diagnosis.

Postobstructive Atrophy

Long-standing obstructive nephropathy results in progressive atrophy and thinning of the cortex, eventually leading to a paper-thin shell surrounding the dilated calyces. The

TABLE 22 ■ Unilateral Decrease in Renal Size

Cause	Comment	Confirmatory test
Congenitally small kidney	Small, but looks like a miniature version of the normal kidney	Isotope scan or IVU shows normal function for size
Renal artery stenosis: ischemic kidney	Structure appears normal; little or no decrease in size in cases of early disease but marked in cases of severe, long-standing disease	Hypertension; Doppler study or angiogram
Renal scarring: reflux nephropathy	Irregular outline with calyceal deformity	
Postobstructive atrophy	Poor function	
Posttraumatic atrophy	History of severe trauma	
Radiation nephritis	History of radiotherapy	
Renal tuberculosis	Often densely calcified	
Heminephrectomy	History of surgery	

Abbreviation: IVU, intravenous urogram.

kidney is initially enlarged but later may shrink in size. If the obstruction, however, occurs in children or in utero, then the kidney does not grow and remains small. Function as assessed by isotope study is disproportionately poor.

Post-traumatic Atrophy

Most cases of renal trauma recover well without intervention, perhaps with some scarring. Significant atrophy usually results from ischemia caused by damage to the vascular pedicle or, occasionally, from chronic compression of the kidney by a perinephric hematoma. The end result is a smooth or irregular kidney, depending on the extent of scarring (150).

Radiation Nephritis

Radiotherapy to the renal area causes a nephritic reaction and may lead to eventual nonspecific reduction in renal size (151).

Renal Tuberculosis

Renal tuberculosis eventually leads to a small, irregular kidney with areas of calcification. The whole small kidney sometimes is calcified, resulting in an irregular, densely shadowing lesion on the ultrasound image (152–154).

Heminephrectomy, Partial Nephrectomy

The diagnosis of heminephrectomy, should be obvious from the clinical history and the presence of an operative scar. The appearance depends on the extent of the surgery. The kidney often looks remarkably normal.

Bilateral Small Kidneys

There are many causes of bilateral small kidneys and renal failure (Table 23). Most have few or no distinguishing features and are classified as end-stage kidneys. It is

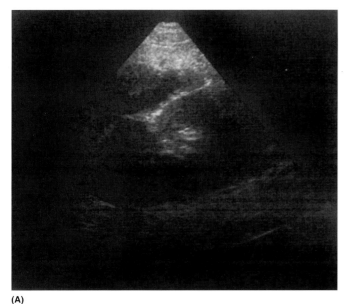

(A)

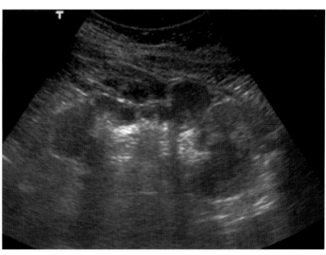

(B)

FIGURE 55 A AND B ■ (**A**) Cortical scarring. An upper pole scar is present. A single scar does not cause reduction in renal size. (**B**) A more extensively scarred kidney.

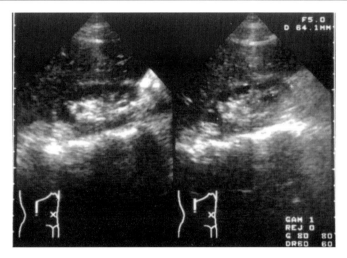

FIGURE 56 ■ Global scarring. There is thinning of the whole cortex, resulting in reduction of renal size.

not productive to discuss each of these individually; the causes are listed in Table 23. In addition, the causes of unilateral small kidney may be bilateral in some patients.

Old Age

It is relevant to discuss old age because, although it results in reduced renal function, it rarely causes overt renal failure. Reduction of renal size with age results from cortical thinning, and is sometimes accompanied by an increase in the renal sinus fat. The degree of atrophy is variable and sometimes results from true age-related atrophy; in other cases, it is caused by additional vascular changes, resulting in further atrophy. The latter patients often are hypertensive. The vascular changes probably vary most. Decrease in renal size with age therefore, although a common condition, often is not a purely normal aging process. It is probably best to report such cases as "age-related cortical loss" or using similar terminology (155). Some patients have kidneys showing a reduced cortex with a normal echo pattern, whereas in other patients, particularly those with additional nephrosclerosis, there is increase in cortical echodensity.

Renal Failure

General Considerations ■ A discussion of renal failure is important even though it does not strictly fit with the image-related approach (Fig. 58).

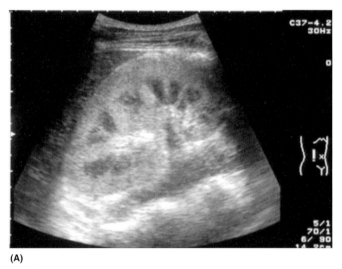

(A)

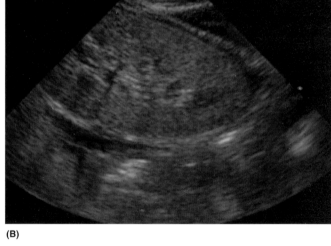

(B)

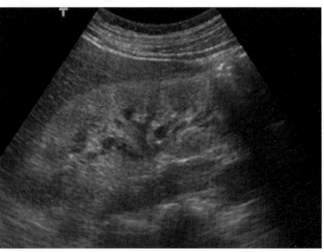

(C)

FIGURE 57 A–C ■ Renal parenchymal disease. (**A**) Type 1 increase in cortical echodensity. The cortex is hyperechoic; the medullary pyramids are normal but appear prominent because of the cortical changes. (**B** and **C**) Type 2 increase in renal echodensity. Both cortex and medulla are hyperechoic so that the medullary pyramids are not seen as separate structures. (**B**) Due to hypoproteinemic renal failure, it also shows perinephric fluid (renal sweat). (**C**) Interstitial nephritis in an AIDS patient.

TABLE 23 ■ Bilateral Decrease in Renal Size

Cause	Comment
As listed in Table 1	Any of the causes of unilateral small kidney may be bilateral
Old age	Variable decrease in cortical width
Hypertensive nephropathy	
Chronic pyelonephritis	
Late papillary necrosis	
Nephrosclerosis	
Hereditary nephritis	
Medullary cystic disease	
Late scleroderma	
Renal cortical necrosis	
Nephropathy of gout	
Chronic lead poisoning	
Any chronic renal parenchymal disease	

Gray-scale ultrasound is the imaging modality of choice in the investigation of acute or chronic renal failure, and is sometimes supplemented by Doppler studies or ultrasound-guided biopsy.

Most cases of renal failure are of clinically undetermined cause. A gray scale ultrasound study determines management.

Calyceal Dilation

In patients with calyceal dilation, obstructive uropathy must be confirmed or excluded, especially because this is a treatable cause of renal failure. Even if the kidneys are small, relief of obstruction may result in a fall in creatinine and avert the need for dialysis or at least reduce the frequency of dialysis. If there is calyceal dilation with a large bladder or a large postmicturition residue, then bladder catheterization is the appropriate initial treatment. A subsequent fall in creatinine confirms that bladder outlet obstruction was the cause for the renal failure. The calyceal dilation may subsequently become less marked, but in severe cases, it may not return to normal. If bladder catheterization does not reduce creatinine levels, then antegrade pyelography and nephrostomy drain insertion, or antegrade or retrograde ureteric stent insertion is necessary. In men with malignant prostatic disease, outlet obstruction may be combined with lower ureteric obstruction from local invasion.

In patients with calyceal dilation and a normal-sized and normally emptying bladder, antegrade studies should be performed immediately. If obstructive uropathy is confirmed, then calyceal drainage should be established during the same session. All pyrexial patients with obstruction should have antegrade puncture to exclude pyonephrosis with drainage if necessary.

Small End-Stage Kidneys

If both kidneys are less than 6cm in length, they are classified as end-stage kidneys, indicating that whatever

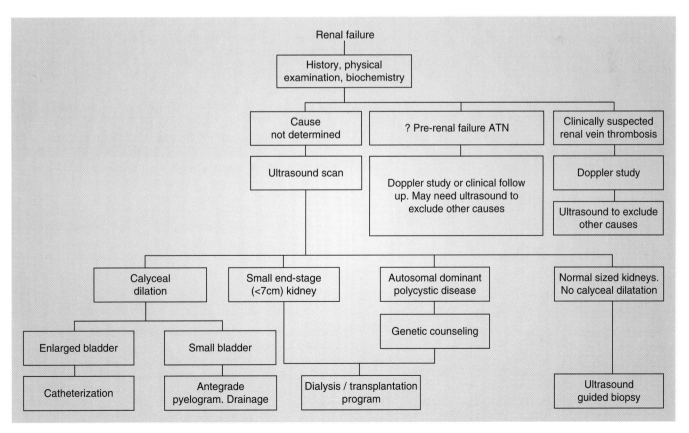

FIGURE 58 ■ Flow chart for the investigation of renal failure.

the cause, insufficient renal cortex remains for adequate function (Fig. 11); the patient then is placed on a dialysis-transplantation program. Some of these kidneys have altered sonodensity, which may indicate a differential diagnosis, but this does not influence management. However, increased sonodensity may make the kidneys difficult to find using ultrasound study since their echodensity is often similar to that of the surrounding fat. With a careful scanning technique, however, they usually are found. Sometimes the distinction between a small and a congenitally absent kidney cannot be made. This affects management only in some hypertensive patients (see the section entitled Hypertension).

Polycystic Kidneys

If autosomal recessive (adult) polycystic kidney disease is found (see the section entitled Cysts), then the patient is offered genetic counseling and placed on a dialysis-transplantation program.

Normal-Sized Kidneys with No Calyceal Dilation

In normal-sized kidneys with no calyceal dilation, a definitive diagnosis is important to decide which patients will respond to medical treatment, principally steroid therapy. This requires a tissue diagnosis. Ultrasound may give some indication of the diagnosis since increased cortical echodensity with normal renal pyramids suggests glomerular disease, and increased cortical and medullary echodensity suggests tubuloglomerular disease (Tables 24 and 25) (156). However, this is not sufficiently accurate for clinical use. In patients with normal-sized kidneys and no calyceal

TABLE 24 ▪ Increase in Cortical Echodensity with No Increase in Medullary Echodensity (Type 1 Change)

Cause	Comment
Acute glomerulonephritis	
Chronic glomerulonephritis	May progress to type 2 change
Nephrosclerosis (hypertension diabetes)	
Acute tubular necrosis	Kidneys and pyramids may be enlarged
Less common causes	
Lupus nephritis	
Alport's syndrome	
Preeclampsia	
Amyloid	
AIDS	
Leukemia	
Beckwith–Wiedeman syndrome	
Myeloglobinurea	
Lipoid nephrosis	
Kawasaki disease	
Acute cortical necrosis	Calcified cortex
Cortical nephrocalcinosis	Pericalyceal calcification

dilation, therefore, renal biopsy is necessary. This is best carried out under real-time ultrasound guidance.

Prerenal Failure or ATN

The clinical history may suggest prerenal failure or ATN. In these cases, an additional Doppler study may distinguish between the two: prerenal failure gives a normal arterial Doppler spectral pattern, whereas ATN, if sufficiently severe to cause renal failure, causes reduced diastolic flow (143b). Many clinicians confidently treat such cases clinically without any imaging. If there is clinical doubt, however, ultrasound is necessary to establish the diagnosis and to exclude other causes; some clinicians argue that an ultrasound study is prudent in all cases.

Vascular Causes of Renal Failure

If renal vein thrombosis or arterial occlusion is suspected, a Doppler study is appropriate (139). Renal vein thrombosis causes a narrow arterial systolic peak and a sharp reversal of diastolic flow. There is absent or reduced venous flow (Fig. 53). However, the opening of collateral channels may cause reversion to a normal waveform, so that Doppler, although highly specific, lacks sensitivity in the native kidney (it is sensitive in the transplanted kidney). Arterial occlusion causes reduced or no flow in the kidney. A normal spectral waveform may be obtained in some cases of ischemia, although more often, low systolic peaks are obtained with absent diastolic flow. In all cases, examination with ultrasound contrast agents shows severely reduced cortical perfusion (Fig. 93).

Changes in Renal Echodensity: General Considerations

Generalized changes in renal echodensity conform to two patterns. There may be increased echodensity of the cortex with normal echodensity of the medullary pyramids and thus enhancement of the corticomedullary differentiation, or increased echodensity of both cortex and the medulla with loss of corticomedullary differentiation. These are sometimes referred to as type 1 and type 2 changes, respectively (Fig. 57). Whereas some diseases typically cause type 1 and others cause type 2 changes, many of the causes of type 1 change progress to type 2 in advanced stages of the disease.

Some diseases cause decreased echodensity of the renal cortex. However, diffuse reduction in cortical echodensity is difficult to appreciate, although focal changes are easier to see. Finally, a few disease processes primarily affect the echodensity of the medullary pyramids (156).

Increase in Cortical Echodensity with Normal Medulla (Type 1 Change)

An increase in cortical echodensity with normal medulla (type 1 change) is the most common change to occur in renal parenchymal disease (Table 24). Numerous disease processes produce this change, many of which also cause an increase in both cortical and medullary echodensity (type 2 change). There is usually little or nothing

TABLE 25 ■ Increase in Cortical and Medullary Echodensity (Type 2 Change)

Cause	Comment
Chronic pyelonephritis	
Chronic glomerulonephritis	Starts as type 1 change
Less common causes	
AIDS	
Autosomal recessive polycystic kidney disease	
Renal tubular ectasia	
Medullary cystic disease	
Autosomal dominant polycystic kidney disease in children	Unusual but occasionally found in this age group
Focal nephronia (acute bacterial nephritis)	Focal change, although may be extensive
Healing infection	Focal change, although may be extensive

on the ultrasound image to distinguish one disease from the other, the diagnosis sometimes being inferred from the history and in other cases being made by renal biopsy. Therefore, a report should be made describing the changes and indicating that they suggest renal parenchymal disease but are not specific for the type of disease.

Increase in Both Cortical and Medullary Echodensity (Type 2 Change)

With an increase in both cortical and medullary echodensity (type 2 change), the whole kidney becomes homogeneously hyperechoic (Table 25). Although many of the diseases that cause type 1 change progress to this pattern, a smaller list of diseases primarily cause this pattern in their early stages. The list is still relatively large, but in these cases, it may be possible to narrow the differential diagnosis. In practice, most cases require biopsy for a definitive diagnosis.

Patchy Increase in Cortical Echodensity

Patchy areas of increased echodensity may be caused by infection (Figs. 56 and 60), scarring, or renal vein thrombosis (Fig. 53) (Table 26). In the latter, there are usually also areas of decreased echodensity and renal enlargement, although the cortical changes may be minimal or absent (148,156). The typical Doppler pattern of sharp reversal of diastolic flow with a narrow systolic peak confirms the diagnosis.

TABLE 26 ■ Patchy Increase in Cortical Echodensity

Cause	Comment
Infection	
Scarring	Increased echodensity beneath an indentation in the renal outline above a calyx
Renal vein thrombosis	Patchy decrease in echodensity with renal enlargement; these changes are not always present

Decreased Cortical Echodensity

Decrease in cortical echodensity is more difficult to appreciate from the ultrasonic scan than increase in echodensity (Table 27). For this reason, the sign is often missed. Most acute disease processes in the early stages may cause some decrease in cortical echodensity, usually accompanied by some renal enlargement. The change presumably results from edema. Edema, however, may cause decreased echodensity or increased echodensity, the latter presumably by enhancing tissue interfaces. This is probably the reason that decreased cortical echodensity in acute disease is so variable. The disease processes in which the sign is most often (although infrequently) seen are listed in Table 27.

Xanthogranulomatous pyelonephritis causes renal enlargement with a general decrease in echodensity, but sometimes also with areas of increased echodensity. There are usually calculi present (61).

Isolated Increase in Medullary Echodensity

The most common cause of isolated increase in medullary echodensity is nephrocalcinosis (Fig. 59) (Tables 28 and 29). This starts as a rim of increased echodensity around the periphery of the medullary pyramids, and later progresses to fill the whole medulla. Shadowing is a late sign. In non-shadowing cases, the calcification usually is not visible on plain radiographs. CT will confirm the diagnosis (157,158). Less common causes are listed in Table 28.

Increased Renal Echodensity in Neonates and Infants

In neonates and infants with increased renal echodensity, the list of causes is relatively small; therefore, the group is discussed separately.

Neonates and Infants: Increased Cortical Echodensity with Normal Medulla

Remember that relative increase in cortical echodensity is the normal pattern in infants up to six months of age (Fig. 3) (Table 29) (4). The most common pathologic causes

TABLE 27 ■ Decreased Cortical Echodensity

Cause	Comment
Acute pyelonephritis	May be generalized or focal areas
Renal vein thrombosis	Also, hyperechoic areas of hemorrhage; characteristic Doppler signals
Acute glomerulonephritis echodensity	Unusual pattern, more often increased
Lupus nephritis	Multiple hypoechoic areas
Lymphoma	Multiple hypoechoic areas
Multicentric renal carcinoma	Multiple hypoechoic areas
Xanthogranulomatous pyelonephritis	Usually calculi; also may be cystic areas and areas of increased echodensity
Many disease in the early acute stage	

in developed countries are glomerulocystic disease, neonatal nephrotic syndrome, and glomerulonephritis, whereas in developing countries, the most common cause is dehydration, which gives a variable increase in cortical echodensity (159,160).

ATN, sometimes combined in postsurgical cases with dehydration, causes enlarged kidneys, with a variable increase in cortical echodensity and a reduction in diastolic flow on Doppler studies, depending on the severity.

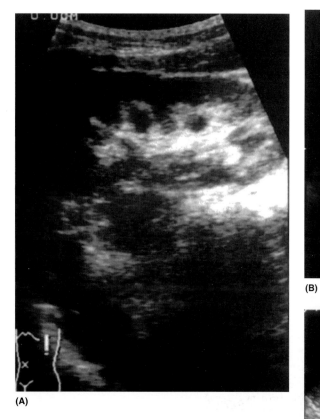

(A)

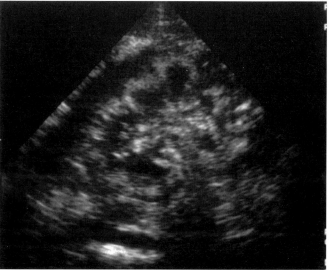

(B)

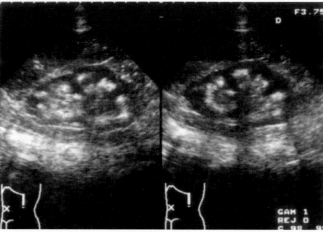

(C)

FIGURE 59 A–C ■ Nephrocalcinosis. (**A**) Early nephrocalcinosis causes an echodense rim around the pyramids. More marked changes are seen with progression of the disease (**B**), whereas later cases. (**C**) show increased echodensity of the whole pyramids.

TABLE 28 ■ Isolated Increase in Medullary Echodensity

Cause	Comment
Medullary nephrocalcinosis	Starts at the periphery of the pyramids and then progresses to fill them in
Renal pyramidal fibrosis	Part of a generalized renal dysplasia
Less common causes	
Medullary sponge kidney	
Tamm–Horsfall proteinuria	
Dehydration	
Pyelonephritis	
Candida infection	
Renal tubular necrosis	
Williams' syndrome	
Sjögern's syndrome	
Gout	
Primary aldosteronism	
Lesch–Nyhan syndrome	
Glycogen storage disease—type 1	
Wilson's disease	
Pseudo-Bartter's syndrome	

Less common causes are oxalosis (Fig. 61), storage diseases, and almost any cause of end-stage renal failure (159,160).

Infants: Increase in Cortical and Medullary Echodensity

An increase in cortical and medullary echodensity in infants results in a homogeneously echodense kidney

TABLE 29 ■ Neonatal and Infant Kidneys: Increased Cortical Echodensity with Normal Medulla

Cause	Comment
Normal	Up to 6 mo; the cortex normally is sonodense
Glomerulocystic disease	Some cysts may be seen; the medulla also may be sonodense
Neonatal nephrotic syndrome	
Glomerulonephritis	
Dehydration	Common in developing countries; there is variable increase in cortical sonodensity
Acute tubular necrosis	Enlarged kidneys with variable increase in cortical echodensity
Oxalosis	Causes calcification, sometimes confined to the cortex, sometimes affecting cortex and medulla
Storage disorders	
Any cause of end-stage renal failure	

with loss of corticomedullary differentiation (Table 30). The main cause is autosomal recessive (infantile) polycystic kidney disease (Fig. 44). Most of the cysts are too small to produce the typical image of an anechoic cyst, although a few may be large enough to be seen. Most produce a generalized increase in echodensity because of the interfaces of the cyst walls (114–116). Autosomal dominant (adult) polycystic kidney disease normally presents after the second or third decades, but rarely presents in infants, in which case, it is often ultrasonically indistinguishable from the infantile form. Glomerulocystic disease (Fig. 46) also may produce increased renal echodensity (119–122). Oxalosis may cause calcifications confined to the cortex or affecting cortex and medulla.

Isolated Changes in Medullary Echodensity in the Infant ■ The most common cause of increased echodensity in the infant is nephrocalcinosis (Table 31). Reduction in medullary echodensity probably does not occur, although increased cortical echodensity causes this impression. Increase in size of the renal pyramids, as occurs in acute cortical necrosis, also gives the impression of reduced echodensity.

Calyceal Dilation (Hydronephrosis)

The term "hydronephrosis" is sometimes used as a synonym for obstruction, but it denotes calyceal dilation of any cause. A hydronephrotic kidney seen ultrasonically contains a group of anechoic fluid-filled spaces within the sinus complex (Fig. 63) (161,162). However, the normal calyceal system is often sufficiently distended to be ultrasonically visible. This is particularly so if there is a high renal output from a fluid load such as is given to fill the bladder, from contrast administration if the ultrasound is carried out after an IVU, from diuretic administration, or in a patient with a single kidney. A full bladder also may cause calyceal dilation, which disappears when the bladder is emptied. In all cases, the normal cupped shape of the calyces is preserved; this is confirmed by careful scanning. Whereas obstruction is the most common cause of hydronephrosis, there are several other causes (Table 32).

Obstruction ■ Ultrasound often is the first imaging modality to be employed in suspected obstruction (163). However, the ultrasound study usually detects only the presence or absence of calyceal and ureteric dilation, and the absence of dilation does not exclude obstruction (Table 33) (164,165). In acute obstruction, the kidney initially may cease to excrete urine, thus delaying the onset of calyceal dilation. In longstanding obstruction, calyceal dilation usually occurs, the exception being retroperitoneal fibrosis where renal failure may ensue with minimal or no calyceal dilation. Conversely, the presence of calyceal dilation does not necessarily indicate obstruction (166,167). It could result from previous obstruction, reflux nephropathy, present or previous pregnancy, megaureter, or other forms of caliectasis (Table 32). Confirmation often requires CT, IVU, antegrade pyelography, or retrograde

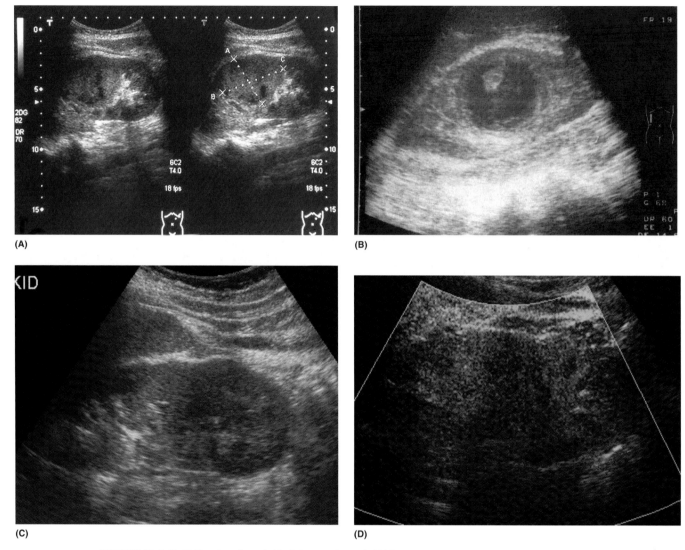

FIGURE 60 A–D ■ Focal pyelonephritis (lobar nephronia). (**A**) There is slight swelling of the mid pole of the kidney with an area of decreased echodensity. In a patient with proven urinary tract infection, this appearance is likely to represent focal pyelonephritis. (**B**) Focal nephronia may progress, as in this case, to a renal abscess. (**C**) Focal nephronia causing a mass lesion simulating a tumor. (**D**) An ultrasound contrast study (Sonovue® with a low MI technique) shows slight hypervascularity but a normal perfusion pattern. A tumor would have a different perfusion pattern.

TABLE 30 ■ Infant Kidneys: Increase in Cortical and Medullary Echodensity

Cause	Comment
Autosomal recessive polycystic kidney disease	
Autosomal dominant polycystic kidney disease	Rarely presents in infancy
Glomerulocystic disease	The cortex may be more echodense than the medulla, and a few cysts may be large enough to be ultrasonically visible
Oxalosis	Causes calcification sometimes confined to the cortex, sometimes affecting cortex and medulla

pyelography. In patients who are allergic to contrast media, however, the ultrasound and KUB radiograph taken in association with the relevant history are often sufficient.

Doppler studies may play a part in the investigation of obstruction. In obstruction, the raised calyceal pressure leads to a complex process involving the production of prostaglandin E_2 and arachidonic acid, causing arteriolar vasoconstriction. This mechanism leads to the reduced and delayed excretion seen in obstructive cases on the IVU. The arteriolar vasoconstriction also causes reduced diastolic arterial blood flow velocities, which may be measured on the Doppler spectral waveform and quantified by RI measurements. An RI above 0.7 or more than 0.1 higher than the opposite normal side is

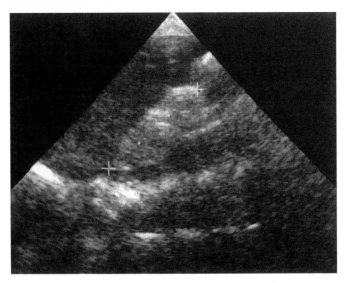

FIGURE 61 ■ Oxalosis. The kidney is typically hyperechoic in this condition.

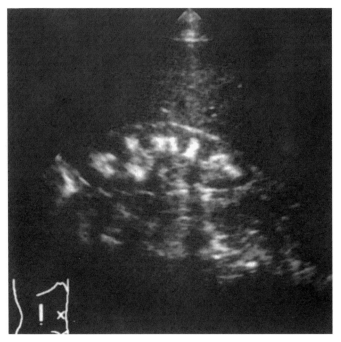

FIGURE 62 ■ Nephrocalcinosis. In this infant, echodense pyramids are seen that are typical of nephrocalcinosis.

significant (17,168). The Doppler study may be used to distinguish a pelviureteric junction obstruction with a high intrarenal pressure from one with a normal pressure. An elevated RI in an obstructed kidney may be increased by the use of furosemide in such cases (110). The study also may be used to distinguish calyceal dilation caused by acute obstruction from other causes. Particular use of this has been made in pregnant patients with loin pain to distinguish dilation of pregnancy from that of obstruction (169).

Relieved Obstruction ■ Previous obstruction with hydronephrosis may result in a permanently dilated system, particularly if the obstructive episode was severe and prolonged.

Reflux Nephropathy ■ Reflux nephropathy causes calyceal dilation, usually confined to, or more marked in, the upper pole calyces. There is usually some cortical scarring over these calyces. This pattern distinguishes reflux nephropathy from obstruction (170). An ultrasound study does not detect all cases of reflux.

Pregnancy ■ Pregnancy causes a variable degree of calyceal dilation, sometimes marked, and maximal at about 38 weeks, and affecting the right kidney more than the left. It is probably mainly caused by hormonal effects, although there also may be some mechanical component. A proportion of cases have flank pain. In these, distinction needs to be made between dilatation of pregnancy and other causes of obstruction, principally ureteric calculus.

TABLE 31 ■ Infants: Isolated Increase in Medullary Echodensity

Cause	Comment
Nephrocalcinosis	Starts at the rim of the pyramids and then progresses to fill them in
Less common causes	
Hereditary tubular ectasia	
Urate deposition	
Vascular congestion	
Renal infection	
Intrarenal reflux	

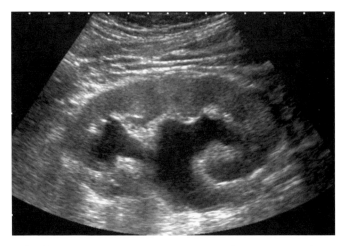

FIGURE 63 ■ Hydronephrosis and hydroureter. There is marked dilation of the calyceal system and upper ureter.

TABLE 32 ■ Calyceal Dilation: Hydronephrosis

Cause	Comment	Confirmatory tests
Obstruction	Absence of dilation does not exclude obstruction	IVU; isotope renogram; antegrade; retrograde; CT
Previous obstruction	If severe, dilation may not return to normal	
Reflux nephropathy	Upper pole calyces more often are affected. Usually dilation is not marked. Scars may be present	Micturating cystogram
Pregnancy	More marked on the right. Greatest at 38 wk. May become permanent, particularly after multiple pregnancies	Doppler study; RI normal in pregnancy and elevated in obstruction. Dilatation down to the level of iliac vessels
Congenital megacalyces		Doppler during pregnancy; IVU if postpregnancy
Papillary necrosis	Causes dilation per se but there also may be obstruction caused by a sloughed papilla	
Postinfective clubbing	Scars over clubbed calyces	
Full bladder	Returns to normal with bladder emptying	
Overhydration IVU contrast media normal	Mild dilation only	

Abbreviations: IVU, intravenous urogram; RI, resistance index.

More dilatation on the left compared to the right favors calculus. In dilatation of pregnancy, the ureter is dilated down to the level that enables it to cross the iliac vessels and not beyond. A level above or below this strongly suggests obstruction. The ureters at the iliac level may be seen in about 70% of pregnant women on a longitudinal oblique scan plane using the posterior uterine wall or placenta as a sonic window (171–176). The distinction between nonobstructive and obstructive dilation may also be made by Doppler studies. The nonobstructed system has a normal diastolic flow, as measured by RI; the obstructed system has a reduced diastolic flow (elevated RI). If doubt remains, an ultrasound-guided antegrade pyelogram with minimal X-ray screening should be performed. Alternatively, some advocate placing an antegrade drain or stent under ultrasound control with no X-ray screening, or a retrograde stent and delaying the contrast study until after delivery. The calyceal system may remain dilated after the pregnancy, particularly after multiple pregnancies.

Congenital Megacalyces ■ Congenital megacalyces may accompany megaureters (Fig. 69). Differentiation from obstruction requires an IVU (177).

Papillary Necrosis ■ Papillary necrosis can cause hydronephrosis per se, the calyces with sloughed papillae becoming clubbed (Fig. 64). Also, the sloughed papillae themselves may obstruct the ureters, leading to hydronephrosis (178).

Postinfective Clubbing ■ Severe, prolonged, or multiple episodes of pyelonephritis may cause calyceal clubbing and cortical scarring similar to that found in reflux nephropathy. Caliectasis of one or more, but not all, the calyces is found in reflux nephropathy, where typically

TABLE 33 ■ Obstruction Without Calyceal Dilation: False-Negative Findings

Cause	Comment
Acute cases	In the first few hours, there may be no calyceal dilation
Renal shutdown	Acute obstruction causes a variable degree of renal shutdown that reduces the degree of dilation
Spontaneous decompression	Renal rupture or, less commonly, backflow
Renal failure	Obstruction occurring in a poorly functioning kidney may not cause dilation
Intermittent obstruction	
Retroperitoneal fibrosis	Dilation occurs late in these cases, often after renal failure is established
Staghorn calculus	There is usually some dilation around the calculus, but this may be difficult to see

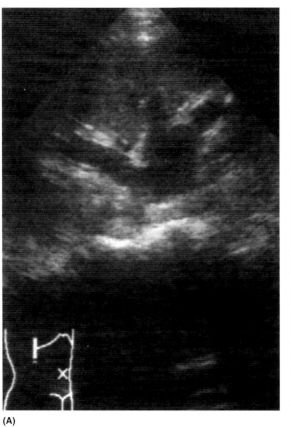

(A)

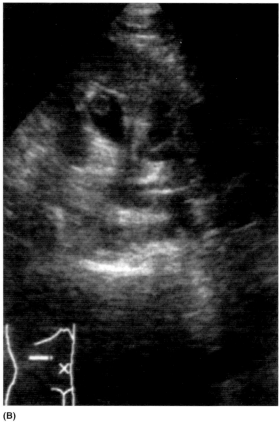

(B)

FIGURE 64 A AND B ■ Papillary necrosis. (**A**) Typically clubbed and deformed calyces are seen. (**B**) Rarely, a sloughed papilla may be seen in one of the calyces.

the upper pole calyces are affected. Renal tuberculosis, calculus or tumor obstructing an infundibulum are other causes.

Uroepithelial Thickening

Generalized Thickening

Generalized thickening of the uroepithelium of the renal collecting system may occur in any form of infection, but it is most marked in opportunist infection occurring in immunocompromised patients, and particularly in fungal infections. It is difficult to detect ultrasonically unless there is a coexisting hydronephrosis or a large renal pelvis (Fig. 65) (179). The normal uroepithelium measures less than 1 mm, but assessment of thickening usually is subjective.

Focal Thickening

Focal thickening usually is caused by a uroepithelial tumor (Fig. 66), although an adherent blood clot may have similar appearances. If in doubt, a repeat scan would reveal a change in the case of a blood clot. Most uroepithelial tumors, however, are not visible on an ultrasound image since they are lost in the renal sinus complex. Contrast CT or IVU studies are better at demonstrating uroepithelial tumors in the calyceal system and ureter.

The Apparently Absent Kidney

An apparently absent kidney on an IVU examination may be truly absent, nonfunctioning, or poorly functioning (Fig. 67). The ultrasound scan shows the morphologic features but not the function of the kidney.

An apparently absent kidney on an ultrasound examination is another matter. When a kidney is not seen, the obvious (although often forgotten) first step is to ask the patient about previous surgery and look for a nephrectomy scar. Apart from a history of previous nephrectomy,

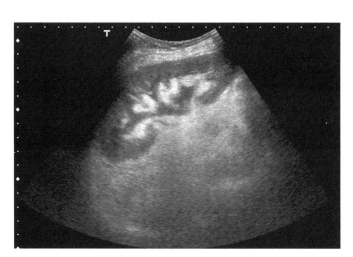

FIGURE 65 ■ Uroepithelial thickening. The thickened uroepithelium, in this case caused by an infection with *Candida albicans*, is seen in the slightly dilated renal pelvis.

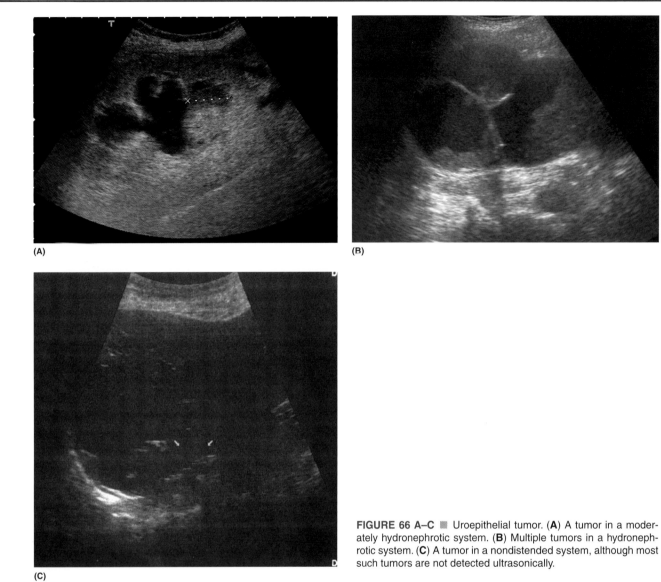

(A)

(B)

(C)

FIGURE 66 A–C ■ Uroepithelial tumor. **(A)** A tumor in a moderately hydronephrotic system. **(B)** Multiple tumors in a hydronephrotic system. **(C)** A tumor in a nondistended system, although most such tumors are not detected ultrasonically.

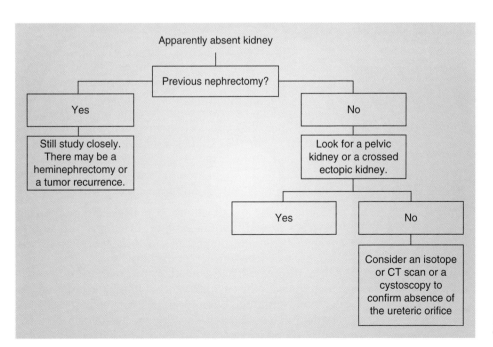

FIGURE 67 ■ Flow chart for the investigation of an apparently absent kidney.

many patients know that they have an absent, small, or ectopic kidney. Such information surprisingly is often omitted from the ultrasound request form.

Failing such a history, a pelvic kidney should be sought. If no kidney is found, then it is either absent or small. Small kidneys may become hyperechoic and are difficult to differentiate from the surrounding fat. If the patient is hypertensive, the presence of a small kidney must be excluded and other tests such as an isotope scan or CT may be necessary. The most accurate indication of an absent kidney is the lack of a ureteric orifice at cystoscopy.

Spina bifida patients are screened regularly by ultrasound for hydronephrosis. In these patients and in others with spinal deformities, the severe scoliosis often causes one of the kidneys to lie close to the spine and lower costovertebral areas. These kidneys are difficult to find. The patients often know that one of the kidneys is in a difficult position to scan from previous examinations. A study of previous ultrasound images often reveals the best approach. Although in most cases, diagnostic images eventually are obtained, in a few, an IVU is necessary.

Perinephric Collections

Collections of fluid in the perinephric space may consist of blood or urine, resulting from trauma, renal biopsy, antegrade procedure, or pus in a perinephric abscess. Although a pure urinoma is anechoic, when caused by trauma, it often is mixed with blood and is of medium echodensity. Apart from the history, little on the ultrasound image definitely characterizes perinephric fluid collections. Abscesses usually are associated with a pyonephrosis or other signs of pyelonephritis (Fig. 68). Diagnostic aspiration is the usual method of distinguishing the nature of a collection.

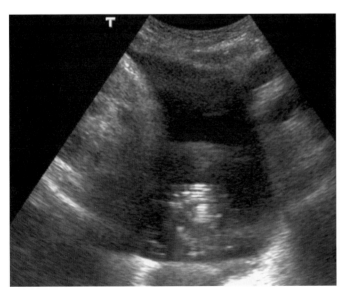

FIGURE 68 ■ Perinephric abscess. There is a collection around the lower pole of the kidney with a drain in situ, shown as multiple parallel lines.

Perinephric fat occasionally may be hypoechoic and may simulate a collection. The appearances in these cases are similar on both sides. In some cases of acute renal failure, particularly if there is hypoproteinemia, there may be an echo-poor rim of fluid around the kidney. This has been called renal sweat (Fig. 57b) (180,181).

The Ureters: General Considerations

Ultrasound has a small but increasing role in imaging the ureters. Contrast studies are more appropriate in most cases. Nevertheless, ultrasound often is the first imaging modality to be used as part of an ultrasound renal study.

Suspected Ureteric Obstruction: The Dilated Ureter

If a dilated calyceal system is seen, the ureter should be carefully studied (Table 34). The mid-ureters, unless dilated, usually are not visible on ultrasound. The upper and lower ureters, however, are well seen (182–184). Thus, a normal upper ureter with calyceal dilation suggests a pelviureteric junction obstruction; a dilated upper but normal lower ureter suggests mid-ureteric obstruction; and a dilated lower ureter suggests vesicoureteric junction or trigonal or bladder outlet obstruction.

Most causes of ureteric obstruction have been discussed in the section entitled Hydronephrosis. Obstruction is the most common cause of ureteric dilatation, but there are other causes. When obstruction is relieved, a dilated ureter may never return to a normal caliber. Vesicoureteric reflux may cause ureteric dilation, although not all refluxing ureters are dilated. The pattern of dilation is indistinguishable from obstruction. The reflux may be caused by a congenital anomaly of the intramural portion of the ureter, with lack of longitudinal muscle fibers and decreased obliquity of its course through the bladder wall, or secondary reflux from bladder outlet obstruction or a high-pressure neurogenic bladder.

Congenital megaureter is a unilateral or bilateral condition caused by the absence of peristalsis in the lower ureter. The ureter becomes grossly dilated and tortuous, often giving the spurious ultrasonic appearance of multiple cystic areas (Fig. 69), as the tortuous loops pass across the ultrasonic plane. The urine dribbles from the ureteric orifice, so that the normal ureteric jet is often not seen. In early cases, there may be little or no calyceal dilation, although later, hydronephrosis may occur (185).

Calculus Obstruction

Although an obstructing calculus may be shown by ultrasound as a crescentic shadowing lesion (Fig. 70), most often, the calculus is not demonstrated by ultrasound and requires a KUB radiograph, CT, or IVU study for diagnosis.

Uroepithelial Tumor

Tumors within the ureter are not usually demonstrated ultrasonically (186), although uroepithelial tumors often are multiple and the presence of tumor in the renal pelvis or the bladder suggests the cause for obstruction (Fig. 71). Tumors at the trigone of the bladder causing obstruction

TABLE 34 ■ Causes of Ureteric Dilation

Cause	Comment
Ureteric obstruction	
Bladder outlet obstruction with reflux	
Residual dilation from relieved obstruction	
Megaureter: congenital, prune-belly (Eagle–Barrett syndrome)	
Ureteric obstruction	
Calculus	May be seen ultrasonically, but more often requires contrast studies
Uroepithelial tumor	Tumor usually is not seen, but coexisting tumors may be seen in the renal pelvis and bladder
Intraureteric endometriosis	Obstructing endometriosis is not often seen ultrasonically
Retroperitoneal fibrosis	Characteristic findings on ultrasound, but CT and MRI are better at delineating the extent
Pelvic and lower abdominal tumors	The tumor may be seen on abdominal ultrasound; secondary image procedures may be necessary to complete the diagnosis
Appendicitis (especially retrocecal)	Characteristic ultrasonic features may be seen
Postsurgery ligation	Rarely seen

Abbreviations: CT, computed tomography; MRI, magnetic resonance imaging.

of the ureteric orifices usually are well demonstrated (186–191).

Other Intraureteric Pathologic Conditions

Tuberculosis, schizosomiasis, and intraureteric endometriosis all cause ureteric obstruction. The ureteric lesions cannot be seen ultrasonically, but associated features may be seen. Endometriosis may cause ureteric obstruction and hematuria caused by the rare entity of intravesical endometrioma. Endometriosis is invariably present elsewhere in the pelvis, which may be demonstrated ultrasonically. Even if it is shown, intraureteric endometriosis is so rare and pelvic endometriosis so common that a coincidental cause for hematuria is likely. Diagnosis is made by ureteroscopy. The bladder is involved more often than the ureter, and this may accompany ureteric involvement (192,193).

Extraureteric Causes

Retroperineal fibrosis classically causes ureteric obstruction, with only late dilation of the proximal ureter and pelvicalyceal system. Renal failure may occur when there is only mild or even no dilation. The causes and appearances of retroperitoneal fibrosis are discussed elsewhere in this text.

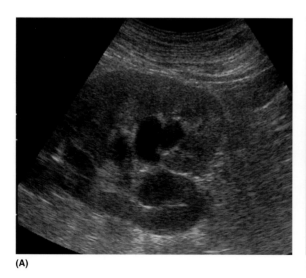

(A)

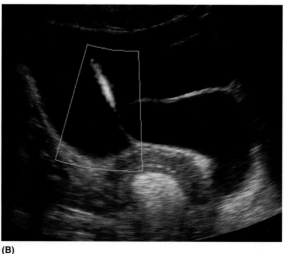

(B)

FIGURE 69 A AND B ■ Megaureter. The ureter is very wide and tortuous. (**A**) The upper end; (**B**) the lower end with, in this case, a strong ureteric jet shown on color Doppler. (The jet is often weak.)

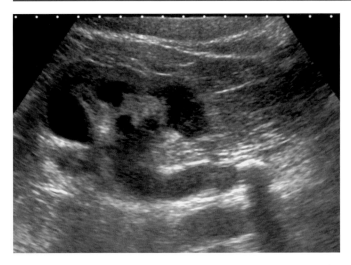

FIGURE 70 ▪ Midureteric calculus. The ureter is dilated down to the shadowing calculus.

Appendicitis, particularly if the appendix is retrocecal, may cause functional obstruction, resulting in dilation of the ureter and pelvicalyceal system. This entity may be confused with ureteric colic. The ultrasound appearances of appendicitis are well described and should be sought in such cases (194–196).

Pelvic and retroperitoneal tumors may cause ureteric obstruction by involving the ureters. Here, the lumen usually is not occluded, but the ureteric walls are involved, causing functional obstruction, and the lumen may be compressed. In the male patient, invasive prostatic cancer, and in the female patient, invasive cervical cancer are the most common causes, although any pelvic or lower abdominal tumor may obstruct the ureters. Retroperitoneal tumors act in a similar manner to retroperitoneal fibrosis, and retroperitoneal fibrosis itself may result as a desmoplastic reaction to other tumors.

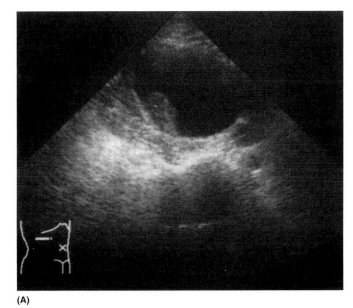

(A)

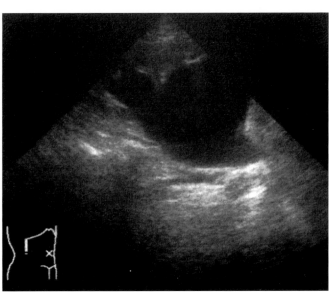

(B)

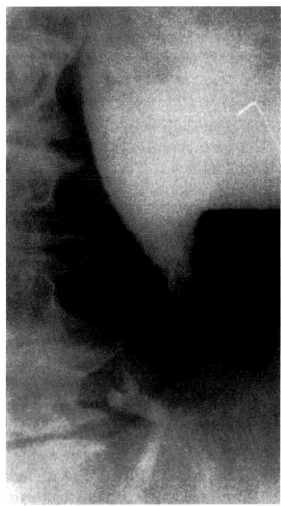

(C)

FIGURE 71 A–C ▪ Uroepithelial tumors. Tumor is shown in the dilated renal pelvis (**A**) and at the pelviureteric junction (**B**). (**C**) The findings were confirmed by an antegrade pyelogram. *Source*: From Ref. 43.

The Vesicoureteric Junction: General Considerations

The vesicoureteric junction comprises the intramural portion of the ureters and the ureteric orifices.

Protrusions of the Ureter into the Bladder

Ureterocele ▪ A ureterocele is a balloon-like dilation of the intramural portion of the ureter that usually bulges into the bladder. The ureterocele itself is thin walled, sometimes with only a mucosal layer, and sometimes with a mucosal layer and a thin muscularis layer. The ureteric orifice, which is narrowed, usually opens at the tip, although occasionally, it opens at the base; sometimes a portion of the ureter extends distal to the ureterocele to open in an ectopic position in the bladder or urethra (197,198).

Ureteroceles may be orthoptic, that is, occurring in a normally situated and otherwise normal ureter, in which case they are usually asymptomatic and are found incidentally for other reasons. Alternatively, they may be ectopic, occurring on duplex ureters, in which case they are often ectopic in location, opening distal in the urinary tract to the normal position, often distal to the proximal sphincter. Ectopic ureteroceles opening outside of the bladder are not normally visible ultrasonically.

Ureteroceles in duplex systems often occur on the ureter, draining the upper pole moiety, and are often imperforate, so that the upper moiety is an atrophic hydronephrotic sac with little or no cortex or function (Fig. 72). Other renal anomalies such as crossed renal ectopia often coexist.

Ureteroceles opening into the bladder appear as thin-walled sac-like structures that often fluctuate in size with ureteric peristalsis (Fig. 72). Some variations in normal appearances are important to recognize. In children, large ureteroceles may completely fill the bladder and cause outlet obstruction. These may be difficult to diagnose ultrasonically. In a full bladder, varicoceles may occasionally invert, in which case, they give an appearance similar to diverticula (Fig. 73). If in doubt, partial emptying of the bladder allows the uretcrocele to revert to its more usual appearance.

Pouting Ureters ▪ Ureters may pout slightly into the bladder as a normal variant. The protuberances, unlike ureteroceles, have a normal wall thickness.

Ureteric Nipples ▪ One method of surgical reimplantation of the ureters results in the ends of the ureters projecting into the bladder like nipples. Their appearance is similar to pouting ureters.

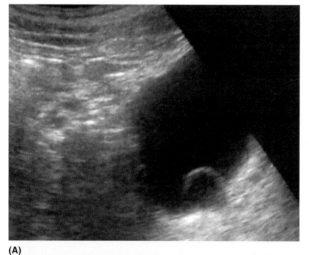

(A)

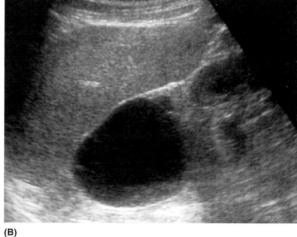

(B)

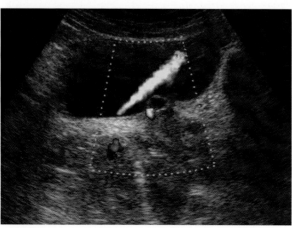

(C)

FIGURE 72 A–C ▪ Ureterocele. (**A**) A typical balloon-like dilatation is seen projecting into the bladder. (**B**) In this case, the ureterocele is in a duplex ureter and there is a hydronephrotic upper pole moiety. (**C**) In this case, the ureteric orifice is at the base of the ureterocele as shown by the position of the ureteric jet, which is weak. Compare the jet on the right, which is normal.

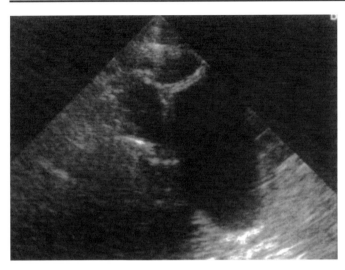

FIGURE 73 ■ Inverted ureterocele. An inverted ureterocele is shown on the left in this full bladder. On partial emptying, it gave the more usual appearance of bulging into the bladder. *Source*: From Ref. 43.

Narrowing of the Vesicoureteric Junction

Schizosomiasis ■ Although rare in the Western world, schizosomiasis is the most common cause of renal failure worldwide. Strictures of the lower ends of the ureters are common. The ultrasonic appearances are identical to other causes of stricture, with dilation of the proximal ureter and calyceal systems. Strictures of the mid-ureter also are common (Makar's stricture). The only differentiating features in these cases, apart from the history of residence in an endemic area, is the coexisting thickening of the bladder wall, often with polypoid projections into the bladder (Fig. 74) (199–200).

Tuberculosis ■ Tuberculosis causes lower ureteric strictures. Coexisting features in these cases are an evenly

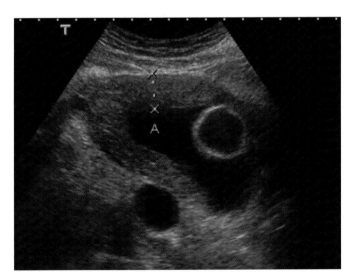

FIGURE 74 ■ Schizosomiasis. The typical bladder wall thickening is shown in this patient who presented with renal failure and bilateral hydronephrosis caused by ureteric strictures. The bladder is catheterized and there is a posterior diverticulum.

thickened bladder wall with a small-volume bladder and, in the kidney, isolated calyceal dilation caused by infundibular narrowing. Renal calcifications may occur later in the disease process (201).

Prostate Cancer ■ Invasive prostate cancer may invade the lower ends of the ureters, causing strictures. The prostatic invasion often is not obvious on transabdominal scans. It is demonstrated on transrectal ultrasound scanning, but better with MRI.

Previous Calculus ■ A ureteric calculus that has passed may cause ureteric narrowing because of edema for a short period and, less often, permanent narrowing from scarring. There are no distinguishing ultrasonic features.

Alteration in the Ureteric Jets

The normal ureteric jet appears as a long jet directed from the ureteric orifice toward the center of the bladder at about 45° (Fig. 5). Spectral Doppler normally shows a biphasic or triphasic pattern. A weak or absent jet suggests obstruction, though correlation is poor. A shallow angle or a monophasic spectral pattern is found in vesicoureteric reflux. An abnormally positioned jet may demonstrate an ectopic ureteric insertion (Figs. 5 and 72) (19–21).

Bladder Wall Thickening

Diffuse Bladder Wall Thickening

Bladder Outlet Obstruction and Neurogenic Bladder ■ Diffuse thickening occurs from muscle hypertrophy in a high-pressure neurogenic bladder and in chronic outflow obstruction (Table 35). The muscle bundles give an irregular outline to the inner bladder wall (trabeculation). Gross trabeculation and an abnormal bladder shape in neurogenic bladders may give the typical "Christmas tree" shape seen on the IVU (Fig. 75) (11,12,202,203).

Cystitis ■ Cystitis gives an edematous, often smooth thickening of the bladder wall, although there may be small excrescences from the bladder wall in early cases that are indistinguishable from bladder tumor, and, in prolonged cases, areas of focal bladder wall thickening (204). In most early or mild cases, however, the bladder appears normal. In tuberculous cystitis, there is marked bladder wall thickening, and the bladder has a small volume. This may only be appreciated when the patient volunteers that the bladder feels full when ultrasonically it appears almost empty (Fig. 76). There may be lower or mid-ureteric strictures and isolated calyceal dilation, as well as renal calcification.

Cyclophosphamide cystitis has no distinguishing features, but the history of cyclophosphamide therapy should be available.

Focal Bladder Wall Thickening

Primary Bladder Tumor ■ The most common cause of focal bladder wall thickening is primary bladder tumor (Table 36). Most bladder tumors in adults are transitional

TABLE 35 ■ Causes of Diffuse Bladder Wall Thickening

Cause	Comment
Neurogenic bladder	Trabeculated bladder; may be typical "Christmas tree" shape
Chronic outflow obstruction	Trabeculated bladder
Cystitis	Smooth thick wall or small excrescences in severe cases
Tuberculous cystitis	Small volume bladder; there may be lower ureteric strictures and renal changes
Cyclophosphamide cystitis	No differentiating features except history
Schizosomiasis	May be polypoidal extension into the bladder. There may be malignant change. There may be lower or mid-ureteric strictures. In early cases, the trigone is affected first

cell carcinomas (95%), although other malignant and benign tumors do occur. Bladder tumors may have varying ultrasonic appearances. Tumors often project into the bladder in a frond-like pattern whereas others are polypoidal or broad based. Massive tumors may obliterate the bladder (Fig. 77). Surface encrustations on large tumors often cast ultrasonic shadows. In general, a broad base suggests malignancy (205), although distinction of benign from malignant tumors with certainty may only be possible by cystoscopy and biopsy. Tumors near the bladder base in the male patient may be confused with prostatic masses, and prostatic enlargement and bladder tumors often coexist. Bladder tumors may also invade the prostate. In cases of doubt, MRI may be helpful. Cystoscopy and biopsy and/or transrectal ultrasound of the prostate and biopsy are usually indicated.

Cystoscopy remains the gold standard in the detection of bladder tumors. Ultrasound has been reported as having sensitivities varying from 64% to 92%, but most studies report a sensitivity between 50% and 90% (206–208). Most series were published some time ago, and it is possible that present-generation equipment may produce better results. Ultrasound is widely used in patients with schizosomiasis to detect malignant change, but apart from in this group, it has not widely replaced cystoscopy for the detection of bladder tumors. The ultrasonic appearance of bladder tumors are nevertheless important to appreciate.

Ultrasound is poor at staging bladder tumors. Some indication of the degree of spread through the wall may be obtained, but accurate staging requires CT or preferably MRI (208).

In children, rhabdomyosarcomas are the most common bladder tumors. They usually cause an irregular mass at the bladder base (Fig. 78) (209).

Other conditions such as focal cystitis or a blood clot may simulate tumors.

Follow-up examination of bladder tumors normally is carried out by flexible cystoscopy. There is, however, a case for using ultrasound instead of cystoscopy in some follow-up studies (210).

Schizosomiasis ■ Schizosomiasis may cause focal and diffuse bladder wall thickening, depending on the stage

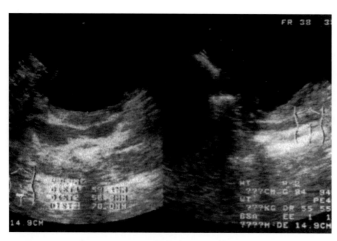

FIGURE 75 ■ Neurogenic bladder. A thick-walled bladder with a "waisted" appearance in the transverse section is shown. Multiple such waists give the "Christmas tree" appearance.

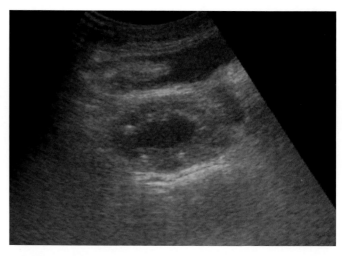

FIGURE 76 ■ Tuberculosis. The bladder is thick walled and of small volume. The patient felt that the bladder was full at the time of this scan. There is some calcification in the wall.

TABLE 36 ■ Focal Bladder Wall Thickening

Cause	Comment
Transitional cell carcinoma	Variable shape. There may be calcific encrustation on the surface
Schizosomiasis	Generalized in late cases, but often there is focal thickening. There may be malignant change. Thickening starts at the trigone
Invasion by adjacent tumor or inflammatory disease	Can be seen to be continuous with the primary disease process
Leiomyoma	
Indwelling catheter	May cause focal thickening where the catheter contacts the bladder wall
Cyclophosphamide	May cause localized wall thickening that simulates bladder cancer

of the disease (Fig. 74). The first part of the bladder to be affected usually is the trigone, and lower ureteric strictures tend to occur early. Later in the disease, diffuse bladder wall thickening occurs and, later yet, focal areas thicken even more and bulge into the bladder. They have a smooth surface. Any irregularity of the surface suggests malignant change (199,200).

Invasion by Adjacent Tumors and Disease ■ The most common invading tumors are prostatic cancer in the male

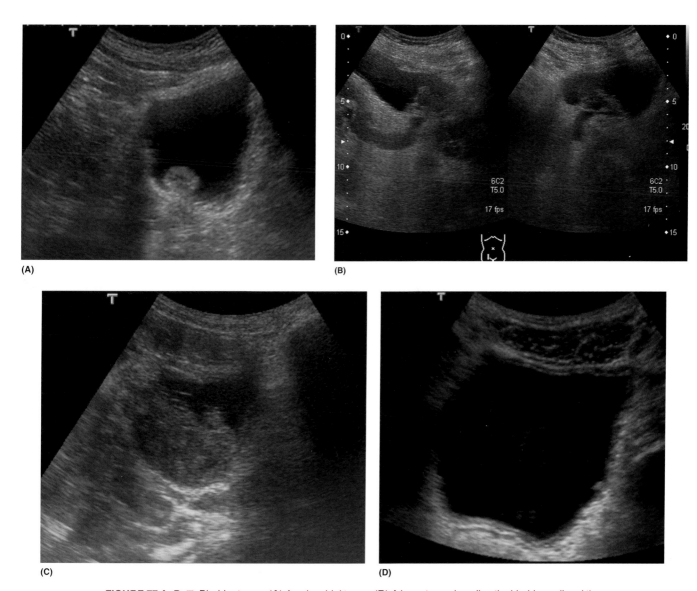

(A)

(B)

(C)

(D)

FIGURE 77 A–D ■ Bladder tumor. (**A**) A polypoidal tumor. (**B**) A large tumor invading the bladder wall and the ureteric orifice. The dilated obstructed ureter is seen. (**C**) A massive tumor almost filling the bladder. (**D**) A small papilloma. This demonstrates that good ultrasound equipment may now find very small tumors.

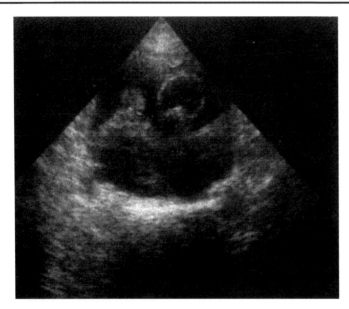

FIGURE 78 ■ Rhabdomyosarcoma. A large tumor is seen at the bladder base of this 12-year-old boy.

patient and uterine cancer in the female patient; however, any pelvic malignancy, particularly of the cervix, uterus, prostate, and rectum, may invade the bladder. Continuity of the abnormal area of the bladder with the mass of the primary tumor may be seen in the early stages, but advanced disease tends to invade the whole pelvis (frozen pelvis), in which case it is impossible to tell where the tumor originates.

Benign conditions may affect the bladder. Loops of inflamed Crohn's bowel may adhere to the bladder wall (Fig. 79), and the inflammation causes thickening of that part of the bladder wall, often progressing to fistula formation (211). Endometriosis also occasionally affects the bladder, either primarily or by involvement in local pelvic disease. The diagnosis is suggested by a history of

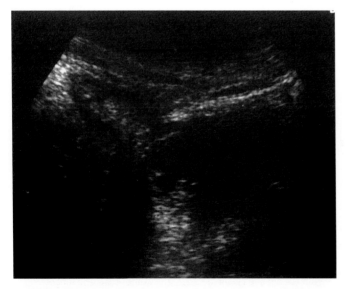

FIGURE 79 ■ Crohn's disease involving the bladder. An inflamed loop of Crohn's bowel is adherent to the bladder, which is locally edematous.

hematuria occurring during the menstrual periods, and by ultrasonic and other evidence of the primary disease (192,193).

Leiomyoma ■ Leiomyomas represent only 0.1% to 0.5% of bladder tumors. Ultrasonically, they are smooth masses of medium echodensity lying within the bladder wall. If the ultrasonic resolution is sufficient, an intact mucosa may be demonstrated over the tumor.

Indwelling Catheter: Catheter Cystitis ■ Localized thickening of the bladder wall may occur where a catheter balloon contacts the bladder wall. This is a nonspecific inflammatory response. It occurs less commonly with modern catheters than with the old rubber variety (212).

Cyclophosphamide ■ The breakdown products of cyclophosphamide produce a cystitis that may cause generalized bladder wall thickening, but sometimes a localized irregular thickening that may simulate a tumor. The history of cyclophosphamide therapy suggests the diagnosis.

Filling Defects and Lesions within the Bladder

Calculi
Bladder calculi, like calculi elsewhere, give a crescentic image and sharp shadowing, and they move when the patient is turned (Table 37). These features, particularly the movement, differentiates calculi from calcification on the surface of bladder tumors (213,214).

Foley Catheter
The balloon of a Foley catheter has a characteristic shape and its nature should be obvious, although confusion does occur. An artifact caused by beam splitting by the rectus abdominis muscle may produce a double image. Visualization of a Foley catheter may be important if it is not draining, to exclude misplacement, usually in the urethra (215), and for guidance of percutaneous balloon puncture in the occasional situation where the balloon does not deflate for the removal of the catheter.

Blood Clot
Blood clots may lie free within the bladder but more often adhere to the bladder wall or an indwelling catheter. They are of medium, slightly speckled echodensity and do not cast shadows. They may be indistinguishable from bladder tumors and often are associated with an underlying bladder tumor, in which case the tumor may merge with the clot. The diagnosis is suggested if there is a history of hematuria and is confirmed as the lesion disappears or changes either spontaneously or with bladder washouts.

Enlarged Median Lobe of Prostate
In some planes, an enlarged prostatic median lobe may appear to lie free within the bladder. On angling the plane caudad, however, it may be seen to be part of the prostate

TABLE 37 ■ Filling Defects Within the Bladder

Cause	Comment
Calculi	Typical crescentic surface with distal shadowing. Moves when the patient is turned
Foley catheter	Should be obvious but occasionally causes confusion
Blood clot	May be mobile but often is adherent to the bladder wall or catheter. Changes or disappears spontaneously or with bladder washouts
Enlarged median lobe prostate	Not really within the bladder but may appear so in some planes
Transitional cell tumor	May project in a polypoidal or frond-like manner into the bladder
Fungus balls	Rare. Occur in diabetics or immunocompromised patients

gland. The median lobe may be smooth but can be irregular and simulate a bladder tumor.

Transitional Cell Tumor

While arising from the bladder wall, tumors may project into the bladder lumen and in some planes appear to lie free.

Fungus Balls

Fungus balls are rare entities occurring in diabetics or immunocompromised patients. More usually seen in the renal pelvis, they may occur in the bladder lumen and appear as medium-echodensity, nonshadowing, rounded mobile defects (Fig. 80) (216).

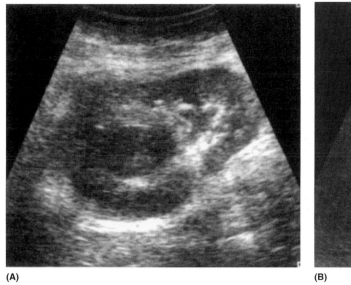

(A)

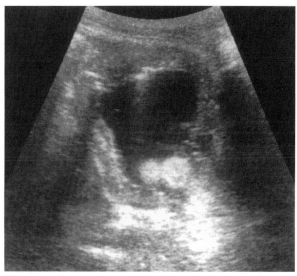

(B)

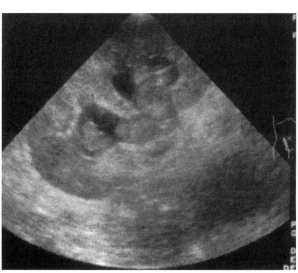

(C)

FIGURE 80 A–C ■ Fungal infection. (**A**) In this case of *Candida* infection, a medium echodensity mass is seen in the upper pole calyx and an upper pole uroepithelium is edematous. (**B**) Typical fungal balls are seen in the bladder. (**C**) Another case with fungal balls in the renal collecting system.

TABLE 38 ■ Cystic Areas Associated with the Bladder Wall

Cause	Comment
Ureterocele	Usually at the trigone but may be ectopic. They vary in size with ureteric peristalsis
Diverticulum	Thin-walled bulging out of the bladder. They vary in size with micturition and bladder filling
Patent urachus	Cyst between bladder and umbilicus
Müllerian duct cyst	These have no communication with the bladder

Cystic Lesions Associated with the Bladder Wall

Ureteroceles

Ureteroceles are discussed in the section entitled The Ureters (Table 38).

Diverticula

Diverticula are outpouchings of the bladder mucosa through defects in the muscle layers (Fig. 81) (Table 38). They are occasionally congenital. Congenital diverticula (Hutch diverticula) lie in a paraureteral position and are

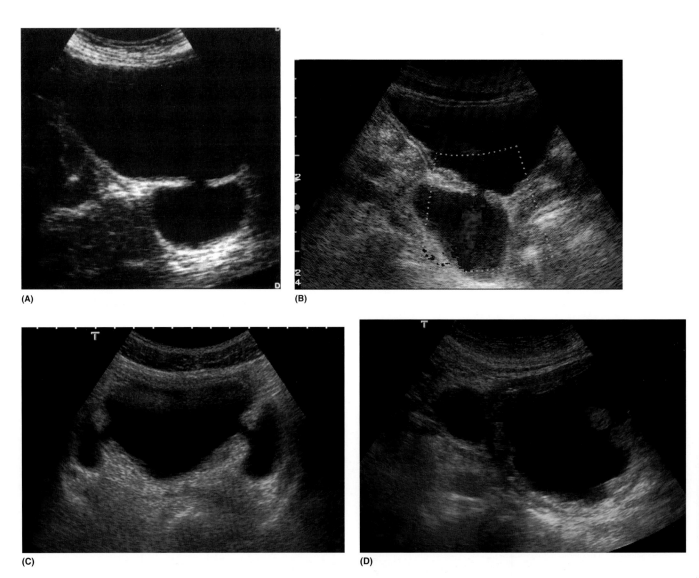

(A)   (B)

(C)   (D)

FIGURE 81 A–D ■ Bladder diverticulum. (**A**) Typical appearances. The neck of the diverticulum is clearly shown. (**B**) A color Doppler scan after a short application of pressure on the bladder by the transducer. The resulting jet may identify a narrow neck not otherwise visible and thus confirm the diagnosis. (**C**) An example of congenital (Hutch) diverticula. In this case, outlet obstruction has caused them to enlarge. (**D**) An urachal cyst.

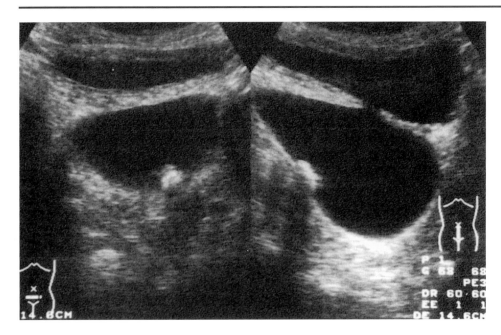

FIGURE 82 ▓ Calculus in a diverticulum.

usually bilateral (Fig. 81). The majority are acquired and are usually associated with weakening of the muscle layers from long-standing outlet obstruction. They may be distinguished from cysts by the demonstration in the appropriate plane of the neck connecting them to the bladder (217). In cases of doubt, the use of color Doppler while pressing sharply on the bladder with the transducer often causes a visible jet of urine through the neck (Fig. 81B). They are most common near the ureteric orifices but may occur anywhere. They vary in size with the degree of bladder filling. Occasionally, diverticula may contain filling defects that may be calculi, hematomas, or tumors (Figs. 82 and 83).

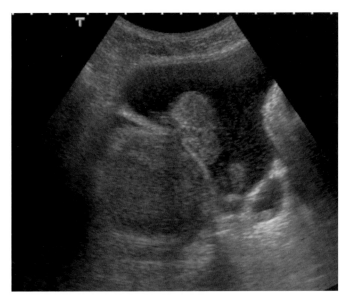

FIGURE 83 ▓ Tumor in a diverticulum. The lesion shown is tumor surrounded by blood clot. The tumor nearly fills the diverticulum and blood clot extends through the neck into the bladder.

Patent Urachus

The urachus is a cord-like embryonic remnant that connects the bladder apex with the umbilicus. Parts of this structure may remain patent, producing cyst-like structures in a line between the bladder and the umbilicus (Fig. 81D). Malignant change may occur, resulting in a complex solid mass (Table 38) (39–42).

Müllerian Duct Cyst

Müllerian duct cysts occur in male patients and often lie adjacent to the bladder. They are frequently misdiagnosed as bladder diverticula, but there is no connection with the bladder and they do not empty with micturition. An IVU shows contrast within a diverticulum but not in a cyst (Fig. 84) (Table 38). Their intraprostatic position and their nature are clearly demonstrated by transrectal ultrasound or pelvic MRI, which demonstrates the neck arising from the verumontanum.

Altered Echodensity of the Urine

Normal urine within the bladder is not truly anechoic but is of low echodensity. Generalized increase in echodensity, often with a swirling pattern, is found in chronic outlet obstruction when the bladder never empties completely. It is caused by cellular debris and possibly crystals. A similar appearance also is found in pyuria and hematuria, although in these cases, the diagnostic sign is layering within the bladder, sometimes with a double fluid–fluid level (Fig. 85). Such appearances should not be confused with reverberation artifact within the bladder, which changes as gain settings change. When a patient is turned, a fluid–fluid level is disturbed and then settles into a new position. Hematuria also may be associated with blood clots and tumor.

Incomplete Bladder Emptying: Bladder Dysfunction

Bladder dysfunction may occur as a result of prostatic enlargement, neurogenic causes, or pelvic floor weakness in the female patient. In addition, children may not empty their bladder completely for no obvious pathologic reasons, and this may be associated with urinary tract infections. As part of the workup of these patients and followup of long-standing cases, the degree of bladder distension, the presence of hydronephrosis, and the ability of the bladder to empty are important considerations (218). Ultrasound is ideally suited to these studies. The patient attends with as full a bladder as possible. The kidneys and bladder are scanned. The patient then empties the bladder, either by normal micturition or, in neurogenic cases, by whatever method the patient normally uses (i.e., self-catheterization, manual expression, incontinence device), and the examination is repeated. The residual bladder volume is estimated by measuring maximal anteroposterior, coronal, and craniocaudal measurements and multiplying by $\pi/6$ (0.52) (Fig. 86). This measurement assumes that the bladder is an ellipsoid. This is not strictly true, and other formulas have been suggested as being more accurate (218–224). In practice, however, extreme accuracy is not necessary, an approximation of bladder volume being adequate for treatment planning. A urine flow rate assessment often is combined with residual volume estimation, and sometimes a full urodynamic study may be preferable. Estimation of residual volume in the surgically augmented bladder is difficult because of the irregular bladder shape. In practice, resolving the bladder shape to the best fit into one, two, or more ovoids and using the same formula is sufficient.

The Augmented Bladder and Incontinence Devices

Bladder augmentation is an operation devised to increase the bladder volume in small- or high-pressure neurogenic bladders. Various techniques involve the use of various loops of bowel. Ultrasonically, they all appear as an irregularly shaped bladder, and often it is not possible from the ultrasound study results to distinguish the different techniques. The bowel mucosal pattern may be identified and peristalsis may be seen. Mucus strands produced by the bowel loop may project into the bladder lumen. The usual reason for examining the augmented bladder ultrasonically is to assess bladder emptying. It is difficult to estimate the bladder volume accurately because of the

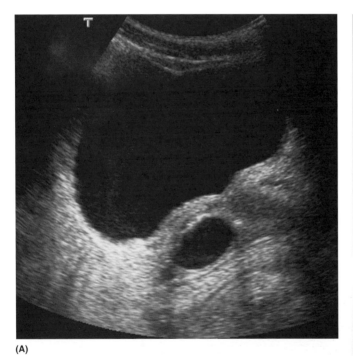

(A)

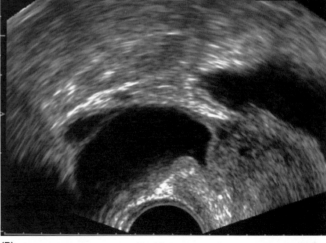

(B)

(C)

FIGURE 84 A–C ■ Müllerian duct cyst. (**A**) A cyst is seen posterior to the bladder, with no communication with the bladder. (**B** and **C**) The transrectal study shows a typical Müllerian duct cyst with its neck at the verumontanum.

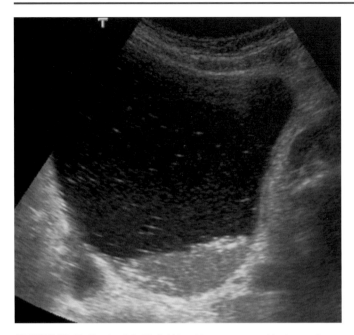

FIGURE 85 ■ Pyuria. A fluid–fluid level is seen caused by layered pus.

irregular shape, but in practice, the method of resolving the shape into the best fit into one or more ovoids is sufficiently accurate.

Incontinence devices consist of a cuff around the vesicourethral junction connected to a reservoir in the pelvis and an activating bulb in the scrotum, labium, or other convenient position. Bladder emptying is assessed in the usual way. The cuff is not easily seen on transabdominal scans but is seen transrectally and transperineally. The reservoir may be seen as a round fluid-filled structure in the pelvis, and in the male patient, the scrotal bulb can be seen as a dense shadowing structure. The importance of this is to recognize these structures for what they are when seen incidentally.

The Urethra: General Considerations

Contrast urethrography is the standard method of studying the urethra. Ultrasound and sonourethrography are viable alternatives in some patients. Filling defects within the urethra are well shown, and in cases of stricture, the tissues around the stricture are demonstrated. These are not shown on a contrast urethrogram. In general, fistulas and false passages are better shown by contrast urethrography. Using sonourethrography images comparable with contrast urethrography can be obtained for the whole of the male urethra.

In micturition disorders, radiographic micturating cystography often combined with urodynamics is the gold standard. Ultrasound is used by some as an alternative.

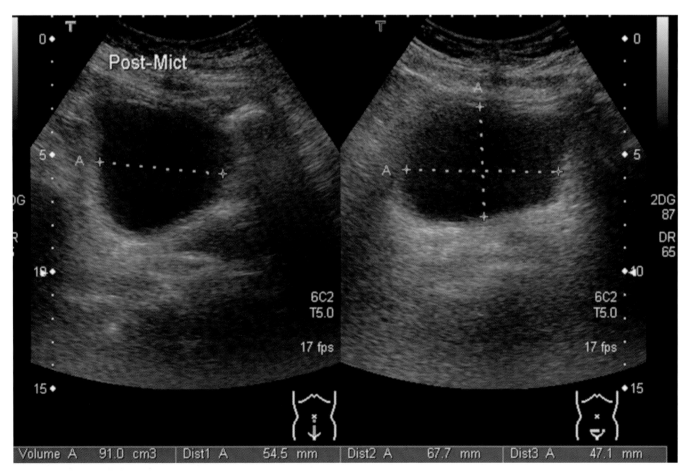

FIGURE 86 ■ Residual bladder volume measurement.

TABLE 39 ■ Cystic Structures Adjacent to the Urethra

Cause	Comment
Urethral diverticulum	Communication with the urethra establishes the diagnosis
Gartner's duct cyst Vaginal inclusion cyst	No communication with the urethra
Ectopic ureterocele	Rarely seen ultrasonically; usually drains a dysplastic obstructed upper pole duplex moiety

The movement of the female urethra during voiding can be shown as described earlier in the chapter.

Cystic Lesions Associated with the Urethra

With cystic lesions associated with the urethra, the only truly urethral abnormalities are urethral diverticula (Table 39). The diagnosis is established by demonstrating, in the appropriate scan plane, the communication with the urethra. If doubt exists, MRI is often a definitive test. If not, a contrast study is indicated (225–227). Gartner's duct cysts and vaginal inclusion cysts do not communicate with the urethra. Ectopic ureteroceles are shown only rarely but when seen have a similar appearance to those seen in the bladder.

Urethral Strictures

Urethral strictures have appearances on sonourethrography that are analogous to the contrast urethrogram image (Fig. 87) (15,228–234).

Prostatic Nodules

Central lobe prostatic hyperplasia compresses the urethra. It is described in Chapter 33. Notice that a small centrally placed nodule may cause severe voiding difficulties without significant change in the rest of the prostate.

Lesions within the Urethra

Urethral Warts

Urethral warts are well demonstrated on sonourethrography as filling defects attached to the wall (Fig. 88).

Urethral Calculi

As elsewhere, urethral calculi have a crescentic shape and distal shadowing. Most are radiopaque (Fig. 89) (235).

Foreign Bodies

Foreign bodies are equally well demonstrated as urethral calculi.

Renal Doppler Studies: General Considerations

With the exception of the investigation of suspected renal artery stenosis, renal Doppler studies are carried out as an adjunct to the gray-scale study. Although there are many subtleties in the interpretation of a Doppler study result, the Doppler spectrum changes in only a few basic ways. Each of these is discussed, but first, the investigation of suspected renal artery stenosis is considered.

Suspected Renal Artery Stenosis

Renal vascular hypertension caused by a hemodynamically significant renal artery stenosis is one of the less common causes of hypertension. It is, however, important to detect it since it is potentially curable by angioplasty or surgery and is a direct contraindication to the use of angiotensin-converting enzyme inhibitors. Also, a number of cases of renovascular hypertension are not diagnosed and progress to renal failure. The traditional simple screening test is the measurement of renal size (8).

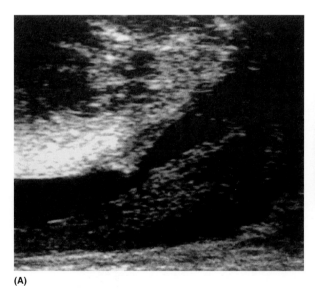

(A)

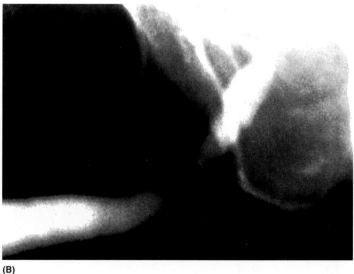

(B)

FIGURE 87 A AND B ■ Urethral stricture. (**A**) A tight bulbar stricture is seen; the corresponding contrast study is shown (**B**). *Source*: From Ref. 43. Courtesy of Drs. Philip Bearcroft and Laurence Berman, Addenbrooks Hospital, Cambridge, U.K.

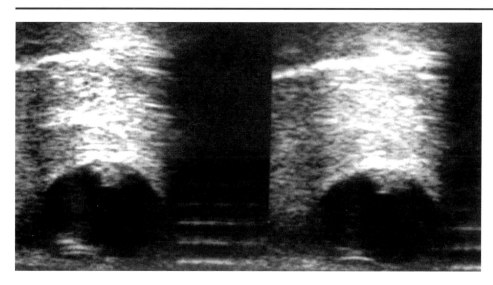

FIGURE 88 ■ Urethral wart. Transverse scan. *Source*: From Ref. 43. Courtesy of Drs. Philip Bearcroft and Laurence Berman, Addenbrooks Hospital, Cambridge, U.K.

The ischemic kidney becomes small, and this is easily assessed ultrasonically. If the right kidney is more than 2 cm smaller than the left, or the left more than 1.5 cm smaller than the right, then there is a high probability of renal artery stenosis. This test, however, has neither a high sensitivity nor specificity. The low specificity is no real problem since all patients believed to have renal artery stenosis on Doppler studies are confirmed or excluded by CT, MR, or contrast angiography. The low sensitivity is, however, problematic. Because of this, more sensitive tests have been sought.

Contrast angiography is the gold standard in the detection of renal artery stenosis. Unfortunately, despite the use of small diameter catheters, it is still invasive and expensive so that it is not suitable as a screening test. Magnetic resonance angiography is noninvasive albeit expensive. It is probably too insensitive to be used as a screening test. Contrasted CT also is a good test but involves a large dose of contrast and a high radiation dose.

Doppler sonography is noninvasive and relatively inexpensive. It is not surprising, therefore, that despite its limitations, it has been extensively investigated as a screening test for renal artery stenosis (236–240).

The following are the three Doppler hallmarks of a renal artery stenosis (Table 40).

- ■ *High systolic peak velocities at the site of the stenosis.* Velocities of more than 3.5 times the aortic peak systolic velocity or more than 2 m/sec are significant. The ratio is preferable since hypertension itself causes increased velocities.
- ■ *Flow disturbance.* Often loosely termed turbulence, flow disturbance is seen for up to 1 cm distal to the stenosis and causes an irregular "spikey" maximum velocity envelope, with irregular powers at different

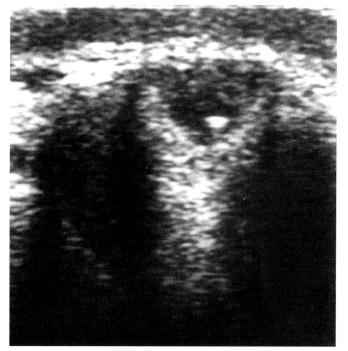

FIGURE 89 ■ Urethral calculus.

TABLE 40 ■ Doppler Criteria of Renal Artery Stenosis

At the stenosis peak systolic velocity	>2 m/sec
Systolic velocity ratio	>3.5 × velocity in the artery proximal to the stenosis, opposite renal artery, aorta, or femoral artery
1 cm distal to the stenosis flow disturbance (turbulence)	
Further distal: damping (tardus parvus)	
Systolic rise time	>100 m/sec
Systolic acceleration	>20 m/sec^2
Resistance index	<0.5
Appearance	Flattened rounded systolic peak

velocities, causing irregularity of the gray scale of the whole waveform and often spikes of reversed flow.

■ *Tardus parvus effect*. Finally, in most cases of hemodynamically significant stenosis, there is dampening of the distal waveform known as the tardus parvus effect. This consists of a lengthened systolic rise time or slow systolic acceleration (tardus) and lowering and rounding of the systolic peak (parvus). The tardus component is measured by assessing the slope of the early systolic curve from the start of the curve to the first systolic peak. This may be expressed as a systolic rise time or systolic acceleration. The parvus component is measured by comparing the height of the systolic peak with end diastole. This is expressed as the RI or a similar ratio (Fig. 90) (Table 40). The stenosis itself may be seen on the color Doppler image where the increased velocity and turbulence are seen as changes in the color pattern. Although this is useful

to rapidly identify the site of a stenosis, the spectral pattern must always be used for confirmation since the color image is notorious for the production of misleading artifacts.

The use of Doppler to screen for renal artery stenosis has problems. The main problem is that it is difficult to visualize the whole of both renal arteries. There are several reasons for this. The kidneys move extensively during respiration, and there is a limit as to how long patients can hold their breath. On color imaging respiratory, transmitted cardiac and aortic pulsations and bowel movements all cause movement artifacts. Achieving a good angle for the Doppler image through the limited sonic window available also is a problem. Finally, between 10% and 20% of patients have multiple renal arteries. Accessory renal arteries usually are missed on Doppler studies, and stenoses of these may cause hypertension. For all of these

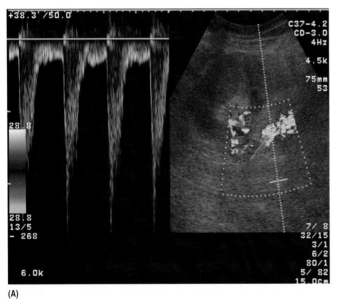

(A)

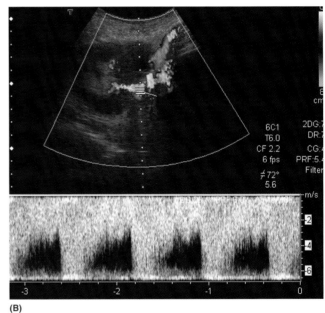

(B)

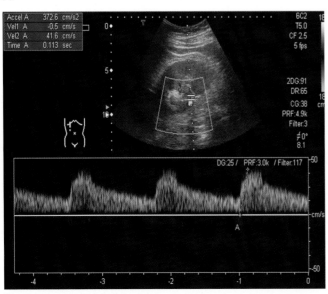

(C)

FIGURE 90 A–C ■ Renal artery stenosis. (A) The stenosis is shown, with increased velocity at the site of the stenosis. (B) Flow disturbance (turbulence) is seen just distal to the stenosis. (C) Damped (tardus parvus) flow is shown within the kidney.

TABLE 41 ■ Reduced Diastolic Flow

Cause	Comment
Acute tubular necrosis	Degree of reduction correlates approximately with the severity
Obstruction	Effect is increased by the use of IV furosemide

Abbreviation: IV, intravenous.

TABLE 42 ■ Reversed Diastolic Flow

Cause	Comment
Acute tubular necrosis	Carries a poor prognosis
Renal vein thrombosis	Sharp reversal with a reversed M pattern and a narrow systolic peak

reasons, Doppler studies of the main renal arteries are difficult (241–243). Although some workers report high success rates, most only achieve good visualization in 60% to 80% of cases. There are two exceptions, the transplanted kidney and children where Doppler studies are sensitive in the detection of renal artery stenosis (172). Some have advocated study of the renal artery origins only, but although most stenoses occur at this site, many (including the important cases of fibromuscular hyperplasia in young women) occur in a more distal part of the artery. Because of the high technical failure rate of studying the main renal arteries, an alternative approach is widely advocated. In this approach, only the renal arteries at the renal hilum or within the kidney are studied and spectral waveforms are analyzed. This technique relies on the fact that a significant stenosis causes a damped tardus parvus waveform in these vessels. This waveform is not produced in all cases of renal artery stenosis, but protagonists of the method argue that the tardus parvus waveform is caused by a pressure drop across the stenosis. Those stenoses without a significant pressure drop do not cause the change. It is argued, therefore, that only stenoses with a significant pressure drop cause renal vascular hypertension, so the test is a good screening test (244). Performing a Doppler study after administering captopril has been suggested to increase the sensitivity of the test. Unfortunately, there are other problems. Measurement of the systolic rise time or acceleration depends on the recognition of a small spike in the ascending waveform (Figs. 12 and 90). This may be difficult or impossible to recognize, making the measurement imprecise. The parvus component is measured by the RI (or some other systolic to diastolic ratio). There is a significant range of normal values in this measurement, and it is generally regarded as being less useful than the systolic rise measurements. Some workers argue that the tardus parvus waveform only occurs in a stenotic but otherwise healthy artery, and that an artery stiffened by atheroma does not produce the waveform. The arguments in both directions continue, but it is clear that these measurements are not as sensitive as previously thought and probably not sufficiently accurate to use as a screening test for renal artery stenosis.

Power Doppler produces little improvement over velocity Doppler: although it is angle independent, movement artifact is increased. Bubble contrast agents imaged with a contrast-specific scanning technique may theoretically solve the problem of motion-induced color artifact. Doppler contrast agents comprising encapsulated microbubbles of 3 to 10 μm in diameter are injected intravenously and they circulate through the vascular bed. When insonated, the bubbles resonate at the insonating frequency and also at a broad band of other frequencies. If the fundamental frequency is then eliminated from the received signal, only the blood vessels containing the bubble contrast agent are imaged. Other moving tissues are not imaged. The remaining problems include finding suitable sonic windows and renal movement, but this technique is promising. Experience at this time however suggests that although the use of contrast-enhanced scanning in difficult cases will reduce the technical failure rate, even with their use, Doppler studies are not a viable screening test.

Changes in the Renal Arterial Waveform

Reduced Diastolic Flow

Reduced diastolic flow is a manifestation of increased renovascular resistance (Table 41). This usually happens when arteriolar vasoconstriction occurs as a response to a

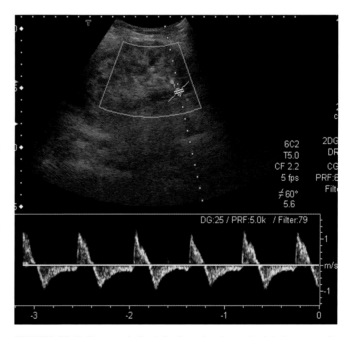

FIGURE 91 ■ Reversed diastolic flow due to acute tubular necrosis (ATN). Reversal of diastolic flow in ATN carries a poor prognosis. Notice the gradual reversal of flow in contrast to the sudden reversal found in renal vein thrombosis and shown in Figure 52.

TABLE 43 ■ Increased Diastolic Flow

Cause	Comment
Any inflammatory condition	
AV fistula	Isolated to the feeding arteries
Renal cell carcinoma	Caused by AV fistulas within the tumor; not all tumors show this change
Recovery from ATN	Hyperemic diuratic phase

Abbreviation: AV, arteriovenous.

TABLE 44 ■ Increased Systolic Velocity

Cause	Comment
Arterial stenosis	Increased at the stenosis only
Arteriovenous fistula	Increased in the feeding arteries
Renal-cell carcinoma	Found in some cases only
Hypertension	Moderate increase only

renal insult or disease or destruction of the arteriolar bed. The change is entirely nonspecific, and determining the cause requires clinical information and possibly further imaging information (18,245,246). The more common causes are discussed here.

Acute Tubular Necrosis ■ ATN causes reduced diastolic flow in severe cases. Doppler study mainly distinguishes between ATN and prerenal failure. In prerenal failure, the Doppler spectral signal is normal whereas ATN causes reduced diastolic flow, the degree of reduction having an approximate correlation with the severity of the disease.

Renal Obstruction ■ Ureteric obstruction has been shown to lead to a complex mechanism, resulting in arteriolar vasoconstriction within the kidney. This in turn leads to

reduction in diastolic velocities, which are measured as an increased RI (247). In acute obstruction, the elevation occurs three hours after the onset of obstruction, so the timing of the study is important. In chronic obstruction, some overlap occurs between obstructed and normal values. The use of furosemide has been shown to increase the RI value in pelviureteric junction obstruction and is likely to do so in any form of chronic obstruction. This would decrease the number of equivocal cases (168).

Perhaps because Doppler renal studies are difficult to perform, Doppler studies in the evaluation of obstruction have not gained universal acceptance. They are used for distinguishing calyceal dilation of pregnancy from obstruction, for distinguishing high-pressure pelviureteric junction obstruction from normal pressure cases, and in a few centers for the evaluation of acute obstruction.

Elevation of the RI to more than 0.7 is the usually accepted criterion of obstruction, although comparison of the two sides in cases of unilateral obstruction is more sensitive (a difference of 0.1 between the two sides being significant).

Other Causes ■ Several chronic renal diseases may cause reduced diastolic flow, although there are no specific Doppler changes that distinguish between them.

Reversed Diastolic Flow

Although reversed diastolic flow may be regarded as a severe form of reduced diastolic flow, it implies poor renal perfusion and as such, whatever the cause, it carries a poor prognosis (Table 42). Severe ATN may cause reversal of diastolic flow (Fig. 91), but these patients, unlike most patients with ATN, rarely recover significant renal function and many progress to cortical necrosis.

Renal vein thrombosis gives a specific pattern of diastolic reversal with a sharp reversal from peak systolic

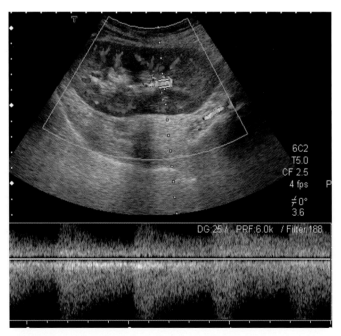

FIGURE 92 ■ Postbiopsy arteriovenous fistula. A complex color pattern is seen at the fistula, which is a combination of turbulence, aliasing, and tissue vibration. The velocity is increased, diastolic flow is increased (resistance index is decreased), and flow disturbance is shown on the spectral signal.

TABLE 45 ■ Decreased Systolic Velocity

Cause	Comment
Arterial stenosis	Only found distal to hemodynamically significant stenoses and not found in all cases
Renal artery occlusion	Flow through collaterals
End-stage renal failure	In some cases, severe destruction of the vascular bed causes this pattern

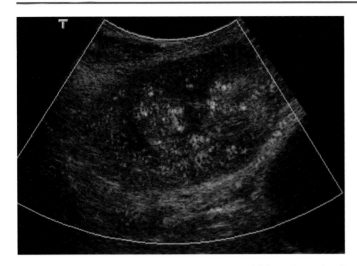

FIGURE 93 ■ Nonperfused kidney due to acute IGA nephropathy. A contrast ultrasound scan (Sonovue® with a low MI and color overlay technique) shows a few patches or perfusion (green patches) but most of the renal tissue is nonperfused.

to maximum reversed diastolic, a biphasic (reversed M) reversed diastolic flow, and a narrow systolic peak (Fig. 53) (138–142). A hematoma compressing the kidney may cause a similar effect resulting from venous compression.

Increased Diastolic Flow

Generalized increase in diastolic flow throughout the kidney indicates reduced renovascular resistance (Table 43). This occurs in the hyperemic diuretic phase of recovery from ATN and in any inflammatory condition of the kidney such as acute pyelonephritis or acute glomerulonephritis.

Arteriovenous (AV) fistulas within the kidney have a similar effect, although systolic velocities also may be increased. AV fistulas rarely occur with no apparent cause (idiopathic, congenital) but more often occur after diagnostic renal biopsy or perforating injuries to the kidney, or they occur within renal tumors. AV fistulas tend to cause Doppler changes, but these are localized to part

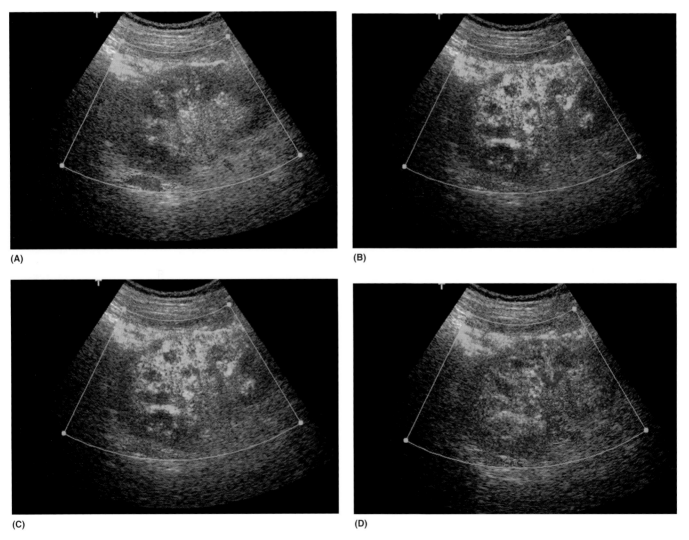

(A)

(B)

(C)

(D)

FIGURE 94 A–D ■ Reduced medullary perfusion. In this case of acute tubular necrosis, the medullary flow is severely reduced, the cortical flow less reduced. The study has been performed using a contrast technique (Sonovue® Low MI with color Doppler overlay). The sequence (A to D) at 15, 20, 30, and 40 minutes shows almost absent perfusion of the medullary pyramids. This is the typical patten of severe acute tubular necrosis (ATN). Compare Figure 95, which shows a normal study.

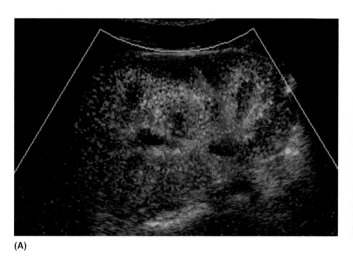

(A)

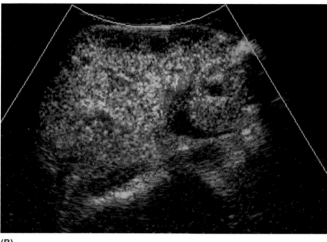

(B)

FIGURE 95 A AND B ■ Normal renal contrast perfusion study (**A**) at 15 seconds after injection shows the larger vessels in red and blue, and good cortical perfusion in green. There is early peripheral perfusion of the medullary pyramids (**B**); at 25 seconds, it shows total perfusion of the pyramids so that they are no longer visible separately from the cortex.

of the kidney instead of appearing as generalized changes. Confirmatory evidence consists of tissue vibration around the fistula, which appears as a mosaic of colors on the color-flow image, pulsatile venous flow and, in larger examples, visualization of the fistula itself (Fig. 92) (248).

Increased Systolic Velocity

Increase in systolic velocities occurs at an arterial stenosis, resulting from the Venturi effect (Table 44). Increase in systolic flow also occurs in AV fistulas. However, some increase in systolic velocity may occur in hypertension because of a central effect.

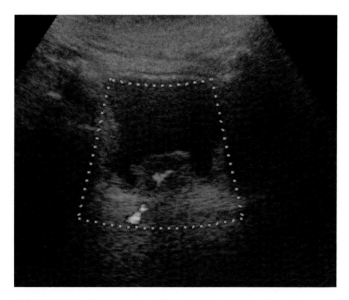

FIGURE 96 ■ Bladder tumor. Vascularity is shown within the mass, thus distinguishing tumor from hematoma.

Decreased Systolic Velocity

Decrease in systolic velocity occurs distal to a significant stenosis (Table 45). This causes a low systolic peak, decreased RI, and a prolonged systolic rise time. End-stage renal failure from any cause may give reduced systolic flow.

Reduced Renal Perfusion

In acute renal vein thrombosis, the whole kidney is underperfused. Arterial signals are seen only at the renal hilum. Collaterals, however, form rapidly, and when this happens, perfusion is reestablished.

Cortical and/or medullary perfusion is known to be reduced in several renal parenchymal conditions. Studies of perfusion using ultrasound contrast agents in these cases are relatively new, and their place in diagnostic studies has not been clearly established. Early experience, however, suggests that ultrasound contrast studies are ideally suited for assessing perfusion. Reduced or absent perfusion may be seen in part or the whole kidney in cases of acute arterial embolus or other causes of arterial occlusion such as dissection after angioplasty or some severe acute nephropathies (Figs. 93–95).

Doppler Studies in the Bladder

Doppler may be used to detect the position and angle of the ureteric jets. This study has limited use in vesicoureteric reflux and the study of ureteroceles, as already discussed. It may also be useful in excluding ureteric obstruction. A strong jet gives evidence against the presence of significant obstruction (20). Tumor flow may sometimes be detected in bladder tumors, and this feature can be used to distinguish tumor from blood clot (Fig. 96). Not all tumors show this feature, so that although detection of flow is useful, nondetection of flow is not helpful.

REFERENCES

1. Dalla Palma L, Bazzocchi M, Cressa C, Tommasini G. Radiological anatomy of the kidney revisited. Br J Radiol 1990; 63(753):680.
2. Patriquin H, Lefaivre JF, Lafortune M, Russo P, Boisvert J. Fetal lobation. an anatomo-ultrasonographic correlation. J Ultrasound Med 1990; 9(4):191.
3. Marchal G, Verbeken E, Oyen R, et al. Ultrasound of the normal kidney: a sonographic, anatomic and histologic correlation. Ultrasound Med Biol 1996; 12(12):999.
4. Haller JO, Berdon WE, Friedman AP. Increased cortical echogenicity: a normal finding in neonates and infants. Radiology 1982; 142:173.
5. Han BK, Babcock DS. Sonographic measurements and appearances of normal kidneys in children. Am J Roentgenol 1985; 145:611.
6. Hayden CK Jr, Santa Cruz FR, Ampara EG, et al. Ultrasonic evaluation of the renal parenchyma in infants and children. Radiology 1984; 152:413.
7. Hricak H, Slovis TL, Callan PW, et al. Neonatal kidneys: sonographic anatomic correlation. Radiology 1983; 147:499.
8. Troell S, Berg U, Johansson B, Wikstad I. Renal parenchymal volume in children. Normal values assessed by ultrasonography. Acta Radiol 1988; 29(1):127.
9. Dremsek PA, Kritscher H, Bohm G, Hochberger O. Kidney dimensions in ultrasound compared to somatometric parameters in normal children. Pediatr Radiol 1987; 17(4):285.
10. Vade A, Lau P, Smick J, Harris V, Ryva J. Sonographic renal parameters as related to age. Pediatr Radiol 1987; 17(3):212.
11. Yang JM, Huang WC. Bladder wall thickness on ultrasonographic cystourethrography: affecting factors and their implications. J Ultrasound Med 2003; 22(8):777.
12. Jequier S, Rousseau O. Sonographic measurements of the normal bladder wall in children. Am J Roentgenol 1987; 148:563.
13. McCullum RW. The adult male urethra: normal anatomy, pathology and method urethrography. Radiol Clin North Am 1979; 17:227–231.
14. Bearcroft PW, Berman LH. Sonography in the evaluation of the male anterior urethra. Clin Radiol 1994; 49:621.
15. Gluck CD, Bundy AL, Fine C, Loughlin KR, Richie JP. Sonographic urethrogram: comparison to roentgenographic techniques in 22 patients. J Urol 1988; 140:1404.
16. Chisholm GD, Innes C, Williams D, eds. Urology: Scientific Foundations. 2nd ed. London: Heinemann, 1982:2.
17. Platt JF, Rubin JM, Ellis JH. Distinction between obstructive and non-obstructive pyelocalyectasis with duplex Doppler sonography. Am J Roentgenol 1989; 153:997.
18. Platt JF, Ellis JH, Rubin JM. Examination of native kidneys with duplex Doppler ultrasound. Semin Ultrasound CT MR 1991; 12:308–318.
19. Jequier S, Paltiel H, Lafortune M. Ureterovesical jets in infants and children: duplex and color Doppler US studies. Radiology 1990; 175(2):349.
20. Burge HJ, Middleton WD, McClennan BL, et al. Ureteral jets in healthy subjects and patients with unilateral ureteric calculi: comparison with color Doppler ultrasound. Radiology 1991; 180:437.
21. Leung VY, Metreweli C, Yeung CK. Immature ureteric jet doppler patterns and urinary tract infection and vesicoureteric reflux in children. Ultrasound Med Biol 2002; 28:873.
22. Djavan B, Roehrborn CG. Bladder ultrasonography. Semin Urol 1994; 12(4):306.
23. Cochlin DL. Urinary system. Ultrasound Med Biol 2000; 26(Suppl 1):S76.
24. Goldberg BB, Lui JB. Endoluminal urologic ultrasound. Scand J Urol Nephrol Suppl 1991; 137:147.
25. Kuo HC, Chang SC, Hsu T. Application of transrectal sonography in the diagnosis and treatment of female stress urinary incontinence. Eur Urol 1994; 26(1):77.
26. Tunn R, Petri E. Introital and transvaginal ultrasound as the main tool in the assessment of urogenital and pelvic floor dysfunction: an imaging panel and practical approach. Ultrasound Obstet Gynecol 2003; 22(2):205.
27. Dietz HP. Ultrasound imaging of the pelvic floor. Part I: two-dimensional aspects. Ultrasound Obstet Gynecol 2004; 23(1):80–92.
28. Dietz HP. Ultrasound imaging of the pelvic floor. Part II: three-dimensional or volume imaging. Ultrasound Obstet Gynecol 2004; 23(6):615.
29. Ninan VT, Koshi T, Nigamthullah MM, et al. A comparative study of methods of estimating renal size in normal adults. Nephrol Dial Transplant 1990; 5:851–854.
30. Hodgson CJ, Edwards D. Chronic pyelonephritis and vesico-ureteric reflux. Clin Radiol 1960; 11:219.
31. Rosenbaum DM, Korngold E, Teele KL. Sonographic assessment of renal length in normal children. Am J Roentgenol 1984; 142:467.
32. Rasmussen SN, Haase L, Kjeldsen H, et al. Determination of renal volume by ultrasound scanning. J Clin Ultrasound 1978; 6:160.
33. Jones TB, Ruddick LR, Harpen MD, et al. Ultrasonographic determination of renal mass and renal volume. J Ultrasound Med 1983; 2:151.
34. Brandt TD, Neiman HC, Dragowski MJ, et al. Ultrasound assessment of normal renal dimensions. J Ultrasound Med 1982; 1:49.
35. King MC, Freedenberg RM, Tena LB. Normal renal parenchyma simulating tumor. Radiology 1968; 91:217.
36. Seppala RE, Hammond DI, Vezina CT, et al. Sonography of the hypertrophied column of Bertin. Am J Roentgenol 1987; 148:1277.
37. Banerjee B, Brett I. Ultrasound diagnosis of horseshoe kidney. Br J Radiol 1991; 64:898.
38. Lubat E, Hernanz-Schulman M, Jenieser NB. Sonography of the simple and complicated ipsilateral fused kidney. J Ulrasound Med 1989; 8:109.
39. Ueno T, Hashimoto H, Yokoyama H, et al. Urachal anomalies: ultrasonography and management. J Pediatr Surg 2003; 38(8):1203.
40. Mengiardi B, Wiesner W, Stoffel F, Terracciano L, Freitag P. Case 44: Adrenocarcinoma of the urachus. Radiology 2002; 222(3):744.
41. Robert Y, Hennequin-Delerue C, Chaillet D, et al. Urachal remnants: sonographic assessment. J Clin Ultrasound 1996; 24(7):339.
42. Holten I, Lomas F, Mouratidis B, Malecky G, Simpson E. The ultrasonic diagnosis of urachal anomalies. Australas Radiol 1996; 40(1):2.
43. Cochlin DL. Basic principles of Doppler. In: Cochlin DL, Dubbins PA, Goldberg BB, et al, eds. Urogenital Ultrasound: A Text Atlas. London: Martin Dunitz, 1994:1.
44. Merritt CRB. Doppler Color Imaging. New York: Churchill Livingstone, 1992.
45. Powis LR, Schwartz RA. Practical Doppler Ultrasound for the Clinician. Baltimore: Williams & Wilkins, 1991.
46. Ascenti G, Gaeta M, Magno C, et al. Contrast-enhanced second-harmonic sonography in the detection of pseudocapsule in renal cell carcinoma. Am J Roentgenol 2004; 182(6):1525.
47. Quaia E, Siracusano S, Bertolotto M, Monduzzi M, Mucelli RP. Characterization of renal tumours with pulse inversion harmonic imaging by intermittent high mechanical index technique: initial results. Eur Radiol 2003; 13(6):1402.
48. Coleman BG, Arger PH, Mulhern CT Jr, et al. Gray scale sonographic spectrum of hypernephromas. Radiology 1980; 168:633.
49. Helenon O, Correas JM, Balleyguier C, Ghouadni M, Cornud F. Ultrasound of renal tumors. Eur Radiol 2001; 11(10):1890.
50. Maklad NF, Chung YP, Doust BD, et al. Ultrasonic characterization of solid renal lesions: echographic, angiographic and pathologic correlation. Radiology 1977; 123:733.
51. Quinn MJ, Hartman DS, Friedman AC, et al. Renal oncocytoma: new observations. Radiology 1984; 153:49.
52. Goiney RC, Goldenberg L, Cooperberg PL, et al. Renal oncocytomas: sonographic analysis of 14 cases. Am J Roentgenol 1984; 143:1001.
53. Hartman DS, Davis CJ, Goldman SM. Xanthogranulomatous pyelonephritis: sonographic pathologic correlation of 16 cases. J Ultrasound Med 1984; 3:481.
54. Kim J. Ultrasonographic features of focal xanthogranulomatous pyelonephritis. J Ultrasound Med 2004; 23(3):409.
55. Tiu CM, Chou YH, Chiou HJ, et al. Sonographic features of xanthogranulomatous pyelonephritis. J Clin Ultrasound 2001; 29(5):279.
56. Kim JC. US and CT findings of xanthogranulomatous pyelonephritis. Clin Imaging 2001; 25(2):118.
57. Rosenfield AT, Glickman M, Taylor KJW, et al. Acute focal bacterial nephritis (acute lobar nephronia). Radiology 1979; 132:553.
58. Hoddick W, Brooke-Jeffrey R, Goldberg HI, et al. CT and sonography of severe renal and perirenal infections. Am J Roentgenol 1983; 140:517.

59. Farmer KD, Gellett LR, Dubbins PA. The sonographic appearance of acute focal pyelonephritis 8 years experience. Clin Radiol 2002; 57(6):483.

60. Arap S, Denes FT, Silva J, et al. Malakoplakia of the urinary tract. Eur Urol 1986; 12(2):113.

61. Shaw PJ, Hartley RB, Fagg NL, Saunders AJ, Saxton HM. Ultrasound and CT in renal parenchymal malakoplakia: report of a case with previous xanthogranulomatous pyelonephritis. Br J Radiol 1985; 58(686):175.

62. Pamilo M, Kulatunga A, Martikainen J. Renal parenchymal malakoplakia. A report of two cases. The radiological and ultrasound images. Br J Radiol 1984; 57(680):751.

63. Siegel CL, Middleton WD, Teefey SA, McClennan BL. Angiomyolipoma and renal cell carcinoma: US differentiation. Radiology 1996; 198(3):789.

64. Hartman DS, Goldman SM, Friedman AC, et al. Angiomyolipoma: ultrasonic pathologic correlation. Radiology 1981; 139:451.

65. Sim JS, Seo CS, Kim SH, et al. Differentiation of small hyperechoic renal cell carcinoma from angiomyolipoma: computer-aided tissue echo quantification. J Ultrasound Med 1999; 18(4):261.

66. Zebedin D, Kammerhuber F, Uggowitzer MM, Szolar DH. Criteria for ultrasound differentiation of small angiomyolipomas (< or = 3 cm) and renal cell carcinomas. [German] Rofo: Fortschritte auf dem Gebiete der Rontgenstrahlen und der Nuklearmedizin 1998; 169(6):627.

67. Taniguchi N, Itoh K, Nakamura S, et al. Differentiation of renal cell carcinomas from angiomyolipomas by ultrasonic frequency dependent attenuation. J Urol 1997; 157(4):1242.

68. Lee TG, Henderson SC, Freeny PC, et al. Ultrasound findings of renal angiomyolipoma. J Clin Ultrasound 1978; 6:150.

69. Totty WG, McClennan BL, Melson GL, et al. Relative value of computed tomography and ultrasonography in the assessment of renal angiomyolipoma. J Comput Assist Tomogr 1981; 5:173.

70. Weyman BJ, McClellan BL, Lee MT, et al. Calcified renal masses. Am J Roentgenol 1982; 138:1095.

71. Choyke PL, White EM, Zeman RK, et al. Renal metastases: clinicopathologic and radiologic correlation. Radiology 1987; 162:259.

72. Bailey JE, Roubidoux MA, Dunnick NR. Secondary renal neoplasms. Abdom Imaging 1998; 23(3):266.

73. Hartman DS, Davis CJ Jr, Goldman SM, et al. Renal lymphoma: radiolgic pathlogic correlation in 21 cases. Radiology 1982; 144:759.

74. Kaude JV, Lacey GD. Ultrasoniography in renal lymphoma. J Clin Ultrasound 1978; 6:321.

75. Hartman DS, Davidson AJ, Davis CJ, et al. Infiltrative renal lesions: CT, sonographic, pathologic correlations. Am J Roentgenol 1988; 150:1061.

76. Zderic SA. Renal and adrenal tumors in children. Urol Clin North Am 2004; 31(3):607.

77. Lowe LH, Isuani BH, Heller RM, et al. Pediatric renal masses: Wilms tumor and beyond. Radiographics 2000; 20(6):1585.

78. Broecker B. Non-Wilms' renal tumors in children. Urol Clin North Am 2000; 27(3):463.

79. Geller E, Smergel EM, Lowry PA. Renal neoplasms of childhood. Radiol Clin North Am 1997; 35(6):1391.

80. Chan HSL, Cheng MY, Mancer K, et al. Congenital mesoblastic nephroma: a clinical radiologic study of 17 cases representing the pathologic spectrum of the disease. J Pediatr 1987; 111:64.

81. Reiman TH, Siegal MJ, Shackleford GD. Wilms' tumor in children: abdominal CT and US evaluation. Radiology 1986; 160:501.

82. Siemer S, Lehmann J, Reinhard H, et al. Prenatal diagnosis of congenital mesoblastic nephroma associated with renal hypertension in a premature child. Int J Urol 2004; 11(1):50.

83. Chen WY, Lin CN, Chao CS, et al. Prenatal diagnosis of congenital mesoblastic nephroma in mid-second trimester by sonography and magnetic resonance imaging. Prenat Diagn 2003; 23(11):927.

84. Cremin BJ. Wilms' tumour: ultrasound and changing concepts. Clin Radiol 1987; 38:465.

85. Jaffe MH, White SJ, Silver TM, et al. Wilms' tumor: ultrasonic features, pathologic correlation and diagnostic pitfalls. Radiology 1981; 140:147.

86. Goske MJ, Mitchell C, Reslan WA. Imaging of patients with Wilms' tumor. Semin Urol Oncol 1999; 17(1):11.

87. Kabala JE, Shield J, Duncan A. Renal cell carcinoma in childhood. Pediatr Radiol 1992; 22:203.

88. Hugosson C, Nyman R, Jacobsson B, et al. Imaging of solid kidney tumours in children. Acta Radiol 1995; 36(3):254.

89. Vujanic GM, Webb D, Kelsey A. B-cell non-Hodgkin's lymphoma presenting as a primary renal tumour in a child. Med Pediatr Oncol 1995; 25(5):423.

90. Gore RM, Shkolnik A. Abdominal manifestations of pediatric leukemias: sonographic assessment. Radiology 1982; 142:207.

91. Glass RBJ, Davidson AJ, Fernbach SK. Clear cell sarcoma of the kidney: CT, sonographic and pathologic correlation. Radiology 1991; 180:715.

92. Sisler CL, Siegel MJ. Malignant rhabdoid tumor of the kidney: radiologic features. Radiology 1989; 172:211.

93. Sahnoun L, Jallouli M, Jouini R, et al. Rhabdoid tumour of the kidney in children. [French] Progres en Urologie 2004; 14(1):55.

94. Han TI, Kim MJ, Yoon HK, Chung JY, Choeh K. Rhabdoid tumour of the kidney: imaging findings. Pediatr Radiol 2001; 31(4):233.

95. Casper KA, Donnelly LF, Chen B, Bissler JJ. Tuberous sclerosis complex: renal imaging findings. Radiology 2002; 225(2):451.

96. Tchaprassian Z, Mognato G, Paradias G, et al. Renal angiomyolipoma in children: diagnositc difficulty in 3 patients. J Urol 1998; 159(5):1654.

97. Marteinsson VT, Due J, Aagenaes I. Focal xanthogranulomatous pyelonephritis presenting as renal tumour in children. Case report with a review of the literature. Scand J Urol Nephrol 1996; 30(3):235.

98. Wiggelinkhuizen J, Mills A, Emms M. Bilateral renal malakoplakia in infancy. Child Nephrol Urol 1988–1989; 9(1–2):101.

99. Marumo K, Horiguchi Y, Nakagawa K, et al. Incidence and growth pattern of simple cysts of the kidney in patients with asymptomatic microscopic hematuria. Int J Urol 2003; 10(2):63.

100. Terada N, Ichioka K, Matsuta Y, et al. The natural history of simple renal cysts. J Urol 2002; 167(1):21.

101. Bowers DL, Ikeguchi EF, Sawczuk IS. Transition from renal cyst to a renal carcinoma detected by ultrasonography. Br J Urol 1997; 80(3):495.

102. Bosniak MA. Problemsin the radiologic diagnosis of renal parenchymal tumors. Urol Clin North Am 1993; 20:217.

103. Bosniak MA, Birnbaum BA, Krinsky GA, Waisman J. Small renal parenchymal neoplasms: further observations on growth. Radiology 1995; 197:589.

104. Warren KS, McFarlane J. The Bosniak classification of renal cystic masses. BJU Int 2005; 95(7):939.

105. Israel GM, Bosniak MA. Calcification in cystic renal masses: is it important in diagnosis?. Radiology 2003; 226(1):47.

106. Ooi GC, Sagar G, Lynch D, Arkell DG, Ryan PG. Cystic renal cell carcinoma: radiological features and clinico-pathological correlation. Clin Radiol 1996; 51(11):791–6.

107. Hammoudi F, Hartani M. Imagariae da Kyste Hydatique du rein. J Radiol Belg 1989; 70:549.

108. Davies F, Coles GA, Harper PS, et al. Polycystic kidney disease re-evaluated: a population-based study. Q J Med 1991; 79(290):477.

109. Demetriou K, Tziakouri C, Anninou K, et al. Autosomal dominant polycystic kidney disease-type 2. Ultrasound, genetic and clinical correlations. Nephrol Dial Transplant 2000; 15(2):205.

110. Levine E, Slusher SL, Grantham JJ, et al. Natural history of acquired renal cysts in dialysis patients: a prospective longitudinal CT study. Am J Roentgenol 1991; 156:501.

111. Heinz-Peer G, Schoder M, Rand T, Mayer G, Mostbeck GH. Prevalence of acquired cystic kidney disease and tumors in native kidneys of renal transplant recipients: a prospective US study. Radiology 1995; 195(3):667.

112. Manns RA, Burrows FG, Adu D, Michael J. Acquired cystic disease of the kidney: ultrasound as the primary screening procedure. Clin Radiol 1990; 41(4):248.

113. Wan S, Cochlin DL. Sonography and computed tomography features of cystic disease of the liver. Gastrointest Radiol 1990; 15:310.

114. Boal DK, Teel RL. Sonography of infantile polycystic kidney disease. Am J Roentgenol 1980; 135:535.

115. Reuss A, Wladimiroff JW, Niermeyer MF. Sonographic, clinical and genetic aspects of prenatal diagnosis of cystic kidney disease. Ultrasound Med Biol 1991; 17(7):687.

116. Nicolau C, Torra R, Badenas C, et al. Sonographic pattern of recessive polycystic kidney disease in young adults. Differences from the dominant form. Nephrol Dial Transplant 2000; 15(9):1373.

117. Kagutt MS, Robichaux WH, Baineau FG, et al. Asymmetric renal size in autosomal recessive polycystic kidney disease: a unique presentation. Am J Roentgenol 1993; 160:835.

118. Saunders AJ, Denton E, Stephens S, Reid C. Cystic kidney disease presenting in infancy. Clin Radiol 1999; 54(6):370.

119. Fitch SJ, Stapleton FB. Ultrasonographic features of glomerulocystic disease in infancy: similarity to infantile polycystic kidney disease. Pediatr Radiol 1986; 16:400.

120. Fredericks BJ, Decampo M, Chow CW, et al. Glomerulocystic renal disease: ulrasonic appearances. Pediatr Radiol 1989; 19:184.

121. Greer ML, Danin J, Lamont AC. Glomerulocystic disease with hepatoblastoma in a neonate: a case report. Pediatr Radiol 1998; 28(9):703.

122. Dedeoglu IO, Fisher JE, Springate JE, et al. Spectrum of glomerulocystic kidneys: a case report and review of the literature. Pediatr Pathol Lab Med 1996; 16(6):941.

123. Patriquin HB, O'Regan S. Medullary sponge kidney in childhood. Am J Roentgenol 1985; 145:315.

124. Blowey DL, Querfeld U, Geary D, Warady BA, Alon U. Ultrasound findings in juvenile nephronophthisis. Pediatr Nephrol 1996; 10(1):22.

125. Garel LA, Habib R, Pariente D, et al. Juvenile nephronophthisis: appearance in children with severe uremia. Radiology 1984; 151:93.

126. Herman TE, Siegel MJ. Pyramidal hyperechogenicity in autosomal recessive polycystic kidney disease resembling medullary nephrocalcinosis. Pediatr Radiol 1991; 21:270.

127. McHugh K, Stringer DA, Hebert D, et al. Simple renal cysts in children: diagnosis and follow up with US. Radiology 1991; 178:383.

128. Strife JL, Souza AS, Kirks DR, et al. Multicystic dysplastic kidney in children: US follow-up. Radiology 1993; 186(3):785.

129. Hendry PL, Hendry GMA. Observations on the use of Doppler ultrasound in multicystic dysplastic kidney. Pediatr Radiol 1991; 20:203.

130. Atiyeh B, Husmann D, Baum M. Contralateral abnormalities in multicystic dysplastic kidney disease. J Pediatr 1992; 121:65.

131. Hartman GE, Smolik LM, Shochat SJ. The dilemma of the multicystic dysplastic kidney. Am J Dis Child 1986; 140:925.

132. Share JC, Lebowitz RL. The unsuspected double collecting system on imaging studies and at cystoscopy. Am J Roentgenol 1990; 155:161.

133. Schaffer RM, Shih YH, Becker JA. Sonographic identification of collecting system duplications. J Clin Ultrasound 1983; 11:309.

134. Mascatello VJ, Smith EH, Carrera CF, et al. Ultrasonic evaluation of the obstructed duplex kidney. Am J Roentgenol 1977; 129:113.

135. Piccirollo M, Rigsby CM, Rosenfield AT. Sonography of renal inflammatory disease. Urol Radiol 1987; 9:66.

136. Edell SL, Bonovita JA. The sonographic appearance of acute pyelonephritis. Radiology 1979; 132:683.

137. Dinkel E, Orth S, Dittrich M, et al. Renal sonography in the differentiation of upper from lower urinary tract infection. Am J Roentgenol 1986; 146:775.

138. Laplant S, Patriquin HB, Robitaille P, et al. Renal vein thrombosis in children: evidence of early flow recovery with Doppler US. Radiology 1993; 189:37.

139. Parvey HR, Isenberg RL. Image-directed Doppler sonography of the intrarenal arteries in acute renal vein thrombosis. J Clin Ultrasound 1990; 18:512.

140. Platt JF, Ellis JH, Rubin JM, et al. Intrarenal arterial Doppler sonography in patients with non obstructive renal disease: correlation of resistive index with biopsy findings. Am J Roentgenol 1990; 154:1223.

141. Hibbert J, Howlett DC, Greenwood KL, Mac Donald LM, Saunders AJ. The ultrasound appearances of neonatal renal vein thrombosis. Br J Radiol 1997; 70(839):1191.

142. Wright NB, Blanch G, Walkinshaw S, Pilling DW. Antenatal and neonatal renal vein thrombosis: new ultrasonic features with high frequency transducers. Pediatr Radiol 1996; 26(9):686.

143a. Erwin BC, Carroll BA, Walter JF, et al. Renal infarction appearing as an echogenic mass. Am J Roentgenol 1982; 138:759.

143b. Izumi M, Sugiura T, Nakamura H, et al. Differential diagnosis of prerenal azotemia from acute tubular necrosis and prediction of recovery by Doppler ultrasound. Am J Kidney Dis 2000; 35(4):713.

144. Tranquart F, Lebranchu Y, Haillot O, et al. The use of perioperative Doppler ultrasound as a screening test for acute tubular necrosis. Transpl Int 1993; 6(1):14.

145. Shultz K, Siffring PA, Forest TS, et al. Serial renal sonographic changes in pre-eclampsia. J Ultrasound Med 1990; 9:415.

146. Feldt-Rasmussen B, Hegedus L, Mathiesen ER, et al. Kidney volume in type 1 (insulin dependent) diabetic patients with normal or increased urinary albumin excretion: effects of long-term improved metabolic control. Scand J Clin Lab Invest 1991; 51:31.

147. Brown JJ, Peart WS, Owen K, Robertson JI, Sutton D. The diagnosis and treatment of renal artery stenosis. Br Med J 1960; 5195:327.

148. Kay CJ, Rosenfield AT, Taylor KJW, et al. Ultrasound characteristics of chronic atrophic pyelonephritis. Am J Roentgenol 1979; 132:47.

149. Gordon I. Urinary tract infection in paediatrics: the role of diagnostic imaging. Br J Radiol 1990; 63(751):507.

150. Furtschegger A, Egender G, Jakse G. The value of sonography in the diagnosis and follow-up of patients with blunt renal trauma. Br J Urol 1988; 62:110.

151. Kim TH, et al. The significance of unilateral radiation nephropathy. Int J Radiat Oncol Biol Phys 1980; 6:1567.

152. Scott RF, Engelbrecht HE. Ultrasonography in the advanced tuberculous kidney. S Afr Med J 1989; 75:371.

153. Schaffer R, Becker JA, Goodman J. Sonography of the tuberculous kidney. Urology 1983 22:209.

154. Vijayaraghavan SB, Kandasamy SV, Arul M, et al. Spectrum of high-resolution sonographic features of urinary tuberculosis. J Ultrasound Med 2004; 23(5):585.

155. Oliver J. Urinary system. In: Cowdry FV, ed. Problems of Aging. Baltimore, Williams & Wilkins, 1952.

156. Huntington DK, Hill SC, Hill MC. Sonographic manifestations of medical renal disease. Semin Ultrasound CT MR 1991; 12:290.

157. Glazer GM, Callen PW, Filly RA. Medullary nephrocalcinosis: sonographic evaluation. Am J Roentgenol 1982; 138:55.

158. Shultz PK, Strife JL, Strife CF, et al. Hyperechoic renal medullary pyramids in infants and children. Radiology 1991; 181:163.

159. Cromer DC, Jequiers S, de Chadervian JP. Factors associated with renal parenchymal echogenicity in the newborn. J Ultrasound Med 1986; 5:633.

160. Brenbridge AN, Chevalier RL, Kaiser DL. Increased renal cortical echogenicity in pediatric renal disease: histopathologic correlations. J Clin Ultrasound 1986; 14:595.

161. Burridge DG, Pereirah H, et al. New quantified echographic features of normal kidneys: hydronephrosis classification. Rontgenblatter 1990; 43:519.

162. Brown MA. Urinary tract dilatation in pregnancy. Am J Obstet Gynecol 1990; 164:641.

163. Bosniak MA. The use of the Bosniak classification system for renal cysts and cystic tumors. J Urol 1997; 157(5):1852.

164. Stuk KJ, White GM, Granke DS, et al. Urinary obstruction in azotemic patients: detection by sonography. Am J Roentgenol 1987; 149:1191.

165. Ellinbogen PH, Scheible FW, Talner LB, et al. Sensitivity of grey scale ultrasound in detecting urinary tract obstruction. Am J Roentgenol 1978; 130:731.

166. Davies P. Ultrasound does not diagnose ureteric obstruction. J R Soc Med 1988; 81:314.

167. Amis ES Jr, Cronan JJ, Pfister RC, et al. Ultrasonic inaccuracies in diagnosing renal obstruction. Urology 1982; 19:101.

168. Renowden SA, Cochlin DL. The potential use of diuresis Doppler sonography in PUJ obstruction. Clin Radiol 1992; 46:94.

169. Stevens PE. Doppler ultrasound in renal disease: not quite "the answer to a maiden's prayer". Ren Fail 1995; 17:89.

170. Jequiers S, Forbes PA, Nogrady MB. The value of ultrasonography as a screening procedure in a first documented urinary tract infection in children. J Ultrasound Med 1985; 4:393.

171. Fried AM, Woodring JH, Thompson DJ. Hydronephrosis of pregnancy: a prospective seqauential study of the course of dilatation. J Ultrasound Med 1983; 2:255.

172. Irving SO, Burgess NA. Managing severe loin pain in pregnancy. BJOG 2002; 109(9):1025.

173. Grenier N, Pariente JL, Trillaud H, et al. Dilatation or the collecting system during pregnancy: physiological vs obstructive dilatation. Eur Radiol 2000; 10:271.

174. Murthy LN. Urinary tract obstruction during pregnancy: recent developments in imaging. Br J Urol 1997; 80(suppl 1):1.

175. Haddad MC, Abomelha MS, Riley PJ. Diagnosis of acute ureteral calculous obstruction in pregnant women using colour and pulsed Doppler sonography. Clin Radiol 1995; 50(12):864.

176. MacNeily AE, Goldenberg SL, Allen EK, et al. Sonographic visualisation of the ureter in pregnancy. J Urol 1991; 146:298.

177. Wood BP, Benami T, Teele RL, et al. Ureterovesical obstruction and megaloureter: diagnosis by realtime US. Radiology 1985; 156:79.

178. Braden GL, Kozinn D, Hampf FE Jr, et al. Ultrasound diagnosis of early papillary necrosis. J Ultrasound Med 1991; 403:405.

179. Bick RJ, Bryan PJ. Sonographic demonstration of thickened renal pelvic mucosa/submucosa in mixed candida infection. J Clin Ultrasound 1987; 15:333.

180. Haddad MC, Hawary MM, Khoury NJ, et al. Radiology of perinephric fluid collections. Clin Radiol 2002; 57(5):339.

181. Haddad MC, Medawar WA, Hawary MM, et al. Perirenal fluid in renal parenchymal medical disease ("floating kidney"): clinical significance and sonographic grading. Clin Radiol 2001; 56(12):979.

182. Mirk P, Maresca G, Fileni A, et al. Sonography of the lower ureters. J Clin Ultrasound 1988; 16:635.

183. Pfister RC, Newhouse JH. Radiology of ureter. Urology 1978; 12(1):15.

184. Holm HH, Torp-Pedersen S, Larsen T, Dorph S. Transabdominal and endoluminal ultrasonic scanning of the lower ureter. Scand J Urol Nephrol Suppl 1994; 157:19.

185. Vereecken RL, Proesmans W. A review of ninety-two obstructive megaureters in children. Eur Urol 1999; 36(4):342.

186. Hadas-Halpern I, Farcas A, Patlas M, et al. Sonographic diagnosis of ureteral tumours. J Ultrasound Med 1999; 18:639.

187. Subramangma BR, Raghavendra BN, Mudambra MR. Renal transitional cell carcinoma: sonographic and pathologic correlations. J Clin Ultrasound 1982; 10:303.

188. Ostrovsky PR, Carr L, Goodman J. Ultrasound of transitional cell carcinoma. J Clin Ultrasound 1985; 13:35.

189. Grant DC, Dee GL, Yoder IC, et al. Sonography in transitional cell carcinoma of the renal pelvis. Urol Radiol 1986; 8:1.

190. Cunningham JJ. Ultrasonic demonstration of renal collecting system invasion by transitional cell cancer. J Clin Ultrasound 1982; 10:339.

191. Mulholland SG, Arger PH, Goldberg BB, et al. Ultrasonic differentiation of renal pelvic filling defects. J Urol 1979; 122:14.

192. Goodman JD, Macchia RJ, Macasaet MA, et al. Endometriosis of the urinary bladder: sonographic findings. Am J Roentgenol 1980; 135:625.

193. Kumar R, Haque CK, Cohen MS. Endometriosis of the urinary bladder: demonstration by sonography. J Clin Ultrasound 1984; 12:363.

194. Puylart JBCM. Acute appendicitis: US evaluation using graded compression. Radiology 1986; 158:355.

195. Jones W, Barie P. Urological manifestations of acute appendicitis. J Urol 1988; 139:1325–1328.

196. Abu-Yousef MM, Bleicher JJ, Maher JW, et al. High resolution sonography of acute appendicitis. Am J Roentgenol 1987; 149:53.

197. Farer LE, Schaffer RM. Transitional cell carcinoma of a simple ureterocele: a specific sonographic appearance. J Ultrasound Med 1990; 9:301.

198. Kahn AM, Boggis CW, Ashleigh RJ. Ultrasonography of calculi in ureteroceles. J Clin Ultrasound 1989; 17:439.

199. Al-Shorab MM. Radiological manifestations of genitourinary bilharziasis. Clin Radiol 1968; 19:100.

200. Abdel-Wahab MF, Strickland GT. Abdominal ultrasonography for assessing morbidity from schistosomiasis. 2. Hospital studies. Trans R Soc Trop Med Hyg 1993; 87(2):135.

201. Premkumar A, Latimer J, Newhouse JH. CT and sonography of advanced urinary tract tuberculosis. Am J Roentgenol 1987; 148:65.

202. Petritsch PH, Colombh TH, Rauchenwald M, et al. Ultrasonography of urinary tract and micturition as an alternative to radiological investigations in the spinal cord injured patient. Eur Urol 1991; 20:97.

203. Hakenberg OW, Linne C, Manseck A, Wirth MP. Bladder wall thickness in normal adults and men with mild lower urinary tract symptoms and benign prostatic enlargement. Neurourol Urodyn 2000; 19(5):585.

204. Goodling JAW. Varied sonographic manifestations of cystitis. J Ultrasound Med 1986; 5:61.

205. Abu-Yousef MM, Narayana AS, Frenken EA Jr, et al. Urinary bladder tumors studied by cystosonography. I. Detection. Radiology 1984; 149:563.

206. Bessette PL, Abell MR, Herwig KR. A clinicopathological study of squamous cell carcinoma of the bladder. J Urol 1974; 112:66.

207. Cronan JJ, Simeone JF, Pfister RC, Newhouse JH, Ferrucci JT Jr. Cystosonography in the detection of bladder tumors: a prospective and retrospective study. J Ultrasound Med 1982; 1(6):237.

208. Denkhaus H, Crone-Munzebrock W, Muland H. Noninvasive ultrasound in the detection and staging of bladder carcinoma. Urol Radiol 1985; 7:121.

209. Bahnson RR, Zaontz MR, Maizels M, et al. Ultrasonography and diagnosis of pediatric genitourinary rhabdomyosarcoma. Urology 1989; 33:64.

210. Malone PR. Transabdominal ultrasound for surveillance of bladder cancer. Urol Clin North Am 1989; 16:823.

211. Boag GS, Nolan RL. Sonographic features of urinary bladder involvement in regional enteritis. J Ultrasound Med 1988; 7:125.

212. Abu Yusef MM, Narayana AS, Brown RC. Catheter induced cystitis: evaluation by cystosonography. Radiology 1984; 151:471.

213. Bree RL, Silver TM. Sonography of bladder and prevesical abnormalities. Am J Roentgenol 1981; 136:1101.

214. Rosenfield AT, Taylor KJW, Weiss RM. Ultrasound evaluation of bladder calculi. J Urol 1979; 121:119.

215. Janus C. Sonographic appearance of the abnormally positioned Foley catheter. J Ultrasound Med 1982; 4:439.

216. McDonald DF, Fagan CJ. Fungal balls in the urinary bladder. Am J Roentgenol 1972; 114:753.

217. Rifkin MD, Needleman L, Kurtz AB, et al. Sonography of nongynecologic cystic masses of the pelvis. Am J Roentgenol 1984; 142:1169.

218. Brandt TD, Neiman HL, Calenoff L, et al. Ultrasound evaluation of the urinary system in spinal cord injured patients. Radiology 1981; 141:473.

219. Naya Y, Kojima M, Honjyo H, et al. Intraobserver and interobserver variance in the measurement of ultrasound-estimated bladder weight. Ultrasound Med Biol 1998; 24(5):771.

220. Hendrikx AJ, Doesburg WH, Reintjes AG, Strijk SP, Debruyne FM. Effectiveness of ultrasound in the preoperative evaluation of patients with prostatism. Prostate 1988; 13(3):199.

221. Griffiths CJ, Murray A, Ramsden PD. Accuracy and repeatability of bladder volume measurement using ultrasound imaging. J Urol 1986; 136:12.

222. Hakenberg OW, Ryall RL, Langois SL, et al. A determination of bladder volume by sonocystoraphy. J Urol 1983; 130:249.

223. Kiely EA, Hartnell GG, Gibson RN, et al. Measurement of bladder volume by realtime ultrasound. Br J Urol 1987; 60:33.

224. McLean GK, Edell SL. Determination of bladder volumes by grey scale ultrasonography. Radiology 1978; 128:181.

225. Wexler JS, McGovern TP. Ultrasonography of female urethral diverticula. Am J Roentgenol 1986; 134:737.

226. Kauzlarie D, Barmear E, Peyer P, et al. Sonographic appearance of urethral diverticulum in the male. J Ultrasound Med 1988; 7:107.

227. Keefe B, Warshauer DM, Tucker MS, et al. Diverticula of the female urethra: diagnosis by endovaginal and transperineal sonography. Am J Roentgenol 1991; 156:1195.

228. McAninch JW, Laing FC, Jeffrey RB Jr. Sonourethrography in the evaluation of urethral strictures: a preliminary report. J Urol 1988; 139:294.

229. Merkle W, Wagner WI. Sonography of the distal male urethra: a new diagnostic procedure for urethral strictures: results of a prospective study. J Urol 1988; 140:1409.

230. Chiou RK, Anderson JC, Tran T, et al. Evaluation of urethral strictures and associated abnormalities using high-resolution and color Doppler ultrasound. Urology 1996; 47:102–107.

231. Heidenreich A, Derschum W, Bonfig R, Wilbert DM. Ultrasound in the evaluation of urethral stricture disease: a prospective study in 175 patients. Br J Urol 1994; 74:93–98.

232. Gupta S, Majumdar B, Tiwari A, Gupta RK, Kumar A, Gujral RB. Sonourethrography in the evaluation of anterior urethral strictures: correlation with radiographic urethrography. J Clin Ultrasound 1993; 21:231–239.

233. Morey AF, McAninch JW. Ultrasound evaluation of the male urethra for assessment of urethral stricture. J Clin Ultrasound 1996; 24:473–479.

234. Nash PA, McAninch JW, Bruce JE, et al. Sono-urethrography in the evaluation of anterior urethral strictures. J Urol 1995; 154:72–76.

235. Solivetti FM, D'Ascenzo R, Oraz C, et al. Ultrasound diagnosis and management of urethral stones. J Ultrasound Med 1989; 8:685.

236. Cohler TR, Zierler RE, Martin RL, et al. Non invasive diagnosis of renal artery stenosis by ultrasonic duplex scanning. J Vasc Surg 1986; 4:450.

237. Dubbins PA, Wells IP. Renal artery stenosis; duplex Doppler evaluation. Br J Radiol 1986; 59:225.

238. Robertson R, Murphy A, Dubbins PA. Renal artery stenosis: use of duplex ultrasound as a screening technique. Br J Radiol 1988; 61:723.

239. Sievers KW, Lohr E, Werner WR. Duplex Doppler ultrasound in determination of renal artery stenosis. Neurol Radiol 1989; 11:142.

240. Middleton MD. Doppler US evaluation of renal artery stenosis: past, present and future. Radiology 1992; 184:307.

241. Desberg AL, Paushter DM, Lammert GK, et al. Renal artery stenosis: evaluation with color Doppler flow imaging. Radiology 1990; 177:749.

242. Handa N, Fukenaga R, Vehara A, et al. Echo Doppler velocometer in the diagnosis of hypertensive patients: the renal artery Doppler technique. Ultrasound Med Biol 1986; 12:945.

243. Hanson KT, Tribble RW, Reeves SW, et al. Renal duplex sonography: evaluation of clinical utility. J Vasc Surg 1990; 12:227.

244. Halpern E, Needleman L, Nack TL, et al. Renal artery stenosis: should we study the main renal artery or segmental vessels? Radiology 1995; 195:799.

245. Kim SH, Kim WH, Choi BI, Kim CW. Duplex Doppler ultrasound in patients with medical renal disease: RI versus serum creatinine level. Clin Radiol 1992; 45:85.

246. Mostbeck GH, Kain R, Mallek R, et al. Duplex Doppler sonography in renal parenchymal disease: histopathologic correlation. J Ultrasound Med 1991 10:189.

247. Platt JF, Rubin JM, Ellis JH, et al. Duplex Doppler US of the kidney: differentiation of obstructive from non-obstructive dilatation. Radiology 1989; 171:515.

248. Renowden S, Blethyn J, Cochlin DL. Duplex and colour flow sonography in the diagnosis of post biopsy arteriovenous fistulae in the transplanted kidney. Clin Radiol 1992; 45:233.

Prostate ● *Ewa Kuligowska and James F. Stinchon*

PROSTATE CANCER

Prostate cancer continues to be the most common lethal malignancy in American men and is the second leading cause of cancer-related death in the male population over the age of 80 in the United States. It is estimated that 232,090 new cases will be diagnosed and 30,350 men will die from the disease. In comparison, breast cancer is diagnosed in approximately 211,000 U.S. women each year with about 44,000 deaths (1). About one man in five will be diagnosed with prostate cancer during his lifetime, and one man in 33 will die of this disease (2). From 1986 to 1991, there was an 82% rise in the incidence rate of prostate cancer in men older than 65 years of age, the largest single increase ever reported for cancer. This increase was related to prostate cancer screening programs. Over the next four years, the age-adjusted incidence rate of prostate cancer decreased dramatically from 240 to 170 cases per 100,000 population following widespread cancer screening. Since 1995, the incidence rate of prostate cancer has increased by 3% among white men and 2.3% among black men (3). This increase may also be attributed to increased screening through prostate-specific antigen (PSA) testing. As the population ages, these numbers are expected to increase.

Prostate cancer incidence and death rates vary considerably among black and white men. For black men, the incidence is 271.3 per 100,000 and death rate 70.4 per 100,000. Comparatively, the incidence rate for prostate cancer in white men is 167.4 per 100,000 and death rate is 28.8 per 100,000 (1). The prevalence rate for prostate cancer in autopsy series is 30% to 50% in men older than 50 years and 35% to 98% above age 90. The natural history of the disease reflects a wide spectrum of potential biologic activity. Some cancers are clinically insignificant and are unlikely to progress and cause morbidity or mortality. Clinically significant prostate cancer is defined as a cancer larger than 0.5 cc, which can progress to cause clinical disease. Whereas an estimated 30% to 50% of men older than 50 years have the disease, only 20% to 25% of prostate carcinomas are estimated to be clinically significant, and only 3% of these men will die from the disease. Several pathologic parameters (tumor grade, extent, and volume) reflect the behavior of the cancer (4). Unfortunately, it is difficult to distinguish at an early stage those cancers that will likely progress and produce clinical disease from those that can be safely observed. Early detection of prostate cancer contributes to reduction in mortality. Treatment of early localized disease is the only chance for cure.

EPIDEMIOLOGY

Studies indicate that American men whose diets are rich in saturated fat from red meat have an approximately 80% greater risk of developing prostate cancer than men with a lower intake of fat. It is believed that these diets do not initiate prostate cancer but influence androgen levels and so promote changes in the gland, leading to clinically significant and possible lethal malignancy. In Japan, for example, prostate cancer is a rare cause of death. However, when Japanese men move to America, their incidence of carcinoma of prostate increases, most likely because of dietary changes.

Another epidemiologic factor for carcinoma of prostate is a positive family history in first- and second-degree relatives. Genetic studies have detected a defect on the short arm of chromosome 8 that is associated with prostate cancer. African-American men have a higher incidence and mortality rate from carcinoma of the prostate than whites. They also develop the tumor at an earlier age. Recent reports also indicate an increased frequency of prostate cancer among relatives of women with breast cancer. Other factors include geography, prior vasectomy, and a history of venereal disease. The role of geography is related to vitamin D, which has potent antitumor properties. Interestingly, eunuchs do not get prostate cancer (5).

SCREENING FOR PROSTATE CANCER

Currently, the PSA test is widely used in the United States. Both the American Cancer Society and the American Urological Association recommend an annual digital rectal examination (DRE) and PSA test beginning at 50 years of age. For high-risk men such as African-Americans and those with a strong family history of carcinoma of the prostate, screening is recommended beginning at 40 years of age (6). DRE, transrectal ultrasound (TRUS), and PSA measurements are limited as screening tests because of insufficient sensitivity, specificity, and cost-effectiveness (7–9). Prostate cancer, hyperplasia, and prostate inflammation elevate serum PSA level to a different extent. This lack of specificity of serum PSA screening has led to a search for the correct combination of the results of PSA, TRUS, and DRE to improve specificity without a reduction in sensitivity (10–12).

Screening studies conducted by Catelona and Saboie detected 8.3 cancers per 1000 men screened. However, the incidence of new fatal cancers is only 1.5 per 1000 in men aged 50 to 69 years, resulting in an overdetection rate of approximately 7 per 1000. The ideal goal using available technology is to detect clinically or potentially significant tumors at a curable stage. Accumulated experience supports screening (13–18). Clinically significant disease may be distinguished from insignificant disease by prognostic features such as the volume of tumor, extent of tumor, Gleason score, and DNA ploidy. Application of these criteria to the cancers detected by DRE, PSA, and TRUS has clearly demonstrated that most detected cancers are clinically significant. In isolation, DRE or PSA results each have positive predictive values (PPVs) of 15% to 30% (19,20). If results from DRE, PSA, and TRUS are positive, the chance of cancer is increased up to 60% (Table 1) (21). This low sensitivity precludes the use of PSA alone as a screening test for prostate carcinoma, but when combined with DRE and TRUS, it can lead to greater sensitivity and specificity. If both DRE and PSA findings are negative, the chance of tumor is only 2% (4). With the addition of PSA,

TABLE 1 ■ PPVs of Various Screening Modalities and Their Combinations

	PPV
DRE+	15–30%
PSA+	10–30%
TRUS+	25%
DRE+ with PSA+	45%
DRE+ with PSA+ and TRUS+	60%

Abbreviations: PPV, positive predictive value; DRE, digital rectal examination; PSA, prostate-specific antigen; TRUS, transrectal ultrasound.

TRUS, and TRUS-guided biopsy, significant cancers may be detected at an early stage.

Digital Rectal Examination

DRE traditionally has been used for detecting prostate cancer. DRE is technically limited. It allows palpation of only the posterior aspect of the prostate gland. Approximately 50% of prostate cancers occur in locations inaccessible to the examining finger, including all cancers occurring in the transitional zone (TZ) and central zone (CZ). The criteria for abnormal DRE results include induration, nodularity, and asymmetry of the gland. Of the palpable masses, only 50% are carcinoma of the prostate and approximately 70% of these already have extended beyond the prostate. The PPV of DRE is 15% to 30%, varying little with age. On average, DRE has a 1% to 2% detection rate when used alone in the population of men older than 50 years (22,23).

Prostate-Specific Antigen

PSA is a blood test that measures the level of PSA in the serum. PSA is a serine protease discovered in 1979 by Wang. The normal level is 0 to 4 ng/mL using the Hybritech monoclonal antibody method (Table 2). With a cutoff level of 4.0 ng/mL, the sensitivity for cancer detection within two years of screening is approximately 73% and specificity approximately 85% (13,17,23–27). Although it is secreted only by epithelial cells in the prostate, it is not specific for prostate cancer; it becomes elevated with any significant derangement of prostate architecture and subsequent leakage of PSA (24,25). Varieties of pathologic conditions cause a leakage of PSA into the stroma of the gland. From there, it enters the circulation by the lymphatics and capillaries (26,27). Causes of elevated PSA include benign prostatic hyperplasia (BPH), prostate cancer, instrumentation,

TABLE 2 ■ Normal PSA Levels

■ Yang polyclonal method	0–2 ng/mL
■ Hybritech monoclonal method	0–4 ng/mL
■ To compare the assay	Hybritech + 1.75 = Yang

Abbreviation: PSA, prostate-specific antigen.

TABLE 3 ■ Causes of Elevated PSA

- Prostate carcinoma
- BPH
- Prostatitis
- Prostatic infarct
- Instrumentation (cytoscopy, Bx, transurethral resection of prostate)
- Sexual activity

Abbreviations: PSA, prostate-specific antigen; BPH, benign prostatic hyperplasia; Bx, biopsy.

TABLE 4 ■ Measurements Used for Interpreting PSA Data

Gland volume	Height × length × width × 0.523
Estimated PPSA	Height × length × width × 0.523 × 0.12
Tumor volume estimation	$\dfrac{PSA - Predicted\ PSA}{2}$
PSA density	$\dfrac{PSA}{Volume}$

Abbreviations: PSA, prostate-specific antigen; PPSA, predicted PSA.

prostatitis, infarction, biopsy, and transurethral resection of the prostate (TURP) (Table 3). Other factors affecting the PSA level include antiandrogen therapy, sexual activity, ambulation, and exercise (5). The incidence of prostate cancer is significantly higher in black men. The PSA often is elevated in these men at an earlier age and may provide an early warning mechanism for prostate cancer. To confound matters, approximately 20% of men with prostatic carcinoma have normal PSA levels.

Serial PSA testing reveals a direct correspondence of the PSA level with the tumor volume and growth rate. PSA levels do not increase significantly until the tumor reaches a volume of 1 cc. Stamey et al. (27,28) discovered that 1 g of BPH elevates the PSA by only 0.3 ng/mL, whereas 1 g of cancer generates 10 times more PSA, elevating the PSA to 3.0 ng/mL. Continued elevation or significant interval increases in PSA over time may be more important indicators of cancer than absolute PSA values. The PPV of PSA varies from 17% to 28% and depends on the degree of elevation. Elevation of the PSA is a better indicator of clinically significant tumor with extracapsular spread than is provided by DRE. Elevated levels of PSA are correlated with increasing clinical stage and the pathologic grade of prostate cancer. Intermediate values between 4 and 9.9 are difficult to interpret (4,26). The PPV for cancer is only about 22% with an elevated PSA level between 4 and 9.9. This increases to approximately 67% with PSA levels greater than 10. Five measurements provide guidelines for interpreting PSA data, especially for levels in the ambiguous 4 to 10 ng/mL range: PSA velocity (PSAV), PSA density (PSAD), predicted PSA (PPSA), age-specific PSA, and investigation of different circulating forms of PSA molecules (Tables 4 and 5) (11,29).

PSA Velocity

The PSAV is based on the rate of change of the annual PSA level. An increase of the PSA level by more than 0.75 ng/mL per year or by more than a 20% each year is highly (90%) suspicious for cancer and is less likely to be from benign causes. PSA variation greatly limits the use of PSAV unless a patient has had at least three PSA values measured over several years. PSAV does not predict future tumor behavior or metastatic potential (Table 5) (30,31).

PSA Density

The PSAD is a method that accounts for the portion of the serum PSA related to BPH. It is obtained by dividing the PSA serum level by the prostate volume. The mean PSAD of BPH is 0.04, and for prostate cancer, 0.58. It can be reasonably assumed that if the PSAD is greater than 0.1, the patient has cancer, and if PSAD is less than 0.1, the patient has a benign cause for the elevated PSA (Table 5). The American Cancer Society National Prostate Cancer Detection Project (NPCDP) determined patients with PSAD above 0.1 ng/mL had six- to ninefold increased risk of prostate cancer (32–34).

Predicted PSA

Lee and Littrup (12) developed a concept of a PPSA value based on the individual prostate volume estimation from TRUS. The PPSA is calculated by multiplying the gland volume by 0.12. The PPSA value is then compared with the measured serum PSA level to generate a value for excess PSA level (11,12,21). The often significant contribution of prostatic hyperplasia is thus taken into account (29,33,35). If the PSA is too high for the gland volume, the presence of cancer should be highly suspected. By dividing the excess PSA (PSA–PPSA) by two, it is possible to estimate the approximate size of the underlying tumor (Table 5) (21).

TABLE 5 ■ Cancer Prediction Using PSA

$PSAD = \dfrac{PSA}{Volume}$	BPH: density <0.1
	Cancer: density >0.1
PPSA = volume × 0.12	BPH: excess PSA ≤0
	(Excess PSA = PSA – PPSA)
	Cancer: excess PSA ≥0
	(Excess PSA ÷ 2 = estimate of tumor volume)
PSAV = rate Δ PSA	BPH: <0.75 ng/mL/yr
	<20% increase
	Cancer: >0.75 ng/mL/yr
	>20% increase

Abbreviations: PSA, prostate-specific antigen; PSAD, prostate-specific antigen density; PPSA, predicted prostate-specific antigen; PSAV, prostate-specific antigen velocity; BPH, benign prostatic hyperplasia.

TABLE 6 ▪ Age-Specific PSA

Age (yr)	Level (ng/mL)
40–49	0.0–2.5
50–59	0.0–3.5
60–69	0.0–4.5
70–79	0.0–6.5

Abbreviation: PSA, prostate-specific antigen.

Age-Specific PSA

As PSA levels increase with age, certain authors believe that using age-specific reference ranges results in an improved sensitivity for younger men and specificity for older men. Osterling et al. (36) defined the age-specific reference range for normal values as seen in Table 6.

Free PSA

Measurement of free PSA has been postulated to provide additional discrimination between men with prostate cancer and men with BPH. Christensson et al. (37) demonstrated that each patient has a unique ratio of free PSA to total PSA. Patients with advanced prostate cancer have been observed to have less circulating free PSA. Most of the PSA is bound to serum protease inhibitors when compared with patients with BPH. Thus, a low free PSA (<20%) increases the PPV for cancer and enhances the ability to distinguish cancer from benign conditions (38–40).

PSA Level as an Indicator for Staging

There is a good correlation between PSA levels and staging of prostate carcinoma. PSA levels of 10 ng/mL or less are seldom associated with metastatic lesions. Only when the PSA value is significantly over 40 ng/mL will the bone scan result be positive for metastases. PSA parameters for positive pelvic nodes are being developed and could potentially replace computed tomography (CT) and magnetic resonance imaging. When the PSA is greater than 50 ng/mL, there is a 90% chance of invasion of the seminal vesicles (8).

ANATOMY OF THE PROSTATE ON TRUS

The prostate is shaped like an inverted pyramid. It lies behind the inferior arch of pubic symphysis and in front of the rectal ampulla (Fig. 1). The apex rests on the superior aspect of the urogenital diaphragm and is attached to the posterior aspect of the pubic bone. The superior region, called the base of the gland, is the largest portion and is adjacent to the inferior margin of the bladder base. There is a thin, fibrous capsule surrounding the anterior

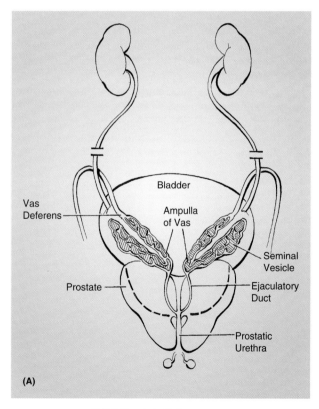
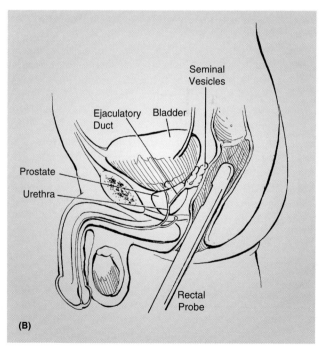

FIGURE 1 A AND B ▪ Normal anatomy of the prostate. (**A**) Prostate located in true pelvis, inferior to bladders, rests on levator ani sling accompanying diagnostic representation of the coronal view of the prostate, which demonstrates the ductal system. (**B**) Sagittal view of the normal prostate gland demonstrates the relationship of the rectum, levator sling, and bladder. The probe is in the rectum on the diagnostic view.

and lateral portion of the prostate that is continuous with the anterior fibromuscular zone. The prostate is separated from the rectum by periprostatic fat and a membrane called Denonvillier's fascia. The venous plexus of Santorini is located within the connective tissue surrounding the prostate anteriorly and anterolaterally. In the posterior lateral regions of the prostate, there are paired vessels and nerves called the neurovascular bundles that run obliquely into the prostate. Branches from the neurovascular bundles perforate the capsule and enter the prostate (9).

ZONAL CONCEPT OF PROSTATIC ANATOMY: CLINICAL APPLICATIONS

A zonal concept of prostate anatomy was described by McNeil (41) in 1968. There are three glandular zones—TZ,CZ, and peripheral zone (PZ)—and one nonglandular region, the anterior fibromuscular stroma (Figs. 2 and 3). The urethra and ejaculatory ducts pass through these zones. New high-resolution transducers have made it possible to use the McNeil zonal concept of the prostate to develop criteria for early cancer detection. Tumors can be more readily identified, size can be better estimated, and tumor volume more objectively calculated. By using this zonal system of prostate anatomy, it is also easier to assess subsequent growth, response to therapy, or both (41,42).

Transitional Zone

Before the onset of benign enlargement of the prostate, the TZ constitutes approximately 5% of the glandular tissue. It is located on both sides of the proximal urethra. This is the site of BPH in older men. There are two types of BPH. The first is a proliferation of homogenous stroma

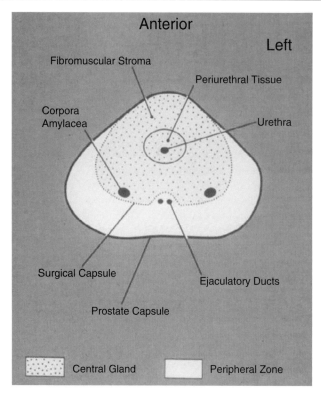

FIGURE 3 ▓ Zonal anatomy of the prostate, axial view.

or fibromuscular hyperplasia, which is hypoechoic. The second is glandular hyperplasia, which can be mixed in echogenicity and appears hypoechoic or hyperechoic, depending on the size of the prostate (19). Calculi often develop within this zone in a periurethral location. The TZ is separated from the adjacent PZ by the surgical capsule (Figs. 2 and 3).

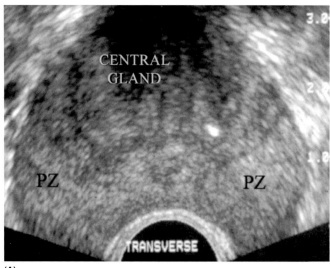

(A)

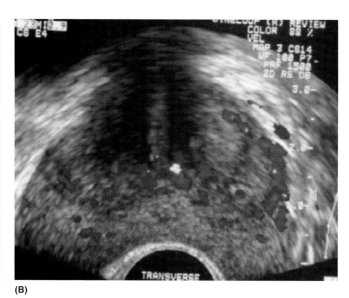

(B)

FIGURE 2 A AND B ▓ Transrectal ultrasound of normal prostate. (**A**) The peripheral zone (PZ) constitutes the peripheral and apical portion of the prostate and is easily recognized as homogenous and hyperechoic compared with the central gland. Note punctuate calcification in the central gland. (**B**) Color Doppler image of normal prostate.

According to McNeal, the TZ is the site of origin of approximately 20% of prostate cancer. Transurethral resection of the prostate (TURP) occasionally shows the cancer tissue and is designated as stage A by the Whitmore–Jewett staging system (41,42).

Central Zone

The CZ is pyramidal and is located at the base of the prostate. It constitutes approximately 25% of prostatic glandular tissue. It is not present below the verumontanum. The seminal vesicles and the vas deferens enter into the CZ. This confluence forms the bilateral ejaculatory ducts. The entrance of the seminal vesicles and vas deferens into the CZ produces a site of anatomic weakness at the base of the prostate caused by the absence of an encompassing capsule, thus providing little resistance to tumor spread. The echogenicity of the CZ is indistinguishable from that of the PZ. Only a thin band of connective tissue separates them (Fig. 4).

Prostatic calculi may form in the CZ in the corpora amylacea. These calculi are thought to be secondary to reflux of urine into the ducts. Less than 5% of prostate cancer originates in the CZ. However, the CZ offers poor resistance to the spread of cancer from the PZ because of the absence of an anatomical barrier between the two zones.

Peripheral Zone

The PZ makes up 70% of the normal gland volume. It is composed of acinar tissue and constitutes the postero-lateral and apical portion of the gland (Figs. 2 and 3).

In young men, it is isoechoic compared with the CZs and TZs and so is poorly seen. However, when the TZ becomes hypoechoic because of the changes of BPH, the PZ appears relatively hyperechoic and is more easily recognized (Fig. 2A).

Approximately 70% to 80% of prostate cancer occurs in the PZ. Most of the cancers are located within 3 mm of

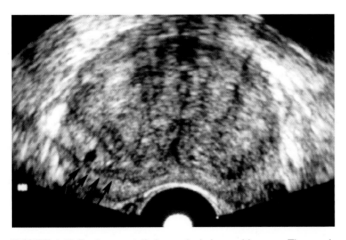

FIGURE 4 ■ Benign prostatic hyperplasia in an older man. The surgical capsule outlines the border between the peripheral zone and the enlarged central gland. The peripheral zone (indicated by the *arrows*) is compressed by the enlarged central gland.

the capsule, most commonly at the apex and base of the gland, and laterally where the neurovascular bundles penetrate the capsule. Of tumors in the PZ, 25% arise anterior to the level of verumontanum and are not palpable on DRE (9,10,12).

There are several sites of anatomic weakness in the gland through which either CZ or PZ cancers may penetrate.

1. The capsule of the prostate is open at the apex; thus, cancers occurring here can extend directly into the trapezoid area.
2. Another site of weakness is the invaginated extraprostatic space along the course of the seminal vesicles and ejaculatory ducts.
3. There is also a low resistance to cancer spread along the neurovascular bundles at the site of their penetration into the posterolateral aspect of the apical region.

Anterior Fibromuscular Stroma

The anterior fibromuscular stroma is a nonglandular region that forms the anterior surface of the prostate. It is resistant to disease (Fig. 3).

PROSTATE CANCER ON TRUS

The use of ultrasound for evaluation and biopsy of the prostate gland has increased dramatically since 1990. TRUS is a relatively noninvasive, inexpensive, and easily available technique for examining the prostate gland. High-frequency transducers provide a detailed view of internal prostate anatomy. The entire gland may be visualized, including the anterior portion, which is beyond the reach of DRE. The detection of early prostate cancer has dramatically improved with the development of high-frequency transducers (5–9 MHz).

Ultrasonography, like fluoroscopy, is operator dependent. The quality of the examination and interpretation depend on the clinical skill and interpretive experience of the radiologist. If a technician performs the examination following a protocol and the radiologist only reads static films, the diagnostic accuracy will not be the same as when the examination is performed by a well-trained radiologist. The average examination requires 15 to 30 minutes. During this time, abnormal areas can be identified. If they are compressible, they are usually caused by BPH; if not, cancer is more likely. Color Doppler imaging (CDI) is used then to assess the vascularity and identify the patterns of blood vessels suggestive of tumor. Suspicious areas then systematically undergo biopsy to identify possible tumors. One of the most common presentations of cancer missed is the presence of a large, infiltrative tumor that looks like normal prostate. The diagnosis of cancer in these cases requires the recognition of subtle changes in the architecture of the PZ, slight asymmetry of the surgical or prostatic capsule, and careful analysis of the periprostatic tissue adjacent to these suspicious areas to detect abnormal thickness or the possible extension of a tumor.

Color Doppler ultrasound has been shown to be an important adjunct to conventional gray-scale TRUS, improving the accuracy of cancer detection, especially for isoechoic cancer (43–51). It has also been suggested that color Doppler ultrasound is important for evaluation of tumors with high Gleason grades (50–52).

TRUS EXAMINATION

TRUS examination is indicated in patients with an abnormal finding on DRE, an elevated PSA, or both. It is also used routinely to examine patients with positive family history of prostate cancer, evaluation of BPH, infertility, and prostatodynia (Table 7). Optimal evaluation of the prostate gland by TRUS requires images in multiple planes, including transverse, sagittal, and oblique. The most effective transducer is the end-fire transducer in which two planes are directly centered along the long axis of the transducer. Rotation of the transducer allows multidirectional imaging. The patient is placed in the left lateral decubitus position with legs in the knee–chest position (51). No preparation such as a cleansing enema is usually necessary. A DRE always should be performed by the radiologist to identify abnormalities reported by the patient's physician and to correlate DRE results with the TRUS examination. The TRUS examination is then performed. The seminal vesicles and vas deferens are evaluated for symmetry. Special attention must be paid to the fat plane between the prostate and the seminal vesicles; obliteration of the fat planes suggests tumor invasion. The entire gland is scanned in the transverse plane from the base to the apex. Special attention is paid to the symmetry and echogenicity of the PZ. Next, the gland is viewed in the sagittal and parasagittal planes. The volume of prostate is calculated using the three

TABLE 7 ■ Indications for TRUS of Prostate

For detection of cancer	Positive DRE
	Elevated PSA
	Family history of prostate cancer
Others	Pre-TURP
	BPH
	Infertility
	Prostatodynia

Abbreviations: DRE, digital rectal examination; PSA, prostate-specific antigen; TRUS, transrectal ultrasound; TURP, transurethral resection of the prostate; BPH, benign prostatic hypertrophy.

dimensions (Fig. 5). PPSA for the patient is calculated and compared with the laboratory results of PSA. If the PSA level is greater than the PPSA for the prostate volume, the probability of cancer is increased. The volume of suspected tumor can be predicted by dividing the excess PSA (PSA–PPSA) by two (Tables 4 and 5) (9–12). During the examination, any suspicious-appearing hypoechoic area should be compressed by the probe to determine its elastic properties. This maneuver helps to expel fluid from the normal gland, making an infiltrating tumor more visible. Atrophy and BPH are compressible whereas prostate cancer is not (52).

Of all prostate cancer, 95% is adenocarcinoma (Table 8). Early tumors can be classified by three growth patterns: nodular, nodular with infiltrating components, and predominantly infiltrative (Table 9). Small, nodular, prostate cancers are always hypoechoic and are located in the PZ, adjacent to or in close proximity to the capsule. When neoplasms enlarge, they tend to invade the adjacent parenchyma in a pattern of least resistance, engulfing adjacent tissue and becoming relatively isoechoic (18). The presence of a hypoechoic lesion is not diagnostic of prostate cancer, and its absence does not rule out the disease. In our experience, the use of gray-scale ultrasound

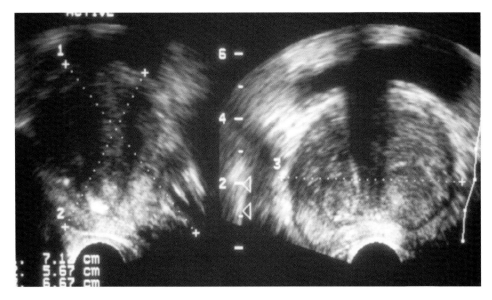

FIGURE 5 ■ The prostate volume is calculated using three dimensions (height × weight × width × 0.523). Calculated volume 140 cc.

TABLE 8 ■ Histologic Types of Prostate Cancer

- Adenocarcinoma 95%
- Others
- Transitional cell cancer
- Squamous cell cancer
- Sarcoma
- Carcinosarcoma
- Endometrioid cancer
- Small cell anaplastic cancer

alone in diagnosing prostate cancer resulted in a sensitivity of 41%, specificity of 81%, PPV of 52.7%, negative predictive value of 72%, and accuracy of 67% (51). Cancer must be suspected when the PZ architecture is distorted. CDI should be used to detect disorganized blood vessels and increased vascularity (Fig. 6) (43–48). The isodense echogenicity observed in certain tumors may reflect diffuse infiltration of the normal prostate by the tumor cells. The contours of both the prostatic and the surgical capsules may reveal bulging or asymmetry caused by these isodense tumors (Fig. 7).

Variations in histologic features and clinical staging are reflected in the ultrasound appearance (53,54). There is a direct relation between tumor volume, size, differentiation, and stage of disease. Tumors as small as 0.5 cc may be identified by TRUS. While they cannot be detected by palpation until they obtain a size of at least 1 cm (9–12,19,20,52).

Occasionally, cancers can be hyperechoic. Hyperechogenicity may be caused by the presence of dystrophic calcification in a necrotic tumor. These cancers usually are cribriform adenocarcinomas. On TRUS, they present as fine, often intense hyperechoic foci surrounded by a hypoechoic mass.

In summary, a meticulous search for abnormal masses is the most important part of any ultrasound examination of the prostate. Negative results may be encountered in patients with microscopic disease, diffuse multicentric involvement, or large infiltrative tumors. When tumor echogenicity is not helpful in identifying a

TABLE 9 ■ Tumor Patterns

Nodular (40%)
Hypoechoic caused by paucity of interfaces within the tumor mass.

Nodular infiltrating (30%)
Only nodular portion is recognized early.
Often, real size is not appreciated on TRUS.
Look for asymmetry of gland and architecture of PZ.
Use color Doppler.

Infiltrating (30%)
Nonvisible on TRUS.
Permeates normal tissue.
Look for asymmetry and subtle change in architecture.
Use color Doppler.

Abbreviations: PZ, peripheral zone; TRUS, transrectal ultrasound.

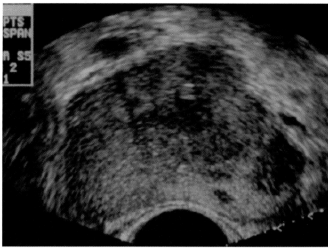

(A)

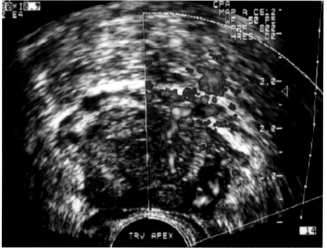

(B)

FIGURE 6 A AND B ■ (**A**) 53-year-old man with prostate volume 47 cc, predicted prostate-specific antigen (PSA) 5.2 (Table 4). (**B**) Hypoechoic, hypervascular mass is identified in the left apex using color Doppler.

lesion, additional findings may alert the radiologist to the presence of malignancy. Secondary signs described earlier may be the result of a space-occupying tumor producing a bulge of the prostatic capsule, asymmetry in the capsular contour, capsular disruption, loss of the seminal vesicle angle, or asymmetry of the neurovascular bundles (Fig. 7).

Color Doppler ultrasound (CDI) is a convenient and integral adjunct to gray-scale ultrasound. The recognition of increased or abnormal vascularity may improve both the depiction and the prediction of malignancy (Fig. 6) (Table 10). CDI is especially useful in detecting nonvisible infiltrating tumors. When CDI is added to transrectal gray-scale ultrasound findings, prostate cancer detection improves 10% to 20%. Transrectal CDI also improves the detection of higher-grade prostate cancer, and depicts hypervascularity, which is a marker for more aggressive tumors (Fig. 8B) (9,43–45,55–59).

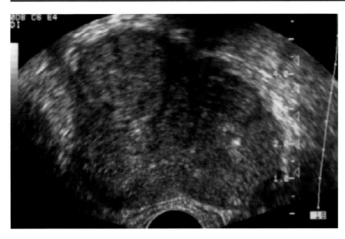

FIGURE 7 ■ Isodense, infiltrating tumor in a 60-year-old man with prostate-specific antigen (PSA) 9, gland volume 50 cc, predicted PSA 6.0, excess PSA 3. This is biopsy-proven adenocarcinoma.

BIOPSY

TRUS–guided biopsy of the prostate is essential for detecting prostate tumors. It is performed using a biopsy attachment on a transrectal probe (5–9 MHz) (Fig. 8). It is a safe, well-tolerated procedure that gives accurate histologic features of suspicious lesions (Table 11). Transrectal biopsy also allows staging by determining whether the cancer is organ confined or extends outside of the gland. Our transrectal-guided routine biopsy includes directed biopsy of abnormal masses (hypoechoic or isoechoic lesion with hypervascularity detected by CDI) and sextant biopsy of the rest of the gland (Figs. 9–11). Biopsy confirmation of the diagnosis is necessary because hypoechoic lesions in the PZ often are nonspecific. The PPV value of a hypoechoic lesion being a cancer is only 25% to 30%. In addition, biopsy of the contralateral PZ and central gland are performed to exclude isodense tumor (9,52–64).

Informed consent is obtained prior to biopsy. Complications of prostate biopsy include hematuria, rectal bleeding, hematospermia, urosepsis, and perineal pain. For analgesia, 20 cc of xylocaine gel is injected into the rectum. Using an 18-gauge automated gun, as many as 12 tissue cores are obtained (9,51–59). All patients take a prophylactic antibiotic such as 500 mg of ciprofloxacin one day prior to biopsy and for two days after. All biopsies are performed using a biopsy guide which permits accurate visualization and control of the needle path (Fig. 11) (51,52). The biopsy gun has a 2.5 cm fire length,

TABLE 10 ■ Differential Diagnosis of Hypervascular Lesions

- Tumor
- Infection
- Vascular malformation
- Postbiopsy arteriovenous fistulas

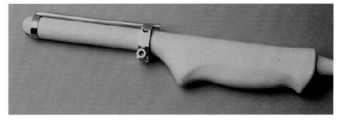

FIGURE 8 ■ Dedicated endorectal probe, broad bandwidth 5 to 9 MHz (Phillips), with biopsy guide attached to transducer.

thus the tip of the needle should be placed proximal to the biopsy site so that an appropriate core can be obtained. The biopsy needle is directed toward the lateral and anterior portion of the prostate parenchyma during sextant biopsy. Two targeted biopsies are added of any suspicious area seen on gray-scale or color Doppler ultrasound (47,55). We retrieve the cords out of the chamber of the needle and place them in sequence on labeled paper. The proximal end of the cord is identified for the pathologist according to the orientation of the specimen type and location (9,51,52,57,58).

TABLE 11 ■ TRUS Pitfalls for Prostate Cancer

Hypoechoic	Acute prostatitis or abscess
	Atypical hyperplasia
	Infarct
	Complex cyst
	Hematoma
	Blood vessel
	Fibrosis
	Periurethral smooth muscle in the anterior part of the prostate
	Muscles inverting into the prostate apex
Anechoic	Benign prostate cyst and ejaculatory cyst
	TURP defect
	Cystic carcinoma
	Cystic degeneration of glandular tissue caused by BPH
	Abscess
	Hematoma
	Abnormal vasculature
Isoechoic	Infarct
	Fibrosis
	Hematoma
	Atypical hyperplasia
	Granulomatous prostatitis
Hyperechoic	Fibrosis
	Chronic prostatitis
	Concentrations
	Comedocarcinoma

Abbreviations: TURP, transurethral resection of the prostate; BPH, benign prostatic hyperplasia; TRUS, transrectal ultrasound.

BIOPSY TECHNIQUE: TRUS+

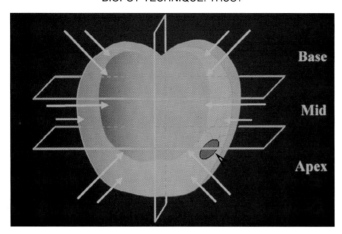

FIGURE 9 ▨ Coronal schematic diagram for targeted and sextant biopsy technique. Sextant biopsy technique includes sampling of both the peripheral and the central zones. *Arrowhead* indicates area for targeted biopsy. A systematic sextant biopsy of the entire gland would follow (*arrows*). TRUS, transrectal ultrasound.

Once the presence of prostate cancer is confirmed with a biopsy specimen, the tumor is staged and assigned a grade (Tables 12 and 13). The most common grading system is the Gleason score. This system is based on the glandular architecture of the most frequently seen histologic patterns. Each pattern is assigned a grade between 1 and 5. Grade 1 is the most differentiated. The sum of the grades or the Gleason score ranges from 2 to 10 (60,65–67).

Sextant biopsy results in dramatic increased sensitivity of sampling for prostate cancer. A substantial number of cancers occult at ultrasound have Gleason scores greater than six. Sextant biopsy is safe and should be mandatory in all patients with abnormal DRE results or elevated PSA levels, regardless of TRUS findings. The primary value of TRUS is to guide the systematic sampling of normal prostate parenchyma and abnormal prostate parenchyma. TRUS, even coupled with color Doppler, is not an adequate screening method for prostate carcinoma. Therefore, targeted biopsy should always be accompanied by complete sampling of the gland with sextant biopsy. Contraindications to biopsy include patients on anticoagulants or those who are taking more than one aspirin tablet (500 mg) per day (Table 14).

CONCLUSION

The traditional DRE gold standard for evaluating prostate carcinoma has been unsuccessful in detecting prostate cancer at a sufficiently early stage for effective treatment with either radical prostatectomy or radiation therapy. No single test, i.e., PSA, DRE, or TRUS coupled with color Doppler ultrasound, is sensitive enough to accurately detect prostate cancer or to predict the tumor's biologic potential. Although serum PSA and DRE findings identify men at high risk of having prostate cancer, progress in early diagnosis of prostate cancer is largely dependent on TRUS, which improves the specificity of PSA and allows accurate

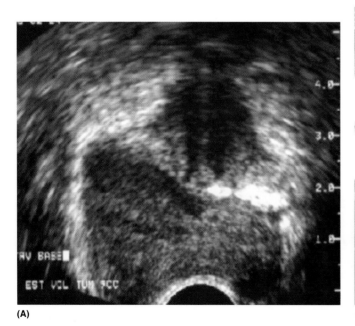

(A)

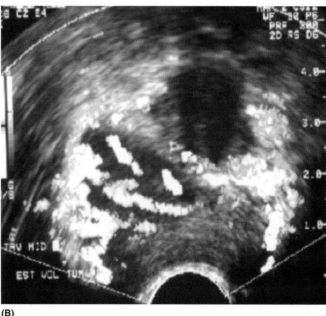

(B)

FIGURE 10 A–C ▨ Ultrasound (US) images in a 57-year-old man with prostate-specific antigen (PSA) level of 27.0 ng/mL, a predicted PSA level of 8.1 ng/mL, and prostatic adenocarcinoma (Gleason score, 8). (**A**) Transverse gray-scale US image shows a homogeneous isoechoic mass bulging from the right apex. (**B**) Color Doppler US image demonstrates increased blood flow within the mass. (*Continued*)

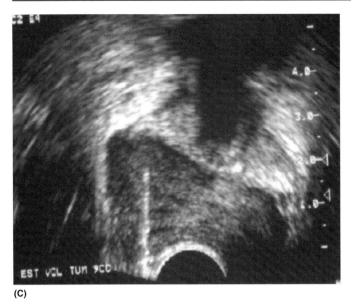

(C)

FIGURE 10 A–C ■ (*Continued*) (**C**) Biopsy of the mass was performed. US image shows the needle within the mass.

staging biopsies of nodules and hypervascular areas. A combination of DRE and PSA followed by TRUS and ultrasound-guided biopsy can detect clinically significant prostate cancers that are still confined to the gland and can be cured (Fig. 12). The false negative biopsy rate for detecting carcinoma is approximately 30% and approximately 25% of biopsies due to abnormal DRE or PSA detect cancer despite normal TRUS findings (7,51,68).

OTHER CLINICAL APPLICATIONS OF TRUS

Benign Prostatic Hyperplasia

BPH is a nonmalignant enlargement of the prostate commonly found in men older than 40 years (Fig. 4). It is caused by an excessive cellular growth of both the glandular and the stromal elements of the gland. It develops almost exclusively in the TZ, although about 5% originate in periurethral glandular tissue (69).

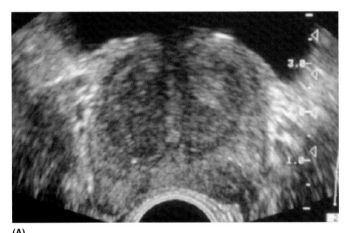

(A)

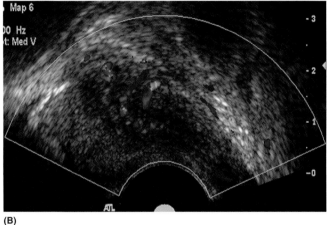

(B)

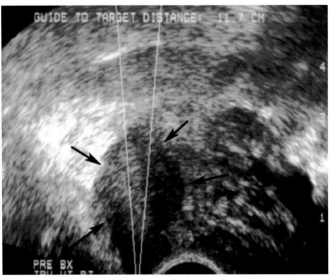

(C)

FIGURE 11 A–C ■ (**A**) 58-year-old with a negative gray-scale ultrasound examination. (**B**) Color Doppler image in sagittal plane showing abnormal vascularity. (**C**) Pre-biopsy cursor for needle guidance. This is biopsy-proven adenocarcinoma, Gleason score 7. *Arrows* show tumor.

TABLE 12 ■ TNM Staging of Prostate Cancer

Stage	Definition
T1	Tumor is an incidental histologic finding
1a	Three or fewer microscopic foci of carcinoma
1b	More than three microscopic foci
T2	Tumor present clinically or grossly limited to the gland
2a	Tumor ≤1.5 cm greatest dimension, with normal tissue on at least three sides
2b	Tumor >1.5 cm in greatest dimension, or in more than 1 lobe
T3	Tumor invades into the prostatic apex or into or beyond the capsule or bladder neck or seminal vesicle but is not fixed
T4	Tumor is fixed or invades adjacent structures other than those listed for T3
N0	No abnormal nodes
N1	Metastasis in a single node ≤2 cm
N2	Metastasis in a single node >2 cm but no more than 5 cm or multiple nodes with none >5 cm
N3	Metastasis in a lymph node, >5 cm in greatest dimension

Abbreviation: TNM, tumor node metastasis.

Glandular hyperplasia may be hyper- or hypoechoic with cystic areas, whereas stromal hyperplasia tends to be hypoechoic. The well-defined nodules that result can compress both the CZ and the PZ but do not infiltrate beyond the confines of the gland (19,20).

Infection

Prostatitis, especially in its acute stage, is primarily a clinical diagnosis and is rarely imaged. Patients with subacute and chronic prostatitis often are referred for imaging.

TABLE 13 ■ Whitmore–Jewett Staging System

A	Incidental findings, clinically nonpalpable and clinically unsuspected
	■ A1 focal
	■ A2 diffuse
B	Palpable but confined to prostate without extension through capsule
	■ B1 small discrete nodule ≤1.5 cm in size and involving one side of gland
	■ B2 single lesion >1.5 cm in size and involving one side of gland orbilateral lesions
C	Palpable and extension is beyond the prostatic capsule
	■ C1 minimal extracapsular involvement, periprostatic fat involvement
	■ C2 extracapsular tumor involvement of seminal vesicle
D	Metastases to distant areas
	■ D1 pelvic lymph node involvement
	■ D2 other organ involvement

TABLE 14 ■ Prostate Biopsy

Before biopsy:

- No aspirin, aspirin-containing products, or nonsteroidal medications [i.e., ibuprofen (Advil, Motrin), Neosporin] for 7 days before the biopsy
- If you are taking warfarin (Coumadin), be sure to notify your physician
- You will be given antibiotics for 4 days. You are to begin taking theantibiotic the day before the scheduled biopsy and will continuetaking the prescribed dosage until they are finished
- If you have a history of heart murmur, heart valve problems, or have any type of prosthesis, be sure to notify your physician because you may need additional antibiotics
- No preparation is required, you may eat breakfast or lunch
- Please attempt to have a bowel movement the morning of examination to ensure an empty rectum
- The biopsy itself may not be painful, but the pressure from the rectal examination may be uncomfortable

After biopsy, what to expect:

- It is vital to take the prescribed antibiotics as directed
- There may be some bleeding for the first few days in the urine and the stool
- It is common to see blood in the semen for the first few ejaculations after the biopsy
- If you experience continuous bleeding in the urine or from the rectum, call your physician
- Do not resume aspirin or nonsteroidal medications for at least 5 days after biopsy
- It is not unusual to have a low-grade fever; if you have a fever of >101°F, call your physician

Most prostatitis occurs in the PZ, where it produces diffuse hypoechogenicity or focal hypoechoic lesions, usually with associated hypervascularity. Chronic prostatitis can cause either band-like foci in the PZ or areas of atrophy.

Prostatitis may also occur in the central gland, most commonly after instrumentation or surgery. Abscess formation is rare, and it appears as a hypoechoic or anechoic lesion with a thick wall and good through transmission (Fig. 13). Abscesses occasionally may be hyperechoic because of gas-forming organisms. These abscesses can be easily drained using a one-stick transrectal approach (70).

Male Infertility

Until recently, the clinical evaluation of male infertility was limited by the inability to visualize directly and noninvasively the distal parts of the vas deferens, seminal vesicles, ejaculatory ducts, and prostate. Vasography was regarded as the best method for imaging these structures for many years. It is an invasive technique, which can cause iatrogenic scarring and occlusion of the vas deferens. Currently, CT and operative vasography have been almost totally replaced by TRUS, which provides superior visualization and identification of the many varieties of anomalies of the distal reproductive system (Fig. 14) (71).

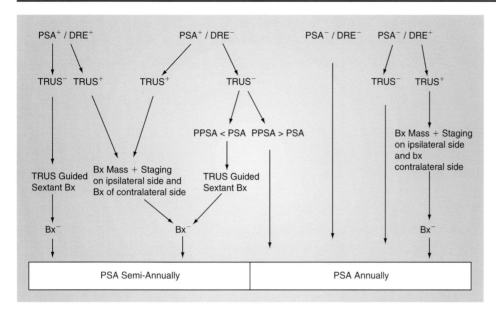

FIGURE 12 ■ Algorithm for detecting prostate cancer based on prostate-specific antigen and DRE. Bx, Biopsy; TRUS, transrectal ultrasound; DRE, digital rectal examination; PSA, prostate-specific antigen.

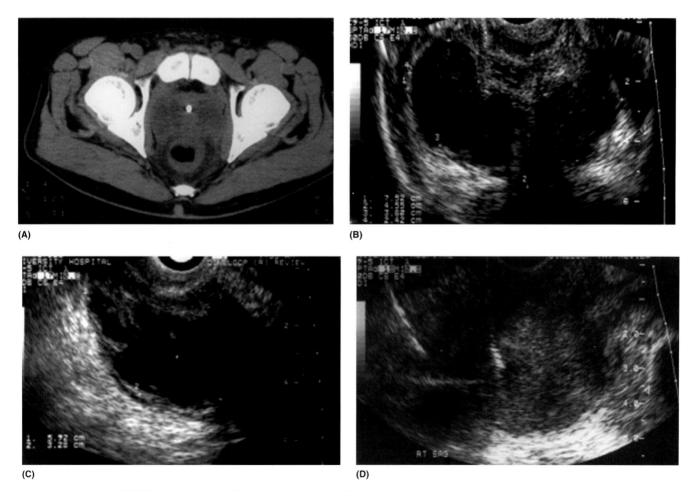

(A)

(B)

(C)

(D)

FIGURE 13 A–D ■ Middle-aged diabetic man with fever and dysuria. (A) Computed tomography of the pelvis showing Foley catheter in the prostatic urethra. (B and C) Gland is heterogeneous with multiple confluent, low attenuation areas. Axial and sagittal ultrasound clearly identifies abscess formation with a shaggy border. (D) 18-gauge needle inserted into the abscess cavity via transrectal route demonstrating complete drainage.

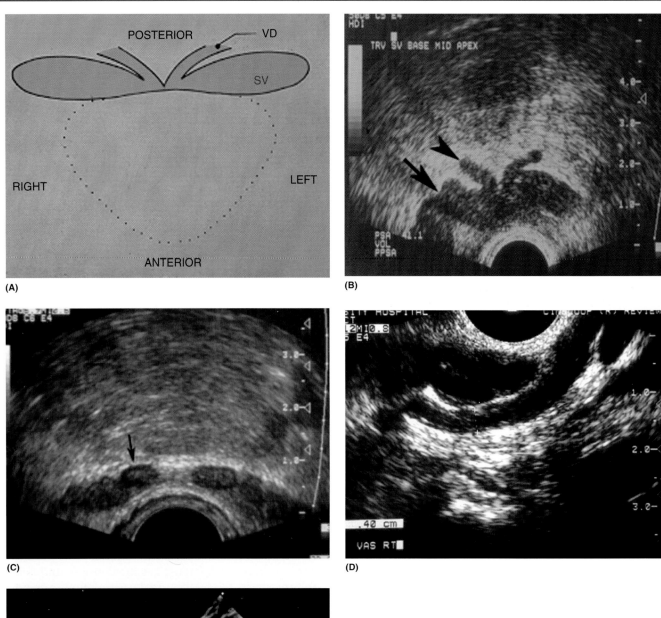

(A)

(B)

(C)

(D)

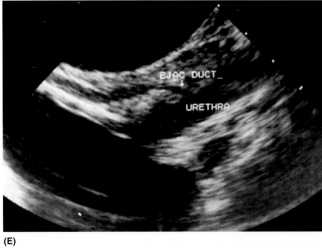

(E)

FIGURE 14 A–E ■ Normal anatomy of the seminal vesicles, vas deferens, and ejaculatory ducts. (**A**) Schematic drawing of seminal vesicles (SV) and vas deferens (VD). (**B**) Axial image showing vas deferens (*arrowhead*) and seminal vesicle (*arrow*). (**C**) Axial image of ampullary region of vas deferens (*arrow*). (**D**) Sagittal image of the vas deferens seen as a tubular structure medial and parallel to seminal vesicle (*cursor*). (**E**) Sagittal view shows ejaculatory duct (*arrow*) extending from the vas deferens to the prostatic urethra.

Anatomy of Seminal Vesicle, Vas Deferens, and Ejaculatory Duct

Superior to the prostate and posterior to the bladder are the seminal vesicles. They are hypoechoic compared with prostate parenchyma, with few fine internal echoes and a network of tubules with septations reflecting their saccular convoluted structure. In the axial plane, they have a bow-tie appearance. The seminal vesicles vary in size, shape, and degree of distention since they act as a reservoir for seminal fluid. They are usually symmetrical and measure no more than 3 ± 0.5 cm in length and 1.5 ± 0.4 cm in width, with an estimated mean volume of 13.7 ± 3.7 mL (41,71).

The vas deferens insert anteriorly and medially, joining the seminal vesicles to form the ampullary region on both sides. The vas deferens, including the ampullary portions, are well imaged in both axial and sagittal planes. In the axial plane, they are seen as a pair of oval, cystic structures located medial to the seminal vesicles and just cranial to the prostate gland. On sagittal planes, they can be identified as tubular structures projected medially to the seminal vesicles. The ejaculatory ducts are formed by the union of the seminal vesicles and the ampullary portion of the vas deferens. They cross the prostate obliquely and terminate in the prostatic urethra near the verumontanum. Normal ejaculatory ducts have a diameter of 2 mm and may be recognized on axial and sagittal planes. The entire course of ejaculatory ducts can be visualized on sagittal images (Fig. 14). The urethra divides the prostate into a proximal part from the bladder neck to the verumontanum and a distal part from the verumontanum to the external sphincter. The proximal and distal urethra form an angulation of approximately 35° at the verumontanum. The entire urethra is surrounded by periurethral glandular tissue.

Causes of Male Infertility

To define the causes of azoospermia, it is helpful to sub-classify patients into those with a low ejaculate (less than 1 mL) or a normal-volume ejaculate (above 1 mL) (68). Low-volume ejaculates may result from stenosis, obstruction, or anomalies of distal sperm transport system. Conditions that produce low-volume ejaculate with azoospermia or oligospermia include agenesis of the vas deferens or seminal vesicles, inflammatory strictures or obstruction of the vas deferens and seminal vesicle, ejaculatory duct obstruction, and urethral strictures. Low-volume ejaculate also can be caused by retrograde ejaculation. Retrograde ejaculation is secondary to neurologic conditions such as spinal cord injury, multiple sclerosis, or diabetes mellitus.

Normal-volume ejaculate with azoospermia or oligospermia is caused by testicular or other scrotal abnormalities (Fig. 15).

Seminal Vesicles and Vas Deferens

The seminal vesicles are important in the elaboration of the seminal plasma, constituting 80% to 90% of the ejaculate volume. They also secrete fructose and prostaglandins and maintain an alkaline pH. Congenital anomalies in the

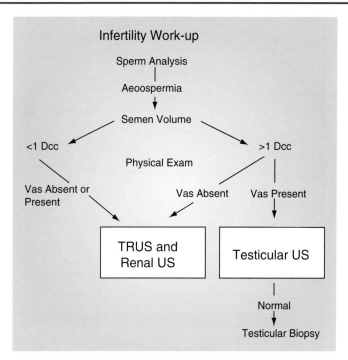

FIGURE 15 ■ Algorithm for management of male infertility. TRUS, transrectal ultrasound; US, ultrasound.

seminal vesicles, as well as obstructive lesions, result in diminished semen volume, low pH, and low fructose levels (72–76).

The congenital defects that produce infertility are caused by developmental abnormalities that occur at approximately 35 days of gestation when the fetus has a crown–rump length of 8 mm. Seminal vesicle abnormalities are reported to occur in 92% of patients with agenesis of the vas deferens. We found seminal vesicle abnormalities in all patients with bilateral or unilateral agenesis of the vas deferens. The incidence of unilateral vasal aplasia in the healthy male population is one to seven per 1000 individuals (Fig. 16) (76–79). Congenital bilateral absence of vas deferens occurs in approximately 1% of infertile men and accounts for between 4% and 17% of cases with azoospermia (Fig. 17). Between 16% and 43% of patients with agenesis of the vas deferens also have renal anomalies such as agenesis, crossed renal ectopia, or an ectopic pelvic kidney, usually on the left side. These patients usually are found to be heterozygous for the cystic fibrosis gene.

Seminal vesicle cysts can be either congenital or acquired secondary to obstructive lesions. Congenital seminal vesicle cysts are rare and usually are associated with either an ectopic ureter draining into the seminal vesicles, with unilateral renal agenesis, or with other genitourinary anomalies. These cysts occasionally become infected or hemorrhagic (Fig. 18).

When an infection involves the seminal vesicles primarily, fibrotic changes may produce cystic dilation or obliteration of the lumen. The seminal vesicles can be identified as echogenic nonhomogeneous structure lacking normal convoluted ductal architecture. Chronic inflammation may decrease seminal vesicle function and cause infertility.

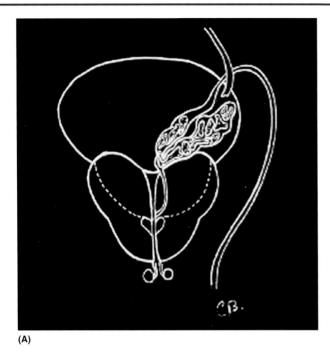

(A)

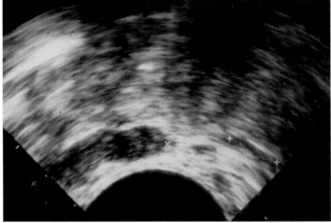

(B)

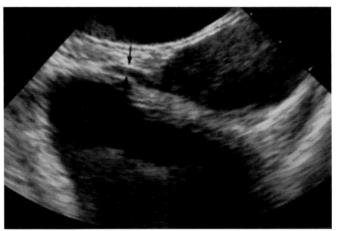

(C)

FIGURE 16 A–C ■ **(A)** Congenital unilateral vasal and seminal vesicle aplasia. **(B)** Axial and **(C)** sagittal images of the same patient show unilateral absence of the left vas deferens.

Stone formation is another sequela of seminal vesicle infection. TRUS readily demonstrates stones as echogenic foci with acoustic shadowing in the seminal vesicles (Fig. 19). Stones and cysts may form in the vas deferens, producing obstruction of sperm and infertility (Figs. 20 and 21).

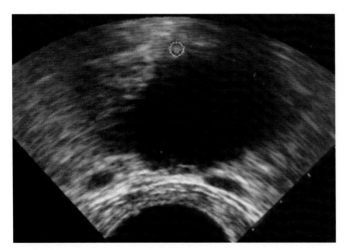

FIGURE 17 ■ Transverse image demonstrates bilateral absence of vas deferens and seminal vesicle.

Ejaculatory Ducts

TRUS is useful in detecting the various anatomic abnormalities associated with complete and partial ejaculatory duct obstruction or stenosis. Because the ejaculatory duct is formed by the confluence of the duct of the seminal vesicle and the terminal ampullary region of the vas in the prostate, an occlusion of the ejaculatory duct results in the diminished semen volume (77). Determining the level of ductal obstruction is critical in managing these patients. With meticulous examination, the ejaculatory duct can be visualized in many cases (Fig. 14e). The entire course of the ejaculatory duct can be visualized only on sagittal images. The precise level and nature of obstructing lesions usually are identified in this view (Fig. 22). This information often is essential for the planning and execution of potentially corrective surgery.

Midline Prostate Cysts

Midline cysts are variably referred to as ejaculatory duct cysts, Müllerian duct cysts, and urogenital sinus cysts. The orifices of the ejaculatory ducts enter into the cyst, and so these cysts contain sperm. They may obstruct the free flow of seminal fluid during ejaculation. The sonographic features of cysts in the ejaculatory duct are

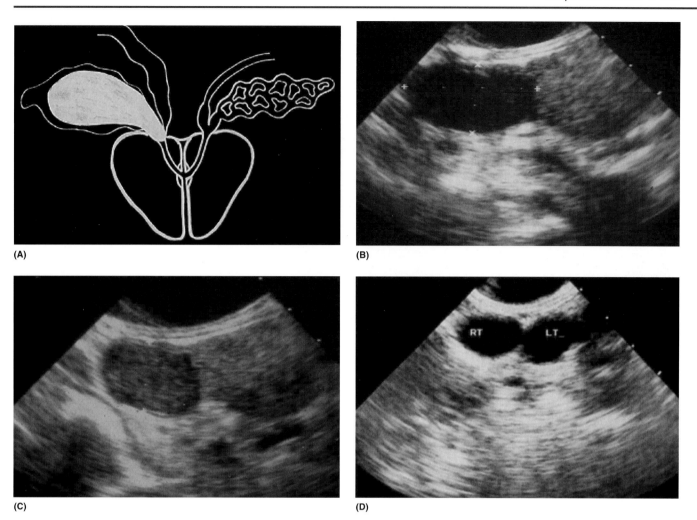

(A)

(B)

(C)

(D)

FIGURE 18 A–D ▓ (**A**) Diagram of a right seminal vesicle cyst. (**B**) Sagittal view demonstrates a right seminal vesicle simple cyst. (**C**) A cyst containing uniform low-level echoes, most likely represents a hemorrhagic cyst (*cursors*). (**D**) Axial view demonstrates bilateral cysts of the vas deferens.

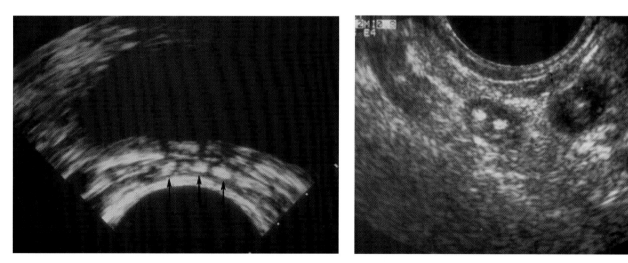

FIGURE 19 ▓ Axial view of seminal vesicle demonstrates multiple stones (*arrows*).

FIGURE 20 ▓ Axial view of the vas deferens. There are two stones in the right vas deferens and one in the left.

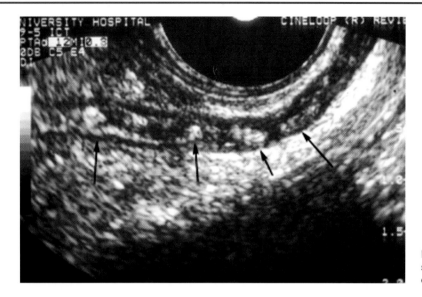

FIGURE 21 ■ 35-year-old infertile male with multiple stones causing obstruction. Sagittal section of vas deferens filled with multiple stones (*arrows*).

variable. Although they are easy to identify, it is not always possible to classify them precisely. When large, they may be difficult to distinguish from prostatic cysts (Fig. 23).

MANAGEMENT

Congenital and acquired ductal anomalies may be amenable to either radiologic or surgical intervention. Determination of the suitability for intervention and the choice of the optimum therapeutic approach demand the precise delineation of the nature and level of each abnormality. In general, distal ductal anomalies can be classified as surgically correctable or nonsurgically correctable depending on the location of the obstruction or occlusion. Surgically correctable causes of infertility are confined to lesions involving the distal two-thirds of the ejaculatory ducts, including ejaculatory duct cysts, calculi, fibrosis, and calcification. Agenesis, obstruction, or occlusion of the duct system above this level is, by definition, nonsurgically correctable, and fertility can be achieved only by epididymal aspiration followed by in vitro fertilization (41,71,80–82).

If a midline cyst or an ejaculatory duct calculus is identified, the optimum surgical approach is simple transurethral resection of the verumontanum. Cysts above the level of prostate can be effectively treated with TRUS -guided needle aspiration. Cyst aspiration may be therapeutic in two ways: Decompression of the cyst may help relieve proximal ductal obstruction, and such cysts may contain spermatozoa, which, if viable, can be used for in vitro fertilization (Fig. 24).

In summary, TRUS is the best method to identify and characterize potentially curable lesions.

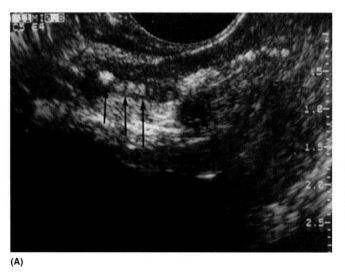

(A)

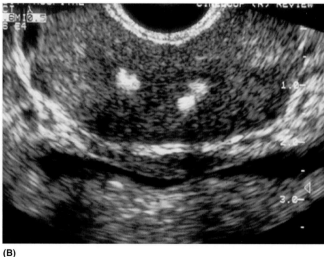

(B)

FIGURE 22 A AND B ■ (**A**) Sagittal section of ejaculatory duct containing multiple stones (*arrows*). (**B**) Transverse image of prostate gland showing heavy calcification in both ejaculatory ducts.

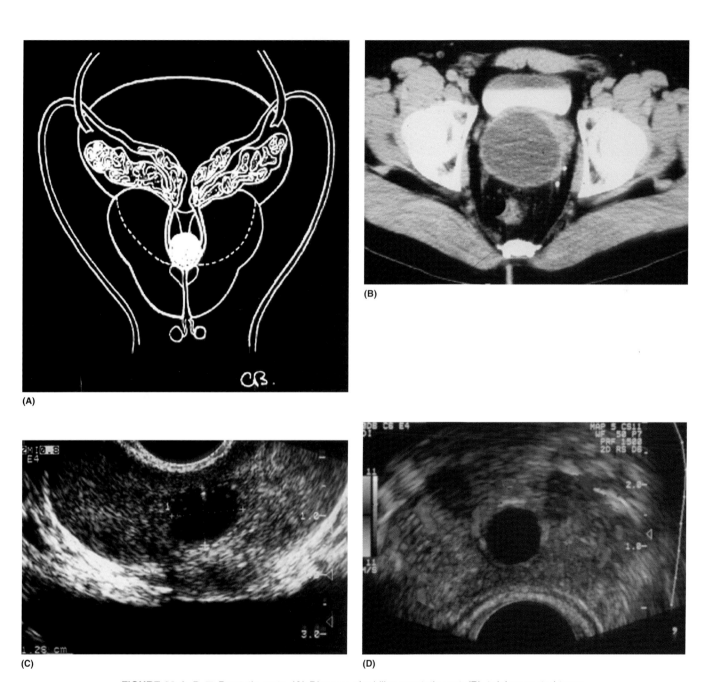

(A)

(B)

(C)

(D)

FIGURE 23 A–D ■ Prostatic cysts. (**A**) Diagram of midline prostatic cyst. (**B**) Axial computed tomography image through prostate showing large midline cyst. (**C**) Prostatic cyst (*cursor*). (**D**) Color Doppler ultrasound of the cyst shows peripheral vascularity.

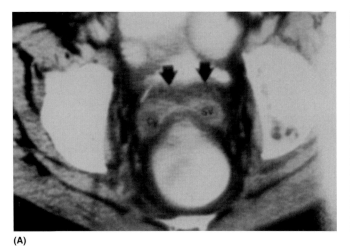

(A)

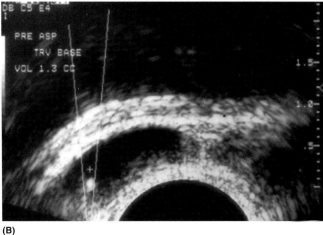

(B)

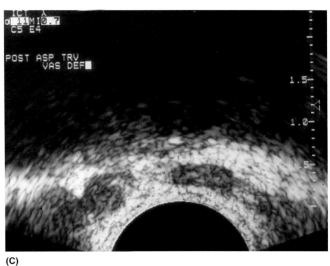

(C)

FIGURE 24 A–C ▨ **(A)** Seminal vesicle cysts noted on computed tomography scan (*arrows*). **(B)** Cyst aspiration performed. 1.3 cc of fluid with sperm was aspirated and sent for in vitro fertilization. The same procedure was performed on the opposite side. **(C)** Post procedure normal seminal vesicle.

REFERENCES

1. Jemal A, Murray T, Ward E, et al. Cancer statistics, 2005. CA Cancer J Clin 2005; 55:10–30.
2. Pienta KJ, Smith DC. Advances in prostate cancer chemotherapy: a new era begins. CA Cancer J Clin 2005; 55:300–318.
3. Weir HK, Thun MJ, Hankey BF, et al. Annual Report to the Nation on the Status of Cancer, 1975–2000, featuring the uses of surveillance data for cancer prevention and control. J Natl Cancer Inst 2003; 95(17):1276–1299.
4. Slawin KM, Ohori M, Dillioglugil O, et al. Screening for prostate cancer: an analysis of the early experience. CA Cancer J Clin 1995; 45:134.
5. Amis ES. Prostate cancer 1995: epidemiology, prognostic factors, diagnosis and imaging. Chicago: RSNA, 1995:course no. 407.
6. Mettlin C, Jones G, Averett H, et al. Defining and updating the ACS guidelines for the cancer related check-up: prostate and endometrial cancer. CA Cancer J Clin 1995; 43:42.
7. McNaughton-Collins M, Ransohoff DF, Barry MJ. Early detection of prostate cancer: serendipity strikes again. JAMA 1997; 278:1516–1519.
8. Benson MC, McMahon DJ, Cooner WH, et al. An algorithm for prostate cancer detection in a patient population using prostate specific antigen and prostate specific antigen density. World J Urol 1993; 11:206–213.
9. Lee F, Torp-Pedersen ST, Siders DB, et al. Transrectal ultrasound in the diagnosis and staging of prostatic carcinoma. Radiology 1989; 170:609–615.
10. Lee F, Littrup PJ, Torp-Pedersen ST, et al. Prostate cancer: comparison of transrectal US and digital rectal examination for screening. Radiology 1988; 168:389–394.
11. Lee F, Littrup PJ, Loft-Christensen L, et al. Predicted prostate specific antigen results using transrectal ultrasound gland volume. Cancer 1992; 70:211–220.
12. Lee F, Littrup PJ. The role of digital rectal examination, transrectal ultrasound, and prostate specific antigen for the detection of confined and clinically relevant prostate cancer. J Cell Biochem Suppl 1992; 16:69–73.
13. Catalona WJ, Smith DS, Ratliff TL, et al. Measurement of prostate-specific antigen in serum as a screening test for prostate cancer. N Engl J Med 1991; 324:1156.
14. Brawer MK, Lange PH. PSA in the screening, staging and follow up of early-stage prostate cancer: a review of recent developments. World J Urol 1989; 7:7.
15. Brawer MK, Beattie J, Wener MH, et al. Screening for prostate carcinoma with prostate specific antigen: results of the second year. J Urol 1993; 150:106.
16. Brawer MK, Beatie J, Wener MH. PSA as the initial test in prostate carcinoma screening: results of the third year. J Urol 1993; 149(suppl):299A.
17. Catalona WJ, Smith DS, Ornstein DK. Prostate cancer detection in men with serum PSA concentrations of 2.6 to 4.0 ng/mL and benign prostate examination. Enhancement of specificity with free PSA measurements. JAMA 1997; 277:1452–1455.

18. Catalona WJ, Richie JP, Ahmann FR, et al. Comparison of digital rectal examination and serum prostate specific antigen in the early detection of prostate cancer: results of a multicenter clinical trial of 6630 men. J Urol 1994; 151:1283.

19. Lee F, Siders DB, Torp-Pedersen ST, et al. Prostate cancer: transrectal ultrasound and pathology comparison. Cancer 1991; 67:1132.

20. Lee F Jr, Bronson JP, Lee F, et al. Nonpalpable cancer of the prostate: assessment with transrectal US. Radiology 1991; 178:197.

21. Rubens DJ, Gottlieb RH, Maldonado CE Jr, et al. Clinical evaluation of prostate biopsy parameters: gland volume and elevated prostate-specific antigen level. Radiology 1996; 199:159.

22. Baran GW, Golin AL, Bergsma CJ, et al. Biologic aggressiveness of palpable and nonpalpable prostate cancer: assessment with endosonography. Radiology 1991; 178:201.

23. Cupp MR, Osterling JE. Prostate-specific antigen, digital rectal examination, and transrectal ultrasonography: their roles in diagnosing early prostate cancer. Mayo Clin Proc 1993; 68:297.

24. Ruckle HC, Klee GG, Osterling JE. Prostate-specific antigen: critical issues for the practicing physician. Mayo Clin Proc 1994; 69:59.

25. Pollack HM, Resnick MI. Prostate-specific antigen and screening for prostate cancer: much ado about something. Radiology 1993; 189:353.

26. Brawer MK. How to use prostate-specific antigen in the early detection or screening for prostatic carcinoma. CA Cancer J Clin 1995; 45:148.

27. Stamey TA. Prostate specific antigen. N Engl J Med 1987; 317:909.

28. Stamey TA, Freiha FS, McNeal JE, et al. Localized prostate cancer: relationship of tumor volume to clinical significance for treatment of prostate cancer. Cancer 1993; 71(suppl 3):933.

29. Benson MC, Whang IS, Pantuck A, et al. Prostate specific antigen density: a means of distinguishing benign prostatic hypertrophy and prostate cancer. J Urol 1992; 147:815.

30. Carter HB, Pearson JD, Metter EJ, et al. Longitudinal evaluation of prostate-specific antigen levels in men with and without prostate disease. JAMA 1992; 267:2215–2220.

31. Easthm JA, Riedel E, Scardino PT, et al. Variation of serum prostate-specific antigen levels. An evaluation of year-to-year fluctuations. JAMA 2003; 289:2695–2700.

32. Bo M, Ventura M, Marinello R, Capello S, Casetta G, Fabris F. Relationship between prostatic specific antigen (PSA) and volume of the prostate in the benign prostatic hyperplasia in the elderly. Crit Rev Oncol Hematol 2003; 47:207–211.

33. Benson MC, Whang IS, Olsson CA, et al. The use of prostate specific antigen density to enhance the predictive value of intermediate levels of serum prostate specific antigen. J Urol 1992; 147:817–821.

34. Kane RA, Littrup PJ, Babaian R, et al. PSA levels in 1695 men without evidence of prostate cancer: findings of the American Cancer Society National Prostate Cancer Detection Project. Cancer 1992; 69:1201.

35. Semjonow A, Hamm M, Rathert P, et al. Prostate-specific antigen corrected for prostate volume improves differentiation of benign prostatic hyperplasia and organ-confined prostatic cancer. Br J Urol 1994; 73:538–543.

36. Osterling JE, Jacobsen SJ, Chute CG, et al. Serum prostate-specific antigen in a community-based population of healthy men. JAMA 1993; 270:860.

37. Christensson A, Björk T, Nilsson O, et al. Serum prostate specific antigen complexed to α1-antichymotrypsin as an indicator of prostate cancer. J Urol 1993; 150:100.

38. Catalona WJ. New PSA assay might avoid three out of four biopsies. Oncol News Int 1995; (suppl):1.

39. Partin AW, Kelly CA, Subong ENP, et al. Measurement of the ratio of free PSA to total PSA improves prostate cancer detection for men with total PSA levels between 4.0 and 10.0 ng/mL. Proc Am J Urol Assoc 1995; 153(suppl):295A.

40. Wang TJ, Hill T, Norton K, et al. Specific immunoassay for free PSA and its clinical relevance. Proc Am J Urol Assoc 1995; 153(suppl):295A.

41. McNeal JE. Regional morphology and pathology of the prostate. Am J Clin Pathol 1968; 49:347.

42. McNeal JE. Normal anatomy of the prostate and changes in benign prostatic hypertrophy and carcinoma. Semin Ultrasound CT MRI 1988; 9:329.

43. Newman JS, Bree RL, Rubin JM. Prostate cancer: diagnosis with color Doppler sonography with histologic correlation of each biopsy site. Radiology 1995; 195:86–90.

44. Alexander AA. To color doppler image the prostate or not: that is the question. Radiology 1995; 195:11.

45. Kelly IM, Lees WR, Rickards D. Prostate cancer and the role of color Doppler US. Radiology 1993; 189:153–156.

46. Rifkin MD, Sudakoff GS, Alexander AA. Prostate: techniques, results, and potential applications of color Doppler US scanning. Radiology 1993; 186:509–513.

47. Halpern EJ, Strup SE. Using gray-scale and color and power Doppler sonography to detect prostate cancer. AJR Am J Roentgenol 2000; 174:623–627.

48. Cornud F, Belin X, Helenon O, et al. Color Doppler US of prostatic nodules: correlation with prostate specific antigen levels and US-guided biopsy [abstr]. Radiology 1998; 209(P).

49. Cornud F, Belin X, Piron D, et al. Color Doppler-guided prostate biopsies in 591 patients with an elevated serum PSA level: impact on Gleason score for nonpalpable lesions. Urology 1997; 49:709–715.

50. Louvar E, Littrup PJ, Goldstein A, et al. Correlation of color Doppler flow in the prostate with tissue microvascularity. Cancer 1998; 83:135–140.

51. Kuligowska E, Barish MA, Fenlon HM, et al. Predictors of prostate carcinoma: accuracy of gray-scale and color Doppler US and serum markers. Radiology 2001; 220:757–764.

52. Lee F, Littrup PJ, Kumasaka GH, et al. The use of transrectal ultrasound in the diagnosis, guided biopsy, staging and screening of prostate cancer. Radiographics 1987; 7:627.

53. Agha AH, Bane BL, Culkin DJ. Cystic carcinoma of the prostate. J Ultrasound Med 1996; 15:75.

54. Lile R, Thickman D, Miller GJ, et al. Prostatic comedocarcinoma: correlation of sonograms with pathologic specimens in three cases. AJR Am J Roentgenol 1990; 155:303.

55. Lavoipierre AM, Snow RM, Frydenberg M, et al. Prostatic cancer: role of color Doppler imaging in transrectal sonography. AJR Am J Roentgenol 1998; 171:205–210.

56. Ohori M, Egawa S, Shinohara K, et al. Detection of microscopic extracapsular extension prior to radical prostatectomy for clinically localized prostate cancer. Br J Urol 1994; 74:72–79.

57. Littrup PJ, Sparshu R. Transrectal ultrasound and prostate cancer risks: the "tailored" prostate biopsy. Cancer 1995; 75:1805–1813.

58. Littrup PJ, Klein RM, Gross M, et al. Color Doppler guides prostate biopsies to higher grade cancers; racial implications [abstr]. J Urol 1996; 155(474A):158.

59. Ismail M, Petersen RO, Alexander AA, et al. Color Doppler imaging in predicting the biologic behavior of prostate cancer: correlation with disease-free survival. Urology 1997; 50:906–912.

60. Lee F, Siders DB, Newby JE, et al. The role of transrectal ultrasound-guided staging biopsy and androgen ablation therapy prior to radical prostatectomy. Clin Invest Med 1993; 16:458.

61. Lee F, Littrup PJ, McLeary RD, et al. Needle aspiration and core biopsy of prostate cancer: comparative evaluation with biplanar transrectal us guidance. Radiology 1987; 163:515.

62. Lee F, Torp-Pedersen ST, Siders DB. Use of transrectal ultrasound in diagnosis, guided biopsy, staging, and screening of prostate cancer. Urology 1989; 23(suppl 6):7.

63. Bastacky SI, Walsh PC, Epstein JI. Relationship between perineural tumor invasion on needle biopsy and radical prostatectomy capsular penetration in clinical stage B adenocarcinoma of the prostate. Am J Surg Pathol 1993; 17:336.

64. Narayan P, Gajendran V, Taylor SP, et al. The role of transrectal ultrasound-guided biopsy-based staging, perioperative serum prostate-specific antigen, and biopsy Gleason score in prediction of final pathologic diagnosis in prostate cancer. Urology 1995; 46:202.

65. Olson MC, Posniak HV, Fisher SG, et al. Directed and random biopsies of the prostate: indications based on combined results of transrectal sonography and prostate-specific antigen density determinations. AJR Am J Roentgenol 1994; 163:1407.

66. Littrup PJ. Bailey SE. Prostate cancer: the role of transrectal ultrasound and its impact on cancer detection and management. Radiol Clin N Am 2000; 38:87–113.

67. Dyke CH, Toi A, Sweet JM. Value of random US-guided transrectal prostate biopsy. Radiology 1990; 176:345–349.

68. Stewart CS, Leibovich BC, Weaver AL, Lieber MM. Prostate cancer diagnosis using a saturation needle biopsy after previous negative sextant biopsies. J Urol 2001; 166:86–91.

69. Oesterling JE. Benign prostatic hyperplasia: medical and minimally invasive treatment options. N Engl J Med 1995; 332:99.

70. Kuligowska E, Keller E, Ferrucci JT. Treatment of pelvic abscesses: value of one-step sonographically guided transrectal needle aspiration and lavage. AJR Am J Roentgenol 1995; 164:201.

71. Kuligowska E, Fenlon HM. Transrectal US in male infertility: spectrum of findings and role in patient care. Radiology 1998; 207:173–181.

72. Gevenois PA, Van Sinoy ML, Sintzoff SA, et al. Cysts of the prostate and seminal vesicles: MR imaging findings in 11 patients. AJR Am J Roentgenol 1990; 155:1021–1024.

73. King BF, Hattery RR, Lieber MM, et al. Congenital cystic disease of the seminal vesicles. Radiology 1991; 178:207–211.

74. Ejeckam GC, Govatsos S, Lewis AS. Cyst of seminal vesicle associated with ipsilateral renal agenesis. Urology 1984; 24:372–374.

75. Heany JA, Pfister RC, Meares EM. Giant cyst of the seminal vesicle with renal agenesis. AJR Am J Roentgenol 1987; 149:139–140.

76. Weingardt JP, Townsend RR, Russ PD, et al. Seminal vesicle cysts associated with autosomal dominant polycystic kidney disease detected by sonography. J Ultrasound Med 1995; 14: 475–477.

77. Meacham RB, Hellerstein DK, Lipshultz LI. Evaluation and treatment of ejaculatory duct obstruction in the infertile male. Fertil Steril 1993; 59:393–397.

78. Asch MR, Toi A. Seminal vesicles: imaging and intervention using transrectal ultrasound. J Ultrasound Med 1991; 10:19–23.

79. Costabile RA. Infertility: is there anything we can do about it? J Urol 1997; 157:158–159.

80. Namiki M. Recent concepts in the management of male infertility. Int J Urol 1996; 3:249–255.

81. Madgar I, Seidman DS, Levran D, et al. Micromanipulation improves in-vitro fertilization results after epididymal or testicular sperm aspiration in patients with congenital absence of the vas deferens. Human Reprod 1996; 11:2151–2154.

82. Schlegel PN, Girardi SK. Clinical review 87: in vitro fertilization for male factor infertility. J Clin Endocrinol Metab 1997; 82: 709–716.

Scrotum and Testes ● *Eugenio O. Gerscovich*

35

INTRODUCTION

Since the pioneering work in 1974 by Miskin and Bain (1), who described the ultrasound appearance of the testes with static B-mode methods, the technology and applications of ultrasound have greatly expanded. The incorporation of real-time, "standoff" pads, high-frequency transducers, and pulsed and color Doppler has made ultrasound the most frequently used imaging modality in evaluation of the scrotum. Ultrasound has the advantages of general availability, portability, high resolution, functional information (blood flow), and relatively low cost. Limitations of the technique are its high dependency on the quality of the equipment and the expertise of the operator. Nuclear medicine, computed tomography (CT), magnetic resonance imaging (MRI), and, to a lesser degree, venous angiography play complementary roles in the imaging of special situations. Indications for ultrasound are listed in Table 1.

Regarding the biologic effects of ultrasound on the direct examination of the male gonads, Grunberger et al. (2) studied 10 men undergoing bilateral orchidectomies for prostatic carcinoma on whom the testes were subjected preoperatively to a 15-minute exposure to conventional ultrasound, followed by studies of the specimens under electron microscopy. No ultrastructural abnormalities and no detectable differences were found when compared with healthy testes. Previous studies that demonstrated changes were based on sound intensity and time exposure that far exceed today's accepted standards (3).

ULTRASOUND TECHNIQUE

The examination should be performed in a room that affords privacy. It should be warm, to avoid a cremasteric reflex (more pronounced in children), which pulls the testes upward, possibly outside the scrotal sac. With the patient in a supine position, a sling is made with a small towel between the proximal thighs to hold the scrotum anteriorly. A second small towel holds the penis on the anterior aspect of the lower abdominal wall. Physical examination is used to find the position, size, and consistency of the testes and to locate a possible area of disease. When a second person, or a foot pedal, is available for freezing and printing sonographic images, the examiner is able to immobilize the appropriate part of the patient's scrotum and testes with one hand while scanning with the other.

High-frequency linear transducers in the range of 8 to 15 MHz with color Doppler capability are necessary. Frequencies of 8 and 10 MHz are preferred in adults and 10 to 15 MHz in children. For color Doppler studies, one should use the highest possible power output, lowest scale and wall filter, and optimal gain.

Scanning parameters should be optimized on the supposedly normal testis, which is imaged first. Then, without changing the parameters, the contralateral side should be imaged. This recommendation applies to both gray-scale and color Doppler techniques. Long and short axis views of the testes and scrotum are obtained for documentation (Fig. 1A and B). It is

TABLE 1 ■ Indications for Scrotal Ultrasound

- Pain: trauma, inflammation, torsion
- Mass: testicular, extratesticular
- Evaluation of a possible hernia and its contents
- Search for occult neoplasm in cases of retroperitoneal or mediastinal lymphadenopathy
- Follow-up of previous infections, tumors, lymphoma, leukemia
- Small testes, atrophy
- Location of undescended testes
- Infertility
- Precocious puberty or feminization

important to understand the high mobility of the testes and because of that, the long and short axes of the testes might not correspond to the same planes as in the patient's body. Side-by-side gray-scale and color images of both testes should be made for comparison (Fig. 2). In the case of a nonapparent but suspected varicocele or inguinal hernia,

the patient is scanned during a Valsalva maneuver or while he is standing. If a tumor of the testis is found and no previous abdominal imaging has been done, the peri-aortic and renal hilar regions should be searched for possible lymphadenopathy.

PITFALLS IN SONOGRAPHIC TECHNIQUE

Incorrect Measurements ■ Failure to find the true long and short axes of the testes will result in incorrect and asymmetrical sizes.

Comparison of Both Testes ■ Comparison of the ultrasound texture and vascularity of the presumed normal testis with the testis of clinical concern is important. This comparison is especially important in certain circumstances. For instance, in disease processes that diffusely affect the testis, such as inflammation, or infiltrative processes, such as leukemia, the alteration of echotexture and blood flow may be so subtle that unless comparison is

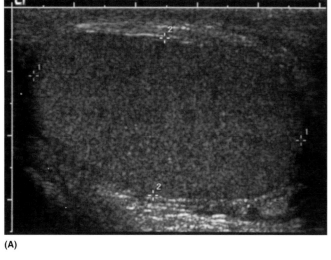

(A)

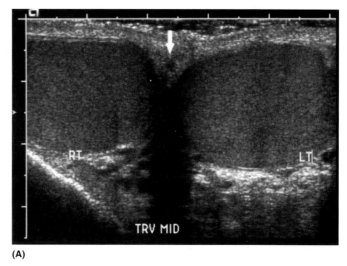

(A)

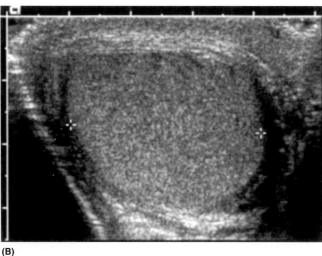

(B)

FIGURE 1 A AND B ■ Normal adult testis (*calipers*). (**A**) Longitudinal view. (**B**) Axial view.

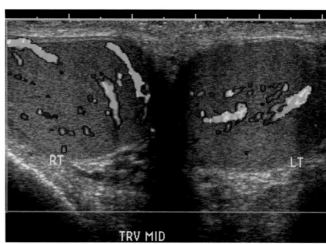

(B)

FIGURE 2 A AND B ■ Comparative view of both testes on axial views. (**A**) Gray scale. (**B**) Color Doppler. *Arrow*, median raphe.

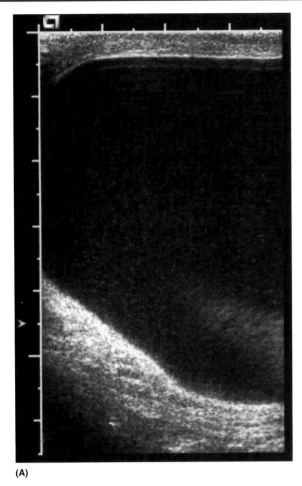

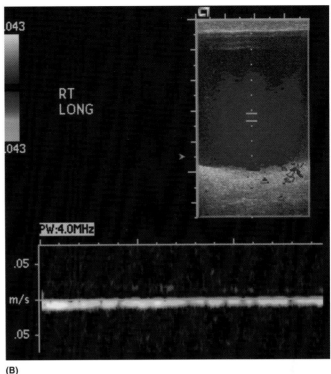

(B)

FIGURE 3 A AND B ■ Phenomenon of acoustic streaming in a large hydrocele. (**A**) Gray-scale image showing fluid with microparticles in suspension, which are energized and displaced away from the transducer resulting in color signal and slow laminar flow tracing on Doppler. (**B**) Color and pulsed Doppler.

(A)

made with the normal testis, it may be missed. This is illustrated in other figures within the text. Comparison might be misleading when the pathology is bilateral.

False-Positive Scrotal Calcifications ■ When examining the scrotum, care must be taken lest the fingers of the operator's hand holding the scrotum mimic scrotal wall calcifications. Foreign bodies may also simulate calcifications within the scrotum. Historical information is important in this regard.

Doppler Color Signal in Scrotal Cysts and Hydrocele ■ It is due to the phenomenon of acoustic streaming and it should not be interpreted as true blood flow (Fig. 3) (4).

SONOGRAPHIC ANATOMY

The testis at birth measures approximately 1.5 × 1 cm. At this time, the epididymis is proportionately larger than in the adult (Fig. 4). At three months of age, the testis slightly increases in size because of the rise in testosterone levels and then slightly decreases at six months. It remains constant until the age of six years, when it slowly starts to enlarge in the pubescent period. In elderly men, the testes again regress and become smaller than in younger men. The adult testis has an ovoid shape and measures 3 to 5 cm in length and 2 to 3 cm in the anteroposterior and

transverse diameters, respectively (Fig. 1). Slight size difference between both sides is normal. The echogenicity of the testis is of medium level. It has been compared to that of the thyroid gland and is thought to result from the presence of the seminiferous tubules. The tubules, which are the site of spermatogenesis, are arranged in

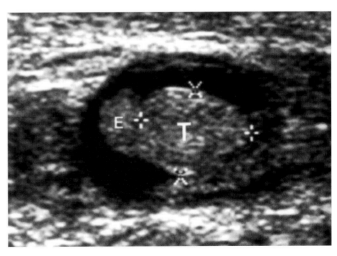

FIGURE 4 ■ Newborn testis showing a proportionally large epididymal head as compared to the testis itself. E, epididymis; T (*calipers*), testis.

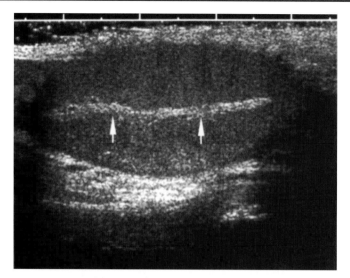

FIGURE 5 ▨ Longitudinal view of a testis at the mediastinum (*arrows*).

approximately 250 to 400 separate lobules that cannot be distinguished individually by ultrasound. The septa that separate them (not visualized) converge toward the posterior aspect of the testis, where the mediastinum (hilum) is identified. It is seen by ultrasound as a linear echogenic structure (Fig. 5). The testis is surrounded by a fibrous capsule, the tunica albuginea, which cannot be seen on ultrasound.

Along the length of the testis, the epididymis lies on the posterolateral aspect. It consists of several meters of coiled tubules that are responsible for transporting the sperm produced in the testis to the vas deferens in the spermatic cord. Anatomically, the epididymis is divided into three portions located from superior to inferior: head or globus major, body, and tail or globus minor. Only the head of the epididymis is visualized in the normal adult on ultrasound (Fig. 9B). It usually does not exceed 1.5 cm in diameter. The echogenicity of the epididymis is similar, or minimally increased, with respect to the testis. Its blood flow is slightly less than that of the testis. The tubules in the testis communicate with the epididymis by an anastomotic network, called the "rete testis," which, in general, cannot be seen on ultrasound.

Two embryologic remnants measuring a few millimeters each are occasionally visualized when the testis is surrounded by fluid, one at the upper pole of the testis and the other at the head of the epididymis. They are called appendix testis and appendix epididymidis, respectively (Fig. 6).

The spermatic cord extends superiorly from the testis into the inguinal canal. Pulsed Doppler tracing can recognize the internal spermatic artery by its low resistance pattern, as opposed to the high resistance pattern found in the cremasteric and deferential arteries (Fig. 7). The spermatic cord contains the vas (ductus) deferens, which is a single tubular structure connecting with the seminal vesicles at the base of the bladder and forming the ejaculatory ducts that carry the sperm to the urethra. The vas deferens connects with the epididymis at the tail (Fig. 8).

The scrotal contents are supplied by several arteries and veins. The internal spermatic (testicular) arteries originate from the aorta immediately below the renal arteries and are responsible for the perfusion of the testes. The deferential arteries originate from the vesical arteries and perfuse the vas deferens and epididymis. The cremasteric arteries originate from the inferior epigastric arteries and perfuse the scrotal wall. Venous drainage of the testes and

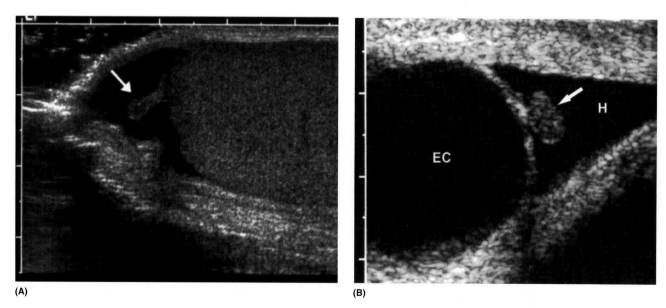

(A)   **(B)**

FIGURE 6 A AND B ▨ Scrotal appendages. (**A**) Appendix testis. (**B**) Appendix epididymis originating from the surface of an epididymal cyst. Both appendages are seen because of the presence of peritesticular fluid. *Arrow,* appendages. EC, epididymal cyst; H, hydrocele.

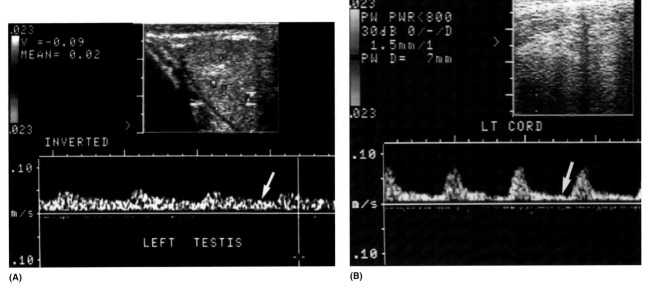

(A)   **(B)**

FIGURE 7 A AND B ■ Arterial Doppler tracing in the scrotum. (**A**) Testicular artery with high diastolic flow. (**B**) Cremasteric or deferential artery in the cord with low diastolic flow as compared to the testicular artery. *Arrow*, diastole.

scrotum is in the form of a net called the "pampiniform plexus," which more proximally becomes the testicular veins. Two more groups of veins drain into the pelvic inferior epigastric and pudendal veins. They anastomose and provide a collateral pathway after high ligation of the internal spermatic veins in the surgical treatment of varicocele. The right testicular vein drains into the inferior vena cava at the level of the renal pedicle, and the left one drains into the left renal vein. Arteries and veins can be easily recognized with color and pulsed Doppler imaging. Lymphatic trunks and nerves (genital branch of the genitofemoral nerve and testicular plexus of the sympathetic trunk) are not visualized as separate structures on ultrasound.

Distribution of arteries in the testis has an unusual pattern (Fig. 9). Beginning at the mediastinum testis, most of

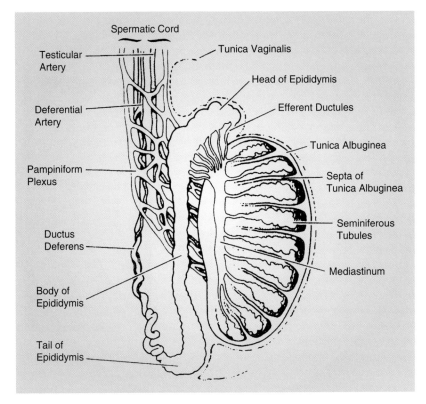

FIGURE 8 ■ Structural anatomy of the testis, epididymis, and spermatic cord. The seminiferous tubules in the testes are connected to the head of the epididymis through the efferent ductules. The epididymis connects with the ductus (vas) deferens to exit through the spermatic cord. *Source*: From Ref. 5.

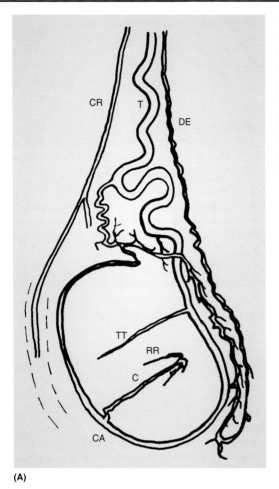

(A)

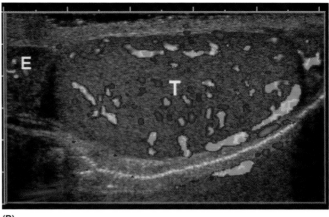

(B)

FIGURE 9 A AND B ■ Arterial perfusion of the scrotum. (**A**) Diagram. (**B**) Color Doppler ultrasound scan of a normal adult testis on sagittal view demonstrates the capsular and intratesticular arteries. C, centripetal artery; CA, capsular artery; CR, cremasteric artery; DE, deferential artery; RR, recurrent rami; T, testicular artery; TT, transtesticular artery; E, epididymis; T, testis. *Source*: (**A**) from Ref. 6.

the branches of the internal spermatic artery run superficially in a circumferential pattern under the tunica albuginea in what is called the tunica vasculosa. From the periphery of the testis, these vessels give origin to *centripetal arteries*, which run in the parenchyma toward the mediastinum. In turn, near the mediastinum, the centripetal arteries give origin to small *recurrent rami*, which run in an opposite, centrifugal direction. This detailed vascular anatomy can best be seen with highly sensitive Doppler equipment. In general, the intratesticular veins are not normally seen (6). More recently, our attention has been drawn to the presence of *transmediastinal* or *transtesticular arteries*, which do not follow the pattern described previously. Instead of running in the periphery at a subcapsular location, they run in a centrifugal direction in the parenchyma itself. Middleton and Bell (7) found these vessels with color Doppler in 52% of the examined testes. In 24 patients, transmediastinal arteries were unilateral in 50%, bilateral in 25%, and absent in 25%. In most cases, these arteries were isolated and occurred in the superior half of the testis. Corresponding veins were found in 26% of the testes, slightly over half of them running with the corresponding arteries. In the remainder, these veins were isolated. Blood flow to the normal epididymis is sometimes not easy to detect.

The scrotal wall is composed of different layers including skin, dartos muscle, external spermatic fascia, cremasteric muscle, and internal spermatic fascia. Sonography

cannot distinguish them separately. The scrotal wall is seen as a single layer measuring 2 to 8 mm in thickness.

The scrotum is divided into right and left halves by a fibrous septum called the "median raphe" (Fig. 2A). Each testis is able to move in the scrotum by the presence of the tunica vaginalis, which has two layers, a visceral layer attached to the surface of the testis and a parietal layer attached to the scrotal wall. A minute amount of fluid is interposed between the two layers. This is similar to the visceral and parietal pleura. The tunica vaginalis does not cover the posterior aspect of the testis at its attachment to the scrotal wall.

ABNORMALITIES

Acute Scrotum

Acute scrotum is defined as sudden, painful swelling of the scrotum or its content. Possible causes with a similar clinical presentation are listed in Table 2. The use of gray-scale ultrasound with its high spatial resolution capabilities combined with color Doppler evaluation of blood perfusion is excellent in the workup of these patients. The proper diagnosis is important, because some of the treatments are surgical. Almost 80% of acute scrotal processes are estimated to be inflammatory and do not require

TABLE 2 ■ Causes of Acute Painful Scrotum

Common
- Epididymitis
- Epididymo-orchitis
- Torsion of the testis
- Torsion of the appendix testis or appendix epididymis
- Trauma
- Strangulated inguinal scrotal hernia

Uncommon
- Acute hydrocele
- Hemorrhage or infarction in a testicular neoplasm

surgery. On the other hand, torsion and traumatic rupture of the testes require emergency surgery. In a study of a group of 20 patients with acute onset of scrotal pain and clinical diagnosis of ischemia, inflammation, or trauma, color Doppler imaging correctly predicted the need for surgery in eight of nine patients (89%). It correctly predicted the outcome in all 11 nonoperated patients (100%) (8). Burks et al. reported an 86% sensitivity and a 100% specificity with color Doppler imaging in distinguishing inflammation from torsion (9).

Acute Inflammation

Epididymo-orchitis is an extremely common clinical problem resulting in an estimated 634,000 medical office visits per year (10). In 80% of cases, a specific organism can be cultured. In heterosexual males under 35 years of age, *Chlamydia trachomatis* and *Neisseria gonorrhoeae* are the most common pathogens. In older men, *Escherichia coli* and *Proteus mirabilis* are found. These infections usually originate in the prostate. *E. coli* is the most frequent organism found in homosexual males (10). An unusual cause of epididymo-orchitis is brucellosis, in which involvement of the scrotum is reported with an incidence from 2% to 20%. Brucellosis is seen in populations that drink unpasteurized milk or eat raw milk products. In children, infection may be due to an underlying congenital or acquired structural urologic abnormality such as obstructive uropathy, caused by urethral stricture or valves with secondary reflux into the ejaculatory ducts. In a study of 238 patients with acute scrotal pain, 39% of the children with epididymitis had either structural or functional urinary tract abnormalities (11). Other abnormalities such as external sphincter dys-synergia with reflux or hypospadias may be found. Instrumentation or surgery of the genitourinary system and indwelling catheters are often responsible for the infections. In children, many cases are viral, resulting from mumps, coxsackievirus, echovirus, and adenoviruses. Parasitic diseases such as malaria, filariasis, and schistosomiasis have also been responsible. In adults, most cases of epididymo-orchitis are a result of sexual or urinary extension of infection. The disorder usually begins as epididymitis at the tail, because it is the portion closest to the urinary tract. Twenty to forty percent of all cases of epididymitis result in secondary orchitis.

Epididymo-orchitis may occur at any age, but most frequently in adolescents and adults. As in any other acutely inflammatory process, fever (usually of low grade), swelling, redness, and tenderness of the scrotum are observed. Urinary signs of dysuria, possible pyuria and urethral discharge, may be found. Patients note spontaneous pain of gradual onset and on palpation (12).

Ultrasound has a spectrum of findings in inflammatory disease. In early cases, no gray-scale findings are seen. As the disease progresses, the examiner sees variable degrees of edema and fluid retention in the different scrotal structures. The inflammation is visible as scrotal wall thickening exceeding the normal maximum of 7 to 8mm, reactive hydrocele seen as a sonolucency surrounding the testis, and an enlarged and hypoechoic epididymis and testis. To some extent, these findings overlap those of acute torsion. For this reason, the diagnosis is made by color Doppler imaging, which demonstrates increased flow to the affected structures as compared with the normal testis, and not decreased, as it would be in cases of torsion. Increased flow to the testis is a sign of orchitis, although it is not specific to the disease. Horstman et al. (13) showed hyperemia on color Doppler in cases of scrotal inflammation, many of which had a normal gray-scale appearance. Epididymitis was focal in one-fourth of the cases, whereas orchitis was most commonly diffuse (Figs. 10 and 11). In this study, the detection of venous flow in the epididymis or testis was notable in many of these patients with inflammatory disease. The authors found that over half the patients with inflammatory changes showed a resistive index in the intratesticular arteries below 0.5 (normal is above 0.5) and in the deferential and cremasteric arteries below 0.7 (normal is above 0.7) (13).

An enlarged epididymis in combination with scrotal wall thickening is the most reliable indicator of a possible benign inflammatory process (14). Additional diagnostic certainty, to differentiate it from torsion, is provided by increased vascularity on color Doppler imaging.

Severe or untreated epididymo-orchitis may progress to pyocele, testicular scrotal abscess, infarction, atrophy, or fulminant fasciitis (Fournier gangrene). Pyocele (Fig. 11A) may look sonolucent as does reactive hydrocele, but it may show some echogenicity when debris or septation is present. An abscess may develop in the testis or external to it, mostly as a complication of epididymo-orchitis, but occasionally in association with mumps, scarlet fever, influenza, typhoid fever, or a distant focus of infection. Sonographically, an abscess is seen as a focal area with an anechoic, hypoechoic, or mixed echo pattern (Fig. 12). In general, blood flow is decreased in the center and is increased in the periphery. Sometimes, a testicular abscess may resemble a tumor. The presence of clinically and sonographically evident inflammation should help in the differential diagnosis. If not, follow-up ultrasound after two weeks of intensive antibiotic treatment is required. Surgery may be required in the absence of clinical and sonographic improvement. A few (10%) neoplasms present with an acute scrotum, which may be secondary to acute infarction or hemorrhage.

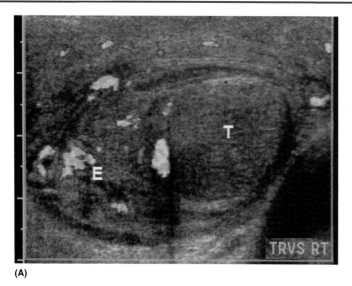

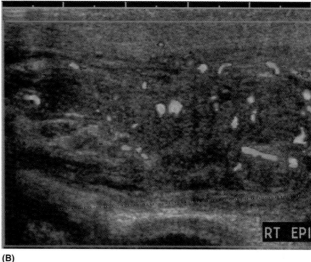

(A) **(B)**

FIGURE 10 A AND B ■ Epididymitis in a 52-year-old patient. (**A**) Axial view of the lower pole of the testes and epididymis. (**B**) Longitudinal view of the epididymis. Observe the presence of scrotal wall thickening (edema), and a large and hypervascular epididymis with a normal testis. E, epididymis; T, testis.

Mumps orchitis occurs in 20% to 30% of patients with the disease. It presents four to six days after the parotitis and it is unilateral in most cases. The sonographic appearance is that of a normal or enlarged testis with diffusely decreased echogenicity. Reactive hydrocele and scrotal wall thickening are frequently seen (15). Atrophy of the testis occurs in about 50% of patients. Infertility is uncommon. Other viral diseases such as infectious mononucleosis, varicella, and coxsackievirus have been associated with orchitis, although orchitis resulting from any of these viruses is rare. For this reason, the diagnosis should be considered only in patients with classic signs and symptoms of the relevant viral disease. Testicular infarction in

inflammation may result from ischemia secondary to epididymal edema and compression of the venous outflow from the testis. It may also result from a similar compression of the internal spermatic artery in the cord (16). The diagnosis of partial or total ischemia of the testis in the inflammatory setting, with edema and hyperperfusion, is extremely difficult. A useful sign reported to assist in the diagnosis consists of the reversal of arterial diastolic flow in the intra-articular arteries as seen with pulsed Doppler (17). This finding is due to increased vascular resistance in the testis with reversal of flow direction in diastole. It is similar to what may be seen in the umbilical artery in extreme cases of fetal distress, and in

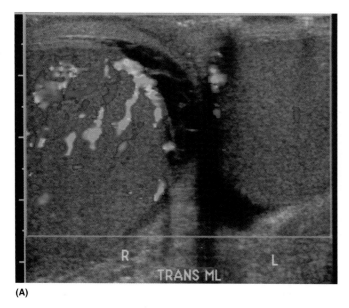

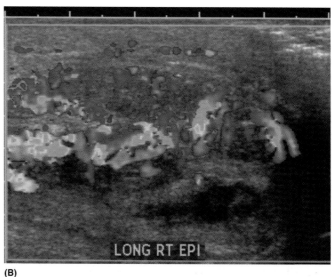

(A) **(B)**

FIGURE 11 A AND B ■ Epididymo-orchitis in a 59-year-old patient. (**A**) Axial view of both testes with enlargement and increased vascularity of the right one. Surrounding organized hydrocele or pyocele on the medial aspect. (**B**) Longitudinal view of the right epididymis showing enlargement and increased vascularity.

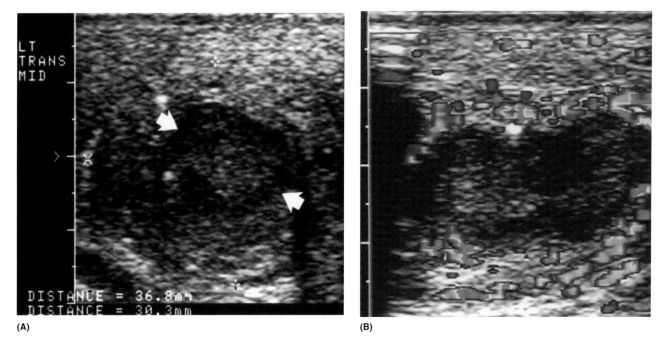

(A)

(B)

FIGURE 12 A AND B ■ Testicular abscess in a 39-year-old patient with acute and chronic epididymal orchitis following trauma one month before. (**A**) Axial view of the testis (*calipers*) shows a focal central area of hypoechogenicity (*arrows*). (**B**) Longitudinal view of the same testis with color Doppler showing a central area of necrosis with peripheral increased vascularity.

renal vein thrombosis. Fournier gangrene results from a scrotal infection by a mixture of anaerobic and aerobic organisms (e.g., *Staphylococcus aureus, Bacteroides fragilis, E. coli,* β-hemolytic streptococci, *B. distasonis, Streptococcus anginosus*). It is seen in patients with diabetes mellitus, immunosuppression, or extensive local trauma. On ultrasound, the hallmarks of the diagnosis are the high reflectivity and reverberation found in the soft tissues of the scrotum secondary to the presence of gas-producing anaerobic organisms (Fig. 13). The scrotal wall is thickened, and, unlike in other forms of epididymo-orchitis, the testes and epididymides exhibit a normal appearance. Treatment is surgical, in addition to antibiotic administration (18). Atrophy of the testis may represent the end stage of infection and epididymo-orchitis.

Epididymitis does not need to be bacterial. Amiodarone is a cardiac antiarrhythmic drug responsible for cases of epididymitis. An acute scrotum was also seen in a case of phlegmon in acute necrotizing pancreatitis (19) in which ultrasound demonstrated an extratesticular mass with increased vascularity. The testes and epididymides were normal in appearance and vascularity, but they were displaced by the mass. Increased extratesticular flow may also be seen in detorsion and chronic torsion of the testis, torsion of the appendix testis, trauma, and extratesticular tumors. Chemical epididymitis arises when urine refluxes into the vas deferens and reaches the epididymis. The head of the epididymis is usually spared, probably by the convoluted nature of the tubules. The reflux of urine results in inflammatory changes. This disorder is usually seen in young males after a sudden increase in intra-abdominal pressure such

as from lifting heavy objects or blunt trauma with a full bladder (20).

Chronic Inflammation with Acute Bouts

In general, chronic inflammation follows an indolent course, but it may cause acute symptoms such as pain and scrotal swelling. The ultrasound appearance of acute epididymitis as it becomes chronic has been described under section entitled "Acute Inflammation." Other specific entities are discussed in the following paragraphs.

Tuberculous epididymo-orchitis is a rare form of genitourinary tuberculosis that clinically manifests with an incidence of less than 3% of all cases with the disease. Prostate, epididymis, and seminal vesicles are the most commonly affected sites. Epididymal tuberculosis is almost always secondary to prostatic involvement. In turn, involvement of the testis is usually by direct extension from the epididymis, with evidence of occasional hematogenous infection. In approximately one-third of the patients with genitourinary tuberculosis, the involvement is solely genital. Tuberculous epididymo-orchitis not only presents as an extension of pulmonary and renal tuberculosis, but also has been reported to be transmitted sexually (21). Clinically, in addition to general symptoms of tuberculosis, patients manifest mild tenderness with induration and nodularity of the epididymis and scrotum. Involvement is usually unilateral. On ultrasound, two forms of presentation have been reported (22): (*i*) an acute form indistinguishable from other types of inflammation and (*ii*) a chronic form with a pattern sometimes similar to the acute form plus confluent, anechoic areas representing necrosis. It also may show a complex mass involving the

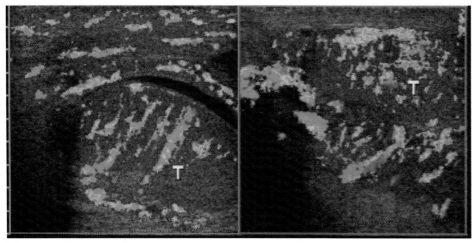

(A)

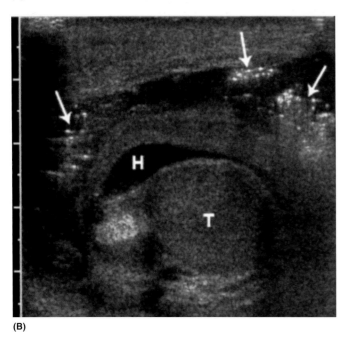

(B)

FIGURE 13 A AND B ▓ Severe epididymo-orchitis with gangrene (Fournier's) in a 31-year-old patient. (**A**) Color Doppler showing very high blood flow to the testes, surrounding structures and scrotal wall. Thickening of the scrotal wall and reactive hydrocele surrounding the testes. (**B**) Axial view of the right hemiscrotum showing the testis with surrounding hydrocele, edema, fluid, and gas in the tissues. *Arrows,* gas in the soft tissues. T, testis; H, hydrocele.

testis and epididymis with areas of increased and decreased echogenicity and an organized hydrocele (Fig. 14).

Occasional areas of calcification are seen as echogenic foci with posterior shadowing in patients with chronic tuberculosis. The sonographic appearance is nonspecific; but in the proper clinical setting, the diagnosis should be considered, and fine-needle aspiration performed. In this way, the patient may avoid orchidectomy (24).

Sarcoidosis of the scrotum is uncommon and occurs in less than 1% of patients with the disease. In 70% of patients, only the epididymis is involved (Fig. 15). Most of the other patients have involvement of the testis only, and even fewer have combined disease (25). Clinically, patients may have acute or recurrent epididymitis, or they may be asymptomatic. Physical examination reveals induration and nodularity of the scrotum. On ultrasound, the epididymis is enlarged and has poorly defined focal areas of hypoechogenicity. Similar areas of hypoechogenicity can be found in an involved testis (15). Occasional

calcifications may be seen. The sonographic appearance is difficult to separate from that of other inflammatory or neoplastic processes.

Fungal involvement of the epididymis has been reported in association with disseminated infections due to *Blastomyces, Coccidioides,* and *Histoplasma* species.

Idiopathic Scrotal Edema
Idiopathic scrotal edema is an unusual cause of acute unilateral or bilateral scrotal swelling and mild pain seen in young boys, usually younger than 10 years. The condition is of unknown origin. The affected site exhibits erythema, which usually extends into the anterior abdominal wall and perineum. The patient is afebrile, with a normal urinalysis and a normal white blood cell count. Peripheral eosinophilia may be seen. It typically resolves on its own in two to five days without sequelae. Ultrasound demonstrates extensive scrotal wall thickening with an "onion-skin" appearance without involvement of the testes. Color

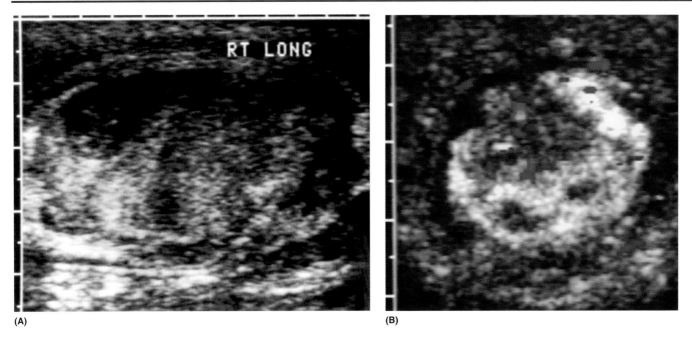

FIGURE 14 A AND B ■ Tuberculous epididymo-orchitis in a 65-year-old patient presenting with an inguinal abscess originating from prostatic involvement by the disease. (**A**) Longitudinal section of the right testis shows a grossly heterogeneous echo pattern. (**B**) Color Doppler axial view of the epididymal head shows increased echogenicity and blood flow. *Source*: From Ref. 23.

Doppler sonography has not demonstrated increased blood flow (Fig. 16) (26).

Torsion of the Testis and Appendages

Torsion of the testis refers to a twist of the spermatic cord or the testis itself on its attachments (Fig. 17). The degree of twisting has been described from partial to several complete turns (28). The degree of ischemia is related to the amount of twisting, beginning with a compromise of the venous flow, progressing to thrombosis, and finally compromising the arterial circulation. Torsion of the testis has been reported from newborns to the elderly. Two peak periods of incidence are described: a small one during the first year of life and a large one at puberty. In one of the largest available series, 65% of cases occurred between the ages of 12 and 18 years. Torsion was as common among men in their 20s as among prepubertal boys (28). Early in life or in utero, the torsion is supratesticular and occurs outside the tunica vaginalis. In many cases, it is asymptomatic, leading to atrophy of the testis. Some patients have a painless scrotal mass associated with mild erythema and edema of the scrotal wall. The testis is always necrotic, and treatment is elective orchidectomy. The contralateral testis does not require orchiopexy

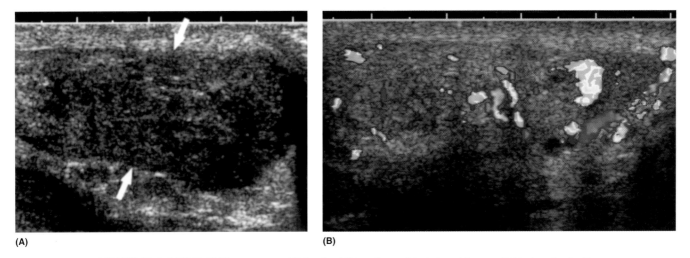

FIGURE 15 A AND B ■ Biopsy-proven bilateral epididymal sarcoidosis in a 15-year-old black patient with pulmonary disease. (**A**) Longitudinal view with gray scale of an enlarged epididymis. (**B**) Longitudinal view with color Doppler of the same epididymis showing increased vascularity. *Arrows*, epididymis.

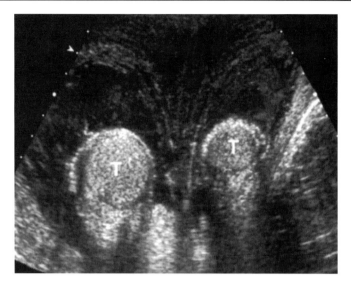

FIGURE 16 ▨ Scrotal edema in a 60-year-old patient with anasarca. Observe the typical "onion-skin" appearance of the scrotal edema. T, testes.

because the patient usually has no associated anatomic defect. Torsion of the testis in older boys and men occurs within the tunica vaginalis. It is due to an insufficient attachment of the testis to the scrotal wall by the tunica vaginalis that results in twisting at this area. The mesorchium joining the testis to the epididymis also may be loose, allowing the twisting of these two structures. These anomalies are always bilateral. A possible factor in the higher incidence at puberty may be the increased weight of the testis, which may facilitate torsion.

Typical clinical presentation of torsion of the testis in the older child and adult is of acute onset of scrotal pain (frequently at night), anorexia, vomiting, and lack of urinary symptoms and fever. Helpful in the distinction between epididymitis and torsion of the testis is the patient's age. In patients younger than 20 years, epididymitis versus torsion occurs at a ratio of 3:2, whereas in patients older than 20 years, the ratio approximates 9:1 (5). Unfortunately, as many as 35% to 50% of patients with testicular torsion have a history of gradual onset of

pain, similar to that seen in epididymitis. As many as one-third of patients have had previous episodes of acute testicular pain that resolved spontaneously. Useful clinical signs, but not pathognomonic, are abnormal elevation of the affected testis, abnormal axis of the testis when the patient is examined in a standing position, abnormal position of the epididymis in the scrotum, and an abnormal axis of the contralateral testis (bilateral poor attachment). A higher incidence of torsion of the left testis has been reported. Torsion is classified on the basis of time elapsed since the onset of pain: acute torsion (when less than 24 hours), subacute (from 1 to 10 days), and chronic (for more than 10 days). This time interval is important because it is associated with the survival rate of the testis. If surgery is performed within five to six hours, the survival rate is 80% to 100%; from 6 to 12 hours, testicular survival is 70%, and after 12 hours, it is 20% (29). Surgical exploration is always indicated to attempt to save the testis, but if salvage is not possible, the necrotic testis should be removed, because its presence may cause the contralateral testis to be damaged by humoral factors (30). It has been reported that unilateral testicular torsion may lead to injury to the contralateral testis. Spermiography is abnormal in 70% of patients after testicular torsion (31). In testes saved by early surgical intervention, reports have shown a direct relationship between the incidence of infertility and the time interval between the onset of pain and surgical detorsion. At surgical exploration for torsion of the testis, contralateral orchiopexy is necessary because torsion-prone anatomy is a bilateral finding.

The sonographic appearance of testicular torsion on gray-scale imaging varies with the time of evolution. Early in *acute* torsion, the testis appears normal (Fig. 18). The testis and epididymis progressively become enlarged and hypoechoic, and variable amounts of peritesticular fluid and scrotal wall thickening are usually observed. These structures may become hyperechoic or may show mixed echogenicity secondary to hemorrhage. In subacute cases of torsion, the testis may be of normal size or enlarged, and it exhibits variable echogenicity. Although the degree of echogenicity may vary, eventually the testis becomes small and hypoechoic. The epididymis becomes enlarged and echogenic. This pattern is characteristic of chronic

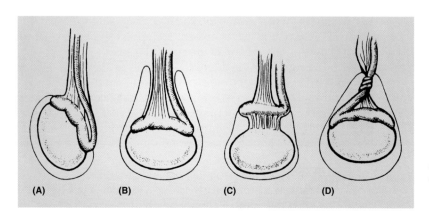

(A)　　**(B)**　　**(C)**　　**(D)**

FIGURE 17 A–D ▨ Schematic illustrations of types of suspension of the testis. (**A**) Normal. (**B**) "Bell-clapper" deformity. (**C**) Loose epididymal attachment to the testis. (**D**) Torsed testis presenting in a transverse line. *Source*: From Ref. 27.

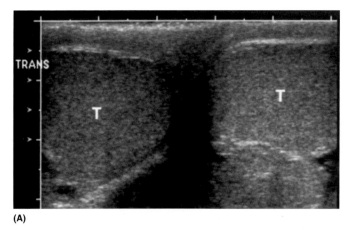

(A)

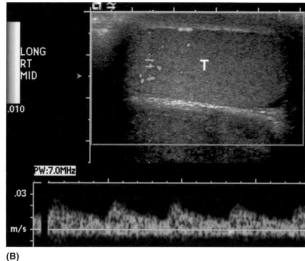

(B)

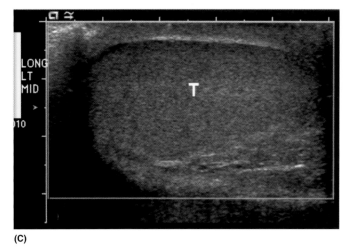

(C)

FIGURE 18 A–C ■ Acute torsion of the left testis in a 16-year-old patient. Exploratory surgery was able to save the testis. (**A**) Axial view of both testes with gray scale showing no abnormalities. (**B**) Right testis longitudinal view. Power Doppler and Doppler tracing show blood flow to the testis. (**C**) Left testis longitudinal view. Power Doppler with no flow to the testis. T, testis.

torsion (32). The described gray-scale findings are nonspecific and are similar to those described in inflammatory disease, scrotal trauma, and testicular neoplasm with hemorrhage or necrosis (Fig. 19). A sonographic sign described as helpful in the diagnosis of torsion is the visualization of the spermatic cord next to the testis, with hyperechogenicity and increased thickness in the range of 1 cm (32). Color Doppler imaging makes the difference in the diagnosis. During the first hours, the patient has no evidence of perfusion to the testis and epididymis on color Doppler ultrasound. As collateral circulation develops with the passing of time, one sees increased vascularity surrounding the testis, which remains hypovascular. Color Doppler imaging has a sensitivity of 86%, a specificity of 100%, and an accuracy of 97% for the diagnosis of torsion of the testis (9). One of the pitfalls in the diagnosis of torsion with this technique is the extremely low flow in infant and prepubertal normal testes, which requires high-frequency transducers in the range of 10 to 15 MHz (Fig. 20). Even in the adult patient, the examiner should ensure that the optimal scanning parameters are able to demonstrate flow in the normal testis before attempting to evaluate the possible abnormal one. Additional pitfalls not related to the technique itself but to the nature of the pathology are (*i*) torsion with spontaneous detorsion in which the testis and epididymis may appear hyperemic, thus leading to a false

diagnosis of epididymo-orchitis (33), and (*ii*) torsion with less than 360° of twist associated with complete venous and incomplete arterial compromise. In the foregoing situation, the examiner can detect intratesticular flow, and this can lead to another false-negative diagnosis (34). Color Doppler imaging compares well with testicular scintigraphy, which was considered the standard until the last few years (34). In addition, ultrasound provides high-resolution anatomic information that is not possible to obtain with scintigraphy.

Once more, the person performing the ultrasound examination should strive to make a diagnosis of testicular torsion at a time when the testis still could be saved. That is to say, when gray scale still shows normal symmetrical findings of both testes and color Doppler shows decreased or absent blood flow in the painful testis.

A significant incidence of torsion of the testis occurs in cryptorchidism (undescended testis) and usually goes clinically undetected. Infarction of a testicle in the absence of torsion may be spontaneous, it may follow epididymo-orchitis or repair of inguinal hernia, or it may be associated with trauma, polyarteritis nodosa, Henoch-Schönlein purpura, or subacute bacterial endocarditis (30).

Torsion of the testicular appendages refers to twisting of embryonic remnants of the testis and epididymis (Fig. 21). This disorder is most common between 7 and 12 years of

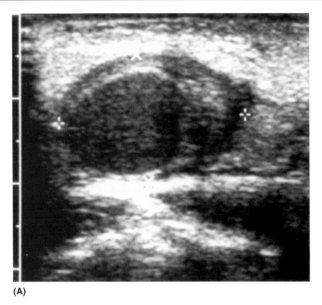

(A)

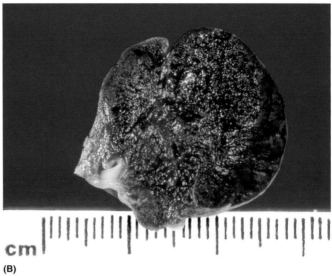

(B)

FIGURE 19 A AND B ■ Subacute torsion of undescended testis in the inguinal canal in a premature one-year-old patient who presented with painful left groin mass. (**A**) Longitudinal view of the abnormal testis in the inguinal canal. (**B**) Pathology specimen showing hemorrhagic infarction.

age, but it may occur at any age. It is the cause of 5% of the cases of acute scrotum (36). Torsion of the appendages is more common on the right side, unlike torsion of the testis. The most common appendage to twist is the *appendix testis* (approximately in 92% of the cases), which is a mullerian duct remnant at the superior pole of the testis. The appendix testis is a 1 to 2 mm pedunculated structure that cannot be recognized normally on ultrasound. It is frequently seen in cases of hydrocele. The second most common incidence of torsion is of the *appendix epididymidis* (7% of the cases). This is another minute pedunculated

structure attached to the head of the epididymis that also is seen when hydrocele is present. This appendix and the vas deferens represent wolffian duct remnants.

Clinically, torsion of the appendages does not cause systemic clinical symptoms. Patients often pinpoint a focal tenderness at the upper pole of the testis that may be acute or gradual, but they have no urethral discharge or other urinary complaint. A history of previous episodes of similar pain is infrequent. On physical examination, inflammatory changes of the scrotal wall are common. In addition, a swollen and cyanotic appendix is sometimes

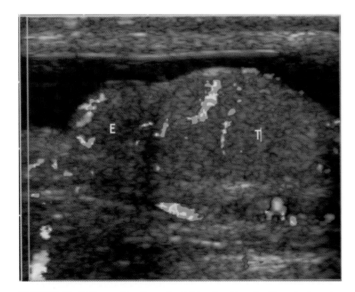

FIGURE 20 ■ Normal testis and epididymis with color Doppler in a six-year-old patient. The excellent depiction of blood flow in this prepubertal testis and epididymis is due to the use of a high-frequency transducer in the range of 10 to 15 MHz. Small hydrocele surrounding the testis.

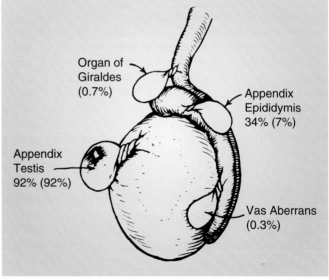

FIGURE 21 ■ Torsion of the scrotal appendages. The schematic illustration shows the anatomic location, incidence of identification in anatomic specimens and (in parentheses) relative incidence of torsion. *Source*: From Ref. 35.

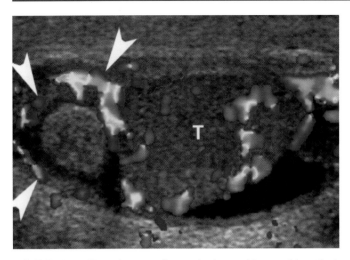

FIGURE 22 ■ Torsed appendix testis in a 10-year-old patient. Longitudinal view of the testis with color Doppler with an enlarged avascular appendix testis surrounded by increased blood flow (*arrowheads*). T, testis. *Source*: From Ref. 37.

visible beneath the scrotal skin and referred to as the "blue dot" sign.

On ultrasound, the swollen hypoechoic appendix attached to the upper pole of the testis or the head of the epididymis is observed surrounded by a reactive hydrocele and increased thickening of the adjacent scrotal wall. The echotexture of the testis and epididymis is normal. On color Doppler imaging, the torsed appendix is hypovascular, but may be surrounded by a rim of hypervascularity. Flow to the epididymis and testis is normal (Fig. 22) (38).

Unlike torsion of the testis, a torsed scrotal appendix is managed conservatively. Pain and swelling usually subside in 2 to 12 days.

A summary of color Doppler findings in acute scrotal conditions is provided in Table 3.

TABLE 3 ■ Color Doppler Ultrasound: Findings in Some Acute Scrotal Conditions

Diagnosis	Intratesticular flow	Peritesticular flow
Acute torsion	—	N
Missed torsion	—	↑
Spontaneous detorsion	N, ↑	↑
Torsion of appendix testis or appendix epididymis	N	↑
Epididymitis	N	↑
Orchitis	↑	N
Epididymo-orchitis	↑	↑
Hematoma (trauma)	↓	Variable

Abbreviations: —, absent; N, normal; ↑, increased
Source: From Ref. 39.

Trauma

The scrotum and its contents may be injured by penetrating or blunt trauma. Surgical exploration is performed after penetrating trauma, whereas ultrasound examination is indicated after blunt trauma (40). Under these circumstances, the main role of ultrasound is in the diagnosis of testicular rupture, which is a surgical emergency and is reported to occur in 50% of victims of blunt scrotal trauma (41). The mechanism of rupture is a direct blow to the testis against a hard surface, such as the symphysis pubis or thigh. Early surgical exploration and repair of a ruptured testis improve testicular survival because the salvage rate is over 80% when the testis is repaired within 72 hours, but it drops to 30% thereafter (42). The need for orchidectomy is 5% to 20% when surgical exploration is performed within the first 72 hours, and it is 45% to 80% thereafter (43). Reported accuracy in the diagnosis of rupture of the testis is in the range of 94% to 100%. Clinical evaluation of a severely traumatized scrotum is difficult. Missed or untreated rupture of the testis may result in an ischemic atrophic testis or secondary infection. In addition, in cases of unilateral testis trauma, which might or might not include orchiectomy as treatment, it has been shown that patients might develop subfertility in association with apoptosis (cell self-destruction by fragmentation of the nuclear DNA) and abnormal sperm. The possibility of a humoral mechanism has been postulated (44,45). Trauma to the testis may result in contusion, edema, hemorrhage, laceration or rupture, and even torsion (by stimulating forceful cremasteric muscle contraction). On ultrasound, the testis shows abnormal echogenicity, either increased or decreased, and either focal or generalized, depending on the degree and extension of the trauma. The appearance varies with the time elapsed since the injury (Fig. 23). Under these circumstances, the finding of a fracture line in the parenchyma in cases of scrotal rupture is unusual. The best criteria for rupture are loss of definition of the margins of the testis, loss of the abnormal oval contour, and protrusion of testicular parenchyma beyond the margins of the testis (Fig. 24) (11). Sometimes, trauma to the testis with its heterogeneous and variable appearance may mimic or overlap with epididymo-orchitis, tumor, post-traumatic pyocele, or scrotal abscess (Fig. 25). Ten to fifteen percent of patients with testicular tumors first seek medical attention after an episode of trauma. In turn, a chronic hematoma may be seen as a solid scrotal mass in a patient with no history of trauma, and it is difficult to distinguish from a tumor, clinically and on ultrasound (11). Color Doppler flow helps to characterize the lesion, which is avascular in the case of hematoma, vascular (variable) in tumor, and hypervascular in inflammation (13). In nonsurgical cases, the ultrasound findings should be followed to resolution to avoid a misdiagnosis. In trauma, all scrotal structures may be affected regardless of the involvement of the testes. Infiltration of the scrotal wall and of the median raphe is seen on ultrasound as an increased thickness that exceeds the normal upper measurements of 7 to 8 mm. Hemorrhage in the tunica vaginalis may have different appearances depending on the time

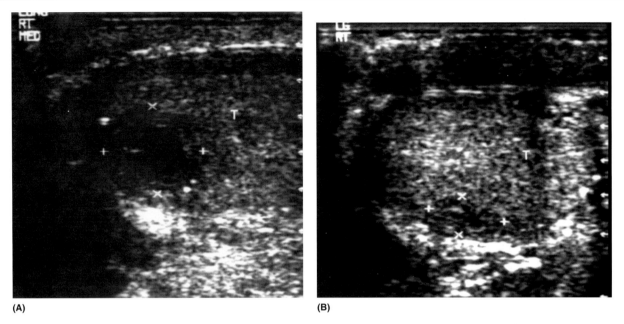

(A) **(B)**

FIGURE 23 A AND B ■ Evolution of hematoma of the testis in a 38-year-old patient who had sustained scrotal trauma three weeks before the first ultrasound examination. (**A**) First ultrasound examination. Longitudinal view shows a poorly defined hypoechoic area representing the hematoma (*calipers*). (**B**) Second ultrasound examination of the testis, longitudinal view, two weeks later. The hematoma (*calipers*) has largely resolved. T, testis.

since the event. If the blood is not coagulated, it is seen as a sonolucent fluid collection, whereas if it is coagulated with different degrees of organization, it shows some echogenicity with possible septations. Hematoma of the epididymis is seen as an enlargement with variable degrees of echogenicity. Lower-frequency curved transducers in the range of 4 to 6 MHz provide better global visualization of the scrotum and identification of the testes in cases of gross scrotal infiltration and large hematoceles. The testes are usually posteriorly displaced; thus, another

way of obtaining better visualization of the enlarged scrotum is by scanning from the posterior aspect. If one or both testes cannot be identified, the infrequent possibility of traumatic dislocation should be considered. Long-standing hematocele results in thickening of the tunica vaginalis with fibrosis and organization, as well as possible calcification. It should be distinguished from abscess or chronic hydrocele (46). Urethral rupture may result in extravasation of urine into the tunica vaginalis that is indistinguishable from a hydrocele (5).

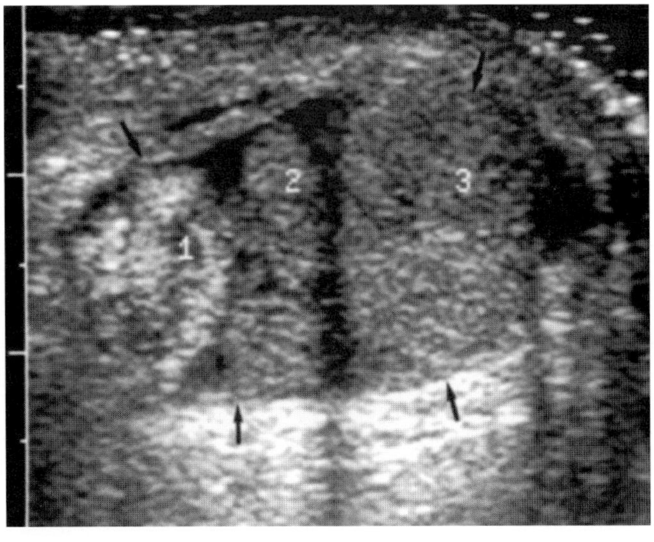

Acute scrotal hemorrhage may occur with or without minor trauma in systemic diseases, such as Henoch-Schönlein purpura (47) and hemophilia.

Testicular Lesions

Scrotal lesions may be divided into intratesticular and extratesticular, and can be further subdivided into solid or cystic (Table 4). Some solid lesions within the testis may, in fact, be partially cystic. For instance, malignant neoplasms may have both solid and cystic components, or they may at first appear solid and then develop an acute hemorrhage or necrosis and appear cystic. Testicular abscesses or hematomas may appear solid, cystic, or mixed, depending on the age of the insult. Other scrotal lesions may be primarily extratesticular. For instance, infection usually starts in the epididymis, but it may also involve the testis, as in epididymo-orchitis. Initially, this disorder is observed as an increase in size of the epididymis. Most extratesticular masses are benign, although some primary and metastatic neoplasms may originate in the extratesticular structures. Common extratesticular cystic lesions include hydroceles and epididymal cysts.

FIGURE 24 ■ Rupture of the testis in a seven-year-old patient who fell in a playground. *Arrows*, testis contour. The numbers 1, 2, and 3 indicate main testicular fractured fragments.

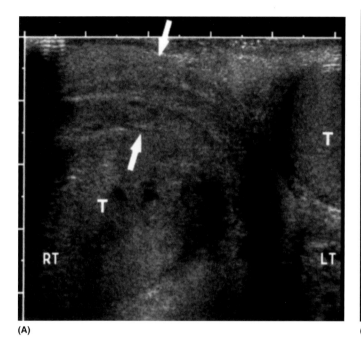

(A)

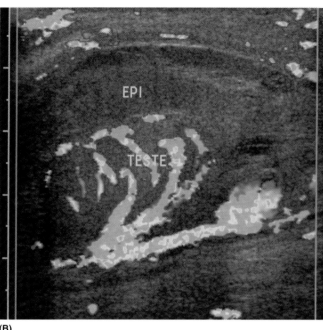

(B)

FIGURE 25 A AND B ■ Scrotal hematoma with testis rupture in a 44-year-old patient who was kicked five days before the ultrasound examination. (**A**) Axial view of both testes showing scrotal wall infiltration (*arrows*) and heterogeneous testis on the right side. The left side is normal. (**B**) Longitudinal view of the right hemiscrotum with color Doppler showing similar findings plus increased vascularity to the viable fragments of the testis. T, testis.

Additionally, multiple tubular extratesticular structures may be encountered in varicoceles. Inguinal hernias may appear as either solid or cystic extratesticular lesions, depending on the content of the sac.

TABLE 4 ■ Scrotal Lesions

Testicular	Extratesticular
Solid	*Solid*
Infection	Infection
Hematoma	Hernia
Infarct (torsion, inflammation, vasculitis)	Hematoma
	Granulomas (postvasectomy)
Malignant neoplasms	Benign neoplasms
Benign neoplasms	Malignant neoplasms
Lymphoma or leukemia	Metastases
Metastases	*Cystic*
Adrenal rests	Hydrocele
Cystic	Epididymal cyst or spermatocele
Simple cyst	Hernia
Abscess	Varicocele
Hematoma	Hematoma
Malignant neoplasm	Abscess
Benign neoplasm	Tubular ectasia (postvasectomy)
Tubular ectasia of the rete testis	
Cystic dysplasia	*Cystic mimicking solid*
	Epidermoid inclusion cysts

Testicular Solid Lesions

Tumors ■ Malignant testicular tumors have a peak incidence of 15 cases in whites and 9 in black and Asians per 100,000 between 15 and 45 years of age. The American Cancer Society estimated that in the year 2005 about 8010 new cases of testicular cancer were diagnosed in the United States with an estimated death rate of 4.9% (390 patients) (American Cancer Society Statistics, National Cancer Institute, SEER). Different factors have been associated with these tumors. Cryptorchidism (undescended testis) is found in the clinical history of approximately 10% of patients with testicular tumors and is the best known of all risk factors (48). A possible explanation is that the testes are exposed to a higher temperature when they are undescended and located in the abdomen or pelvis than when they are located in the scrotum. Even when undescended testes are repositioned, however, the risk of developing a neoplasm is increased, although the risk increases with the length of time that the undescended testis remains untreated. In addition, 5% to 10% of the contralateral and normally located testes in patients with cryptorchidism develop testicular neoplasms. These findings suggest a primary genetic abnormality. The incidence of neoplasia of the testes in these patients is up to 48 times higher than in an age-matched control population (5,48). Any condition associated with abnormal gonadal development, including disorders related to chromosomal abnormalities, may result in an increased incidence of testicular malignancy. An increased incidence of testicular tumors has been reported in patients exposed in utero to diethylstilbestrol, a synthetic estrogen. The incidence of testicular

TABLE 5 ■ Pathologic Classification of Testicular Tumors

Germ cell tumors

Tumors showing a single cell type

Seminoma

   Typical

   Anaplastic

   Spermatocytic

Embryonal carcinoma

   Adult type

   Infantile type

   Polyembryoma

Choriocarcinoma

Teratoma

   Mature and immature

Tumors showing more than one histologic pattern

Embryonal carcinoma plus teratoma (teratocarcinoma)

Embryonal carcinoma plus seminoma

Seminoma and teratoma

Other combinations

Tumors of gonadal stroma

Leydig cell tumors

Sertoli cell, granulosa cell, theca cell tumors

Tumors of primitive gonadal stroma

Mixtures of these three

Source: From Ref. 53.

tumors in the same family is low, although a patient's first-degree relatives are at a sixfold risk of developing these lesions (49). Patients with testicular neoplasms are at an increased risk of developing another primary germ cell tumor on the contralateral side. Most of these lesions develop more than three years after the removal of the first tumor. The frequency of second tumors is 1.5% to 5%, and the risk is 500 to 700 times that of the normal age-matched control population. Overall, the incidence of testicular cancer in young men seems to be increasing

worldwide mostly for seminomas, whereas the mortality is decreasing. With modern treatment, five-year survival rate for stage I is 99%, for stage II 96%, and for stage III 72%. Residual masses often exist after apparently successful treatment of high-stage lesions. Second malignant diseases, most often leukemia, are observed in 30% of patients undergoing successful treatment of primary germ cell neoplasms (50).

Testicular tumors have a geographic and ethnic distribution. One of the highest incidence rates (8 per 100,000) is in Denmark. The lowest incidence (2 per 100,000) is in Israel, Finland, Japan, and in the black population of the United States.

The usual clinical presentation of testicular tumors is a palpable mass on one side of the scrotum. Ten percent of patients present with *acute scrotum*, most likely from intratumoral hemorrhage (51). A history of trauma is found in 6% to 21% of these patients. Another 4% to 14% of patients present with metastatic disease or hormonal changes such as precocious puberty or gynecomastia, with or without a palpable testicular mass (52).

Approximately 90% of testicular tumors are of germ cell origin, 5% are of specialized gonadal stromal origin, and 5% are secondary malignant tumors. A pathologic classification of testicular tumors is given in Table 5 and their relative frequency in Table 6.

Many germ cell tumors and most malignant nonseminomatous tumors produce one or more humoral markers: α-fetoprotein (AFP), human chorionic gonadotropin (hCG), human placental lactogen, $α_1$-antitrypsin, placental alkaline phosphatase, carcinoembryonic antigen, and others. Among these, AFP and hCG have been the most sensitive and specific. They are found in 75% and 60%, respectively, of patients with nonseminomatous germ cell tumors. Elevated hCG levels have been found in approximately 10% of patients with seminomas (Table 7).

Testicular tumors grow locally and extend from the testis into the rete testis, mediastinum testis, and epididymis. Mitotic activity has been found in most germ cell tumors, including seminomas. Metastases occur through lymphatics draining into the retroperitoneal lymph nodes. Inguinal nodes can be involved if the tumor has spread to

TABLE 6 ■ The Frequency of Various Histologic Types of Testicular Germ Cell Tumors

	Percent		**Percent**
Pure seminoma	26.9	ECA + YST + T + SCT	14.3
Spermatocytic seminoma	2.4	Seminoma + SCT	8.1
Embryonal carcinoma	3.1	ECA + YST + T + S + SCT	7.4
Yolk sac tumor	2.4	ECA + YST + teratoma	4.7
Teratoma	2.7	YST + teratoma	2.5
Choriocarcinoma	0.1	ECA + T (TCA)	1.4
ITMGC	0.6	Other combinations	24.0

Abbreviations: ITMGC, intratubular malignant germ cells; ECA, embryonal carcinoma; YST, yolk sac tumor; T, teratoma; SCT, syncytiotrophoblasts; S, seminoma; TCA, teratocarcinoma.
Source: From Ref. 54.

TABLE 7 ■ Tumor Markers Used in Germ Cell Tumors of Testes

Oncofetal substances

α-Fetoproteins

Placental glycoproteins

    β-Fraction of HCG

    Human placental lactogen

    Pregnancy specific antigen (SP$_1$)

    Others

Cellular enzymes

Placental alkaline phosphatase

Lactic dehydrogenase

Others

Abbreviations: HCG, human chorionic gonadotropin.
Source: From Ref. 54.

the scrotal wall or if the retroperitoneal pathways have been blocked by tumor. Hematogenous metastases without retroperitoneal involvement do occur, especially in choriocarcinoma.

In a study of 56 patients with a suspected testicular tumor, comparison of scrotal ultrasound and surgical findings yielded a sensitivity of 94.6%, a specificity of 57.9%, and an overall accuracy of 82.1% (55). The sensitivity and predictive value of the normal sonogram are 100%. With regard to the detection of retroperitoneal lymph node metastases from testicular tumors, abdominal CT is the preferred modality.

A summary of the main unilateral testicular tumors is provided in Table 8.

Color Doppler imaging plays a complementary role to gray-scale ultrasound in the diagnosis of scrotal tumors.

In general, the degree of vascularity seems to depend more on the size than on the histologic features of the tumor. The tumor tends to be hypovascular when under 1.5 cm and hypervascular when larger than 1.5 cm. Distribution of blood vessels in hypervascular tumors may be normal or distorted. Color Doppler has been of help in imaging testicular tumors in children by showing hypervascularity when gray-scale ultrasound showed normal testicular echogenicity (26). Thus, the examiner needs to be careful when interpreting increased vascularity as a sign of inflammation.

Testicular germ cell tumors have a single histologic pattern in 38% of cases and have multiple patterns, in any combination, in 62% of cases (56).

Seminoma, the most common testicular tumor of a single histologic type, accounts for 27% of primary germ cell tumors. Most patients are 30 to 50 years old, the oldest age group for testicular tumors. Most of the tumors manifest with painless swelling or scrotal heaviness. In general, no humoral markers of practical use are found. Tumor extension beyond the testis occurs in fewer than 10% of patients. Most tumors are homogeneous, but foci of necrosis and hemorrhage may be found in large tumors. In most patients, the testis is diffusely enlarged. Seminomas are usually solitary, but they may be multifocal. Sonographically, seminomas (57) are mostly hypoechoic and homogeneous, features that make them easy to distinguish from the normal parenchyma (Fig. 26). Less frequently, seminomas exhibit poorly defined margins or a diffusely infiltrative pattern. Spermatocytic seminoma, which represents 5% of all seminomas, occurs in older men. It is large, does not metastasize, and has not been associated with other germ cell tumors or with cryptorchidism. Macroscopically, this tumor has a homogeneous appearance similar to that described in classic seminoma.

TABLE 8 ■ Adult Unilateral (Occasionally Bilateral) Tumors of the Testis

	Diagnosis	Patient age	Ultrasound findings	Humoral markers
Malignant, homogeneous echotexture, single cell line	Seminoma	30–50 yr	Homogeneous, hypoechoic; large tumors: necrosis, calcifications	
Malignant, heterogeneous echotexture, mixed germ cell tumor	Metastases (15% bilateral)	Older adults	Discrete, hypoechoic	
	Embryonal cell carcinoma	25–35 yr	Large, invasive, heterogeneous, (hemorrhage, necrosis)	α-Fetoprotein Human chorionic gonadotropin
	Teratoma	25–35 yr	Large, heterogeneous (soft tissue, bone, cartilage), cystic areas	
	Choriocarcinoma (early hematogenous metastases)	20–30 yr	Small, heterogeneous (hemorrhage, necrosis, calcifications)	Human chorionic gonadotropin
	Yolk sac	25–35 yr	Large, invasive, heterogeneous (because of combination with other cell tumors)	α-Fetoprotein
Benign (10% incidence of malignancy), stromal tumors	Leydig cell	Adults	Well marginated, homogeneous, hypoechoic, size: 3–5 cm	Sexual steroids (gynecomastia)
	Sertoli cell	Adults	Homogeneous or multicystic, may have heavy calcifications	Sexual steroids (gynecomastia)

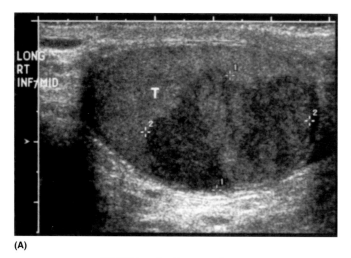

(A)

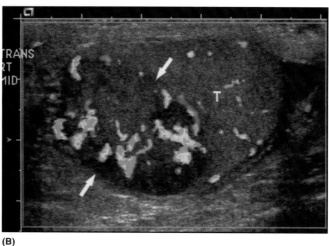

(B)

FIGURE 26 A AND B ■ Classic seminoma in a 46-year-old patient who presented with a right scrotal mass and retroperitoneal metastasis. (**A**) Longitudinal view of the right testis with gray scale showing a mass occupying the lower two-thirds (*calipers*). (**B**) Transverse view with color Doppler of the same testis showing vascularity in the mass (*arrows*). T, testis.

Nonseminomatous tumors comprise different histologic types that mostly appear in a combination, hence the name mixed germ cell tumors. Mixed germ cell tumors are the most common intratesticular neoplasm. The term mixed germ cell tumors, however, refers to different combinations of germ cells, as described in the following paragraphs.

Embryonal cell carcinoma represents 20% to 35% of all testicular tumors. It has a single histologic pattern in only 3.1% of cases. This tumor is most commonly seen in 25- to 35-year-old patients. Clinically, 80% of these patients present with a scrotal mass and 10% have symptoms related to distant metastasis. Elevated serum levels of AFP or hCG are found in 70% of patients with this tumor. These large tumors have poorly defined margins and prominent areas of necrosis and hemorrhage. Local extension to the tunica albuginea, epididymis, and spermatic cord is common. These tumors tend to metastasize early, and, for this reason, it is common to have a small tumor in the testis associated with large retroperitoneal lymphatic metastases. On ultrasound, embryonic carcinoma is seen as a large tumor that often distorts the contour of the testis (Fig. 27). It exhibits a heterogeneous echo pattern, mostly hypoechoic with irregular and poorly defined cystic areas representing necrosis, and focal hyperechogenicity representing hemorrhage (5).

Malignant teratoma represents 5% to 10% of germ cell tumors, and it is almost always seen in combination with other tumors. Teratocarcinoma, a mixture of teratoma and embryonal cell carcinoma, is the most common combination and the second most frequent germ cell tumor (seminoma is the most frequent). It is the most aggressive germ cell tumor, and metastases develop early. Teratomas, like other mixed nonseminomatous germ cell tumors, are most frequently seen in 25- to 35-year-old men. These tumors are large, well demarcated, and grossly heterogeneous. Multiple cystic spaces containing serous, gelatinous, mucous, or sebaceous material are typical. These tumors may contain calcified cartilage or bone. Occasionally, AFP and hCG levels are elevated. On ultrasound, malignant teratomas are large, but occasionally they are small (Fig. 28). The margins are usually well defined. These teratomas exhibit a heterogeneous appearance with clearly defined cystic spaces and strong areas of hyperechogenicity with shadowing that correspond to calcifications. The last two features are typical (5).

Choriocarcinoma accounts for less than 1% of testicular germ cell tumors and is most frequently found in combination with other histologic types. It most commonly affects patients in their 20s and 30s. Unlike other testicular tumors, most patients with choriocarcinoma initially have symptoms related to hemorrhage from distant hematogenous metastases, in addition to lymphatic retroperitoneal spread. These tumors produce large quantities of hCG that result in hormonal changes, such as gynecomastia. Choriocarcinomas are usually small hemorrhagic nodules that do not deform the testis. Margins are poorly defined (5).

"Burned-out" tumors of the testis were originally reported by Azzopardi et al. in 1961 (59). This term refers to retroperitoneal or mediastinal metastatic disease with a histologic pattern corresponding to a germ cell tumor. When studying the testes, no tumor can be found, but a fibrotic scar interpreted as representing necrotic remnants of the original primary tumor is seen. Sometimes, these lesions are found in atrophic testes. Recognition of this tumor is important because, after removal of the primary tumor, metastases respond more favorably to chemotherapy (52). On ultrasound, these tumors exhibit a discrete focal area of echogenicity, often with posterior shadowing (Fig. 29) (5). Residual tumor may or may not be present.

In patients over 50 years of age, *metastatic lesions* to the testis are more common than primary tumors (5).

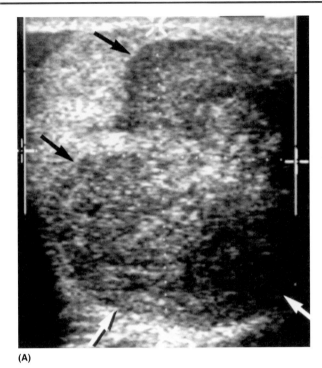

(A)

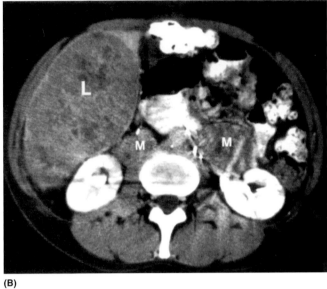

(B)

FIGURE 27 A AND B ■ Embryonal cell carcinoma predominant in a mixed-cell tumor (other components: yolk sac tumor, choriocarcinoma) in a 30-year-old patient with a scrotal mass. (**A**) Axial view of the right testis with a hypoechoic mass (*arrows*) replacing a large part of the testis. *Calipers,* testis contour. (**B**) Single section of an abdominal computed tomography scan showing liver and retroperitoneal metastases in the same patient. L, metastatic liver; M, retroperitoneal metastases. *Source*: (**A**) from Ref. 58.

Although rarely detected clinically, leukemia and lymphoma are the most frequent metastatic lesions. Involvement of the testis is usually bilateral. Testicular involvement occurs in 64% of males with *acute leukemia* (60). Suspected clinical involvement is reported in only 5% to 15% of patients. Involvement of the testes is frequently seen in children with lymphoblastic leukemia who experience a relapse after chemotherapy. This phenomenon has been explained on the basis of the testes representing a "sanctuary" organ where adequate doses of chemotherapy agents do not reach. On pathologic examination, involvement of the testes by acute leukemia is most commonly seen as diffuse infiltration. On ultrasound, the most common pattern is a diffusely infiltrative process with hypoechogenicity (Fig. 30) (61). *Chronic leukemia* involves the testes in up to 24% of patients, most of whom have the lymphocytic type of leukemia (60). On ultrasound, the testes may show a focal multinodular form or a diffuse pattern similar to the one described in acute leukemia. The nodules are hypoechoic or anechoic and well marginated. The testes may be of normal size or enlarged. Of the lymphoproliferative diseases, the nodular pattern is unique to chronic lymphocytic leukemia. It cannot be differentiated from other types of metastatic disease. If the disease is bilateral, however, lymphoproliferative disease should be strongly considered (61).

Non-Hodgkin's lymphoma of the testes is seen in 18.6% of patients. The foregoing described pattern of diffuse infiltration with hypoechogenicity is found on ultrasound (61). Testicular involvement in Hodgkin's disease is extremely rare (60). In lymphoproliferative disease, the correlation between sonographic and biopsy findings is 100% (Fig. 31) (61).

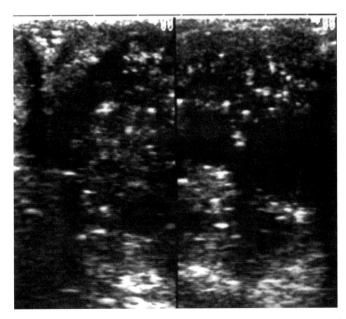

FIGURE 28 ■ Teratocarcinoma predominant in a mixed cell tumor of the testis (other components: seminoma and yolk sac tumor) in a 28-year-old patient with retroperitoneal metastases. A large mass is replacing and expanding the testis with multiple cystic areas and calcification. *Source*: From Ref. 58.

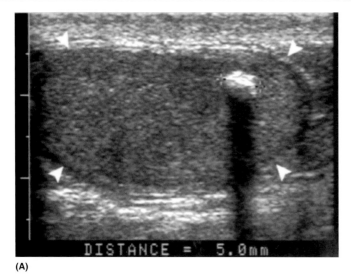

(A)

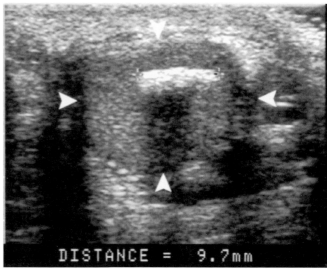

(B)

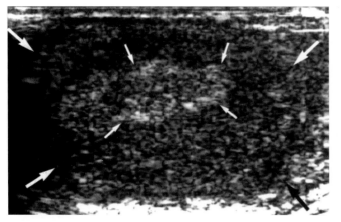

(C)

FIGURE 29 A–C ■ Burned-out nonseminomatous germ cell tumor (combination of embryonal carcinoma and yolk sac tumor) in a 52-year-old patient with scrotal pain and questionable mass on physical examination. (**A**) Longitudinal view of the left testis with a coarse calcification in the lower pole. (**B**) Axial view of the same testis. *Arrowheads*, testis; *calipers*, calcification. (**C**) Axial view of the abdomen with color Doppler from the left flank showing a retroperitoneal mass (*calipers*). *Arrow*, left kidney.

FIGURE 30 ■ Acute lymphocytic leukemia with diffuse infiltration of the testis in a 12-year-old patient. Longitudinal view of right testis showing diffuse hypoechogenicity (infiltration) with a small area of preserved parenchyma in the center (*small arrows*). *Large arrows*, testis contour.

Metastatic carcinoma to the testes is infrequent. Bilateral involvement is recorded in only 15% of patients. In decreasing order of incidence, the following primary tumor sites have been reported in adults: prostate (35%), lung (15%), melanoma (9%), colon (9%), kidney (7%), and stomach and pancreas (4% each). In addition, other less frequent sites have been reported (62). The appearance is variable on ultrasound. It is usually hypoechoic, but it may be either hyperechoic or mixed (Fig. 32) (63).

A summary of the main bilateral testicular tumors is given in Table 9.

Testicular tumors in children are uncommon and represent 1% of all pediatric malignant neoplasms. Germ cell tumors represent 70% of all tumors of the testes developing before puberty. Yolk sac carcinoma constitutes 80% to 85% of them (64). No association with cryptorchidism has been found. Clinical presentation is of a painless mass at about 18 months of age. The tumors exhibit high serum

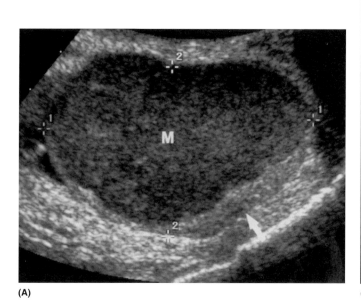

(A)

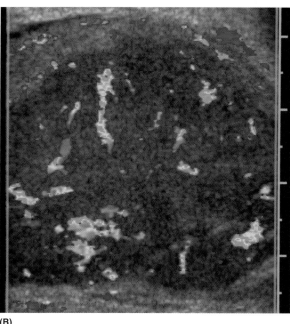

(B)

FIGURE 31 A AND B ■ Non-Hodgkin large B-cell lymphoma in a 66-year-old patient, who presented with a left testis mass. Three years before, he underwent a right orchiectomy for another mass which was reported as seminoma. No other tumor foci were found on imaging. (**A**) Longitudinal view of the right testis (*calipers*) with gray scale showing a mass of uniform hypoechogenicity replacing most of it. M, mass. (**B**) Axial view of the same testis with color Doppler showing blood flow in the tumor.

titers of AFP. They are large, well-marginated lesions that extend into the epididymis. On ultrasound, they are hypoechoic and, in general, homogeneous (Figs. 33 and 34). Fifty percent of these tumors are associated with hydrocele. In adults, yolk sac tumor is usually seen in association with other germ cell lines in mixed tumors.

Benign teratoma is the second most common testicular tumor in children, comprising 15% to 20% of such tumors (64). Unlike teratomas of the adult, these lesions in children are uniformly benign. Like yolk sac tumor, teratoma in children is found as a single germ cell tumor, rather than in combination, as in adults. It does not exhibit

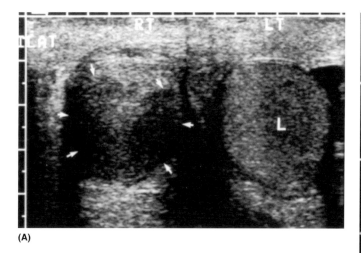

(A)

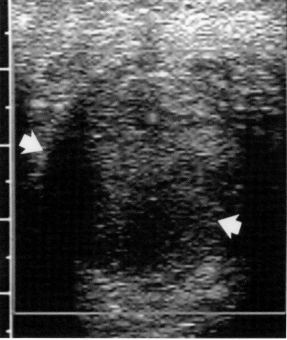

(B)

FIGURE 32 A AND B ■ Metastasis to the testis from a cholangiocarcinoma in a 74-year-old patient. (**A**) Axial view of both testes. The left testis is normal, whereas the normal-sized right testis shows hypoechoic infiltration of most of the parenchyma (*arrows*). (**B**) Axial view of the right testis; color Doppler image. The tumor is hypovascular (*arrows*).

TABLE 9 ■ Adults: Bilateral Tumors and Tumor-Like Masses

Diagnosis	Ultrasound findings
Acute lymphoblastic leukemia, non-Hodgkin's lymphoma	Ill-defined hypoechoic infiltrate (focal or diffuse)
Chronic lymphocytic leukemia	Discrete anechoic masses
Metastases (15% bilateral)	Discrete hypoechoic masses
Adrenal rest hyperplasia	Hypoechoic or hyperechoic, eccentric, variable attenuation, may calcify

elevated AFP. Clinical presentation happens most often when patient is under four years of age, but still older than in yolk sac tumor. On ultrasound, the appearance of the tumor is similar to that described in adults.

Gonadal stromal tumors represent 4% to 6% of all testicular neoplasms (65). No clear association with cryptorchidism or other epidemiologic factors exists. In children, these lesions represent 30% of the tumors of the testis. They are benign in children and in 90% of adults.

Leydig cell tumor represents the majority of gonadal stromal tumors. These tumors, most commonly seen between three and six years of age, produce testosterone and smaller amounts of estradiol, progesterone, corticosterone, and prolactin (66). The presence of these hormones results in precocious puberty as a common form of presentation in children and causes gynecomastia in 30% of the adults. The most common presentation is still that of a mass. Leydig cell tumors are large and homogeneous, with well-defined margins. On ultrasound, they are described as a hypoechoic mass (Fig. 35) (67).

Sertoli cell tumor is rare and accounts for less than 1% of all testicular tumors. It occurs with equal frequency in all ages. Sertoli cell tumors are seen in children at approximately six months of age and have also been found in newborns (67). These lesions are the most common tumors of the testis to result in feminization from hormone secretion. This effect is due to high levels of serum estrogens and gonadotropins and is most commonly seen in malignant disease. These tumors are usually small, but they may become as large as the testis itself. On ultrasound, they are well marginated; small tumors have a uniform hypoechoic appearance, whereas large tumors are heterogeneous, as a result of hemorrhage, necrosis, or calcification (68).

Large cell calcifying Sertoli cell tumor is a subtype with distinct clinical and histologic characteristics. It is often bilateral and multifocal, has a familial pattern, and is associated with complex endocrine abnormalities. Calcium deposits are prominent and may replace most of the neoplasm.

Metastatic tumors in children include the previously described acute leukemia and other primary tumors such as Wilms' tumor, neuroblastoma, histiocytosis, retinoblastoma, rhabdomyosarcoma, and Sertoli cell tumor (69).

A summary of the main testicular tumors in children is provided in Table 10.

Infrequent Tumors and Nonneoplastic Tumor-Like Conditions

Granulosa cell tumor is a rare gonadal stroma tumor that may be hormonally active or inactive and benign or malignant. It appears in two age groups: the adult form, which is extremely rare, and the juvenile form, which constitutes the most common testicular stromal tumor. This tumor has been identified in children with ambiguous genitalia, chromosomal abnormalities, and hormonal

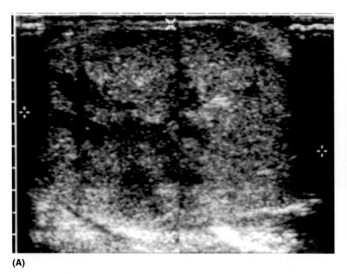

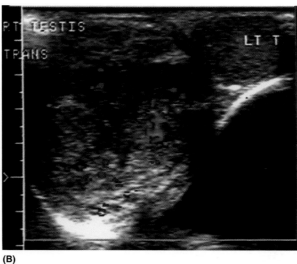

(A) **(B)**

FIGURE 33 A AND B ■ Infrequent single cell line yolk sac tumor of the right testis in a 26-year-old patient. **(A)** Longitudinal view. Large tumor replaces and expands the testis with a heterogeneous echo pattern. **(B)** Axial view of both testes; color Doppler image. The right testis is markedly enlarged and is replaced by a hypervascular tumor with areas of necrosis.

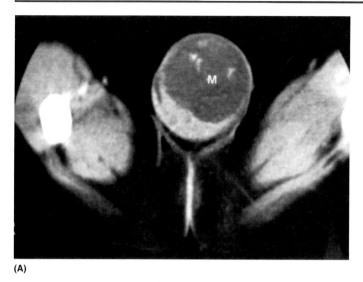

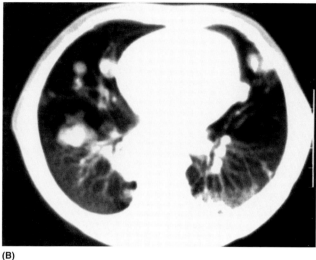

(A)   **(B)**

FIGURE 34 A AND B ■ Yolk sac tumor of the testis in a two-year-old patient presenting with a scrotal mass (M) and regional and distant metastases. (**A**) Contrast-enhanced computed tomography shows a large hypovascular scrotal mass. (**B**) Computed tomography of the chest shows multiple pulmonary metastases. *Source*: From Ref. 58.

imbalance. In newborns, it commonly exhibits elevated AFP. Macroscopically, it appears as thin-walled cysts measuring from 1 to 5 cm in diameter. Ten percent of these tumors are malignant. On ultrasound, one sees diffuse involvement of the testis with a multicystic appearance that may be confused with a teratoma (70).

Gonadoblastoma is a mixed germ cell-stromal tumor that is extremely rare and is mostly found in females with gonadal dysgenesis. It is bilateral in one-third of the cases. Although this tumor is usually small, it may be large and stippled with calcifications. Gonadoblastoma may have diffuse hyalinization or massive calcifications. On ultrasound, it has been reported as a discrete nodule with echogenic foci (71).

Hyperplastic adrenal rests are found in diseases that exhibit a high serum level of adrenocorticotropic hormone, such as Addison's disease, Cushing's syndrome, congenital adrenal hyperplasia, Nelson's syndrome, and adrenogenital syndrome. These lesions are thought to represent hyperplasia of the Leydig cells or adrenal rests from the embryologic time, when the testes were located in the retroperitoneum. They are often bilateral and multifocal, and they may not be palpable. They secrete cortisol, function as hyperplastic adrenal glands, and regress with the administration of prednisone (72). Histologic differentiation of a Leydig cell tumor from hyperplastic adrenal rests can be difficult, and failure of complete regression after steroid therapy does not necessarily prove the presence of

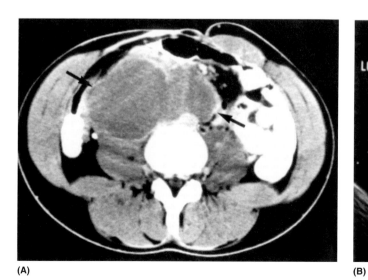

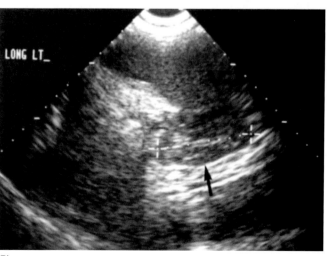

(A)   **(B)**

FIGURE 35 A AND B ■ Malignant Leydig cell tumor in a 20-year-old man with retroperitoneal recurrence. (**A**) Contrast-enhanced computed tomography shows a retroperitoneal mass (*arrows*). (**B**) Abdominal sonogram, in a sagittal section, demonstrates similar findings (*calipers* and *arrow*). *Source*: From Ref. 58.

TABLE 10 ■ Children: Tumors of the Testis

	Diagnosis	Patient age	Ultrasound findings	Humoral markers (comments)
Germ cell tumors (pure cell lines)	Yolk sac (malignant, most frequent)	18 mo	Large, solid, invades epididymis	α-Fetoprotein
	Teratoma (benign, second most frequent)	<4 yr	Large, heterogeneous (soft tissue, bone, cartilage); multiple cystic areas	
Stromal tumors (infrequent, benign)	Leydig cell	3–6 yr	Well-marginated, homogeneous, hypoechoic, size: 3–5 cm	Sexual steroids (precocious puberty)
	Sertoli cell	6 mo	Homogeneous or multicystic; may have heavy calcifications; variable size	Sexual steroids (precocious puberty)
	Granulosa cell	Infants	Thin-walled cysts; size: 1–5 cm	α-Fetoprotein (associated with ambiguous genitalia and chromosomal abnormalities)
Mixed germ cell– stromal tumors (infrequent, usually benign)	Gonadoblastoma (33% bilateral)	<2 yr	Small with stippled calcifications	Associated with intersex problems

a tumor. The importance of the differential diagnosis is that 10% of Leydig cell tumors are malignant. On ultrasound, the testes may or may not be enlarged. They exhibit bilateral solid masses that usually are hypoechoic, but may have a complex appearance with areas of hyperechogenicity and possible shadowing resulting from fibrosis (Fig. 36) (73). The ultrasound appearance of hyperplastic

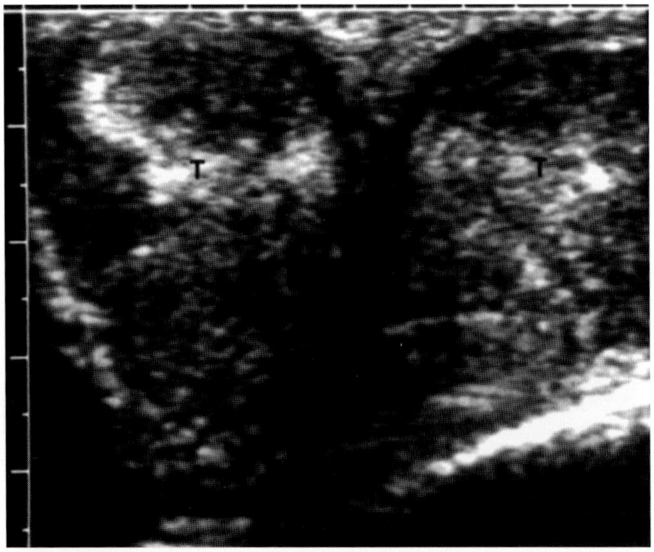

FIGURE 36 ■ Adrenal rests in the testes in a 33-year-old patient with adrenogenital syndrome who had been on steroid medication since early childhood and who had induration of the testes noted on physical examination. Axial view of both testes shows a symmetric pattern of heterogeneous echogenicity. T, testes. *Source*: From Ref. 23.

adrenal rests should be included in the differential diagnosis of other causes of bilateral testicular involvement, such as bilateral germ cell tumor, large cell calcified Sertoli's cell tumor, lymphoproliferative disease, and metastases. Knowledge of the patient's clinical history helps in the differential diagnosis.

When a patient presents with an acute intratesticular event with ultrasound findings consistent with hemorrhage, the examiner should remember that approximately 10% of acute scrotum pathology is due to intratumoral hemorrhage. Therefore, the ultrasound study should be performed so as not to overlook an intratesticular neoplasm.

Necrotizing Vasculitis ■ Necrotizing vasculitis of the testis is a rare manifestation of systemic vascular disease. It is usually part of an autoimmune systemic process. Occasionally, it may be limited to the testis. The most common association is with polyarteritis nodosa, which, on surgical pathology and autopsy studies, is associated with an 85% involvement of the testis. Clinical scrotal symptoms are found in only 2% to 5% of patients. Pathologic examination shows inflammation, fibrinoid necrosis, and aneurysms of small artery walls. Ischemic and hemorrhagic infarcts are seen in the surrounding tissue. This rare entity has been associated even less frequently with rheumatoid arthritis, dermatomyositis, hypersensitivity angiitis (to sulfa drugs and Streptococci infection), Goodpasture's disease, Henoch-Schönlein purpura, Wegener's granulomatosis, typhus, Rocky Mountain spotted fever, and medial fibromuscular dysplasia. Clinically, it may present as acute scrotal disease with swelling, redness, pain, and fever (74), or it may appear as a scrotal mass. In general, routine laboratory findings

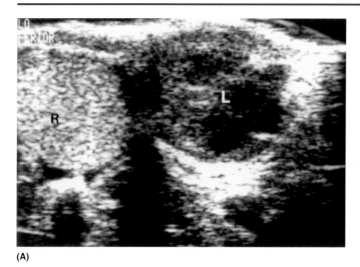
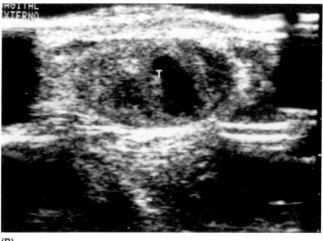

(A)   (B)

FIGURE 37 A AND B ■ Necrotizing vasculitis of the left testis in a 30-year-old man with a three-week history of urinary symptoms and a slightly indurated and tender left testis on physical examination. (**A**) Axial view of both testes shows a diffusely hypoechoic left testis (L) with focal irregular areas of sonolucency (necrosis). The echogenicity of right testis (R) is normal. (**B**) Longitudinal view of the nonenlarged left testis (T) shows similar sonographic findings. With a diagnosis of possible malignant disease, orchidectomy was performed. *Source:* Courtesy of Drs. Bernardo Alanis and Jorge Fernandez de la Torre, Hospital San José, Monterrey, Mexico.

are in the normal range. On ultrasound, a case report of necrotizing vasculitis described the sonographic findings as a 3 cm discrete mass with mixed echogenicity (Fig. 37) (75). Doppler sonography in another case report revealed significantly increased vascularity at the margins of the lesion (76).

Gray-scale findings overlap those of tumor. Therefore, correlation with Doppler findings is important, as is follow-up to complete resolution.

Pitfalls in Diagnosing Solid Testicular Processes

1. *Polyorchidism.* Infrequently, extranumerary testis (polyorchidism) may occur rarely in children. This anomaly may mimic an extratesticular mass. A comparison with the echotexture of the adjacent testis may be a clue in delineating the extranumerary testis (Fig. 38).
2. *False-negative diagnosis of testicular torsion.* Several pitfalls are possible when trying to diagnose testicular torsion. For example, when a patient has torsion with spontaneous detorsion, the testis, instead of showing decreased color flow, may actually appear hyperemic. This hyperemia may occur in both the testis and the epididymis, leading to a false-positive diagnosis of epididymo-orchitis and a false-negative diagnosis of torsion. Moreover, patients with torsion with less than 360° of twist may have complete venous occlusion but normal arterial flow. This situation may also lead to a false-negative diagnosis of testicular torsion.
3. *Hypervascularity of testis from inflammation or tumor.* Color Doppler imaging is usually nonspecific in distinguishing testicular processes such as inflammation versus tumor. Increased color vascularity occurs with

inflammatory response, but it may also be seen in tumors. Follow-up ultrasound is helpful to ensure complete resolution of presumed inflammatory mass. If the mass is tumorous, it will persist over time.

Testicular Cystic Lesions

Nonneoplastic Cysts ■ Testicular cysts are found in up to 10% of the population undergoing ultrasound examination (78). They are usually seen in adults and are infrequent among children. These cysts are classified into two types. Nonneoplastic cysts, more common in older men, may be located in the tunica albuginea or in the testis itself.

Cysts of the tunica albuginea are located in the surface of the testis near the rete testis and the epididymis (Fig. 39). They measure a few millimeters in diameter, are found in middle-aged men, are palpable, and do not change over time. These cysts are thought to represent embryonal remnants.

Intratesticular cysts are located near the mediastinum testis and favor the upper pole and the periphery (Fig. 40) (78). They are found in older adults and are not palpable. They are usually solitary and range from a few millimeters up to several centimeters. They may be bilateral and are associated with epididymal cysts. These cysts are thought to originate in the rete testis from embryonal remnants or to be secondary to inflammation or trauma.

Occasionally, in elderly men, we may see unilateral or bilateral tubular ectasia of the rete testis. In general, this finding is nonpalpable on physical examination. Histology shows dilation of the efferent tubules leading from the testis into the epididymis. On ultrasound, this finding is seen as microtubular or cystic dilation of the testis extending from the mediastinum to a variable distance. It is

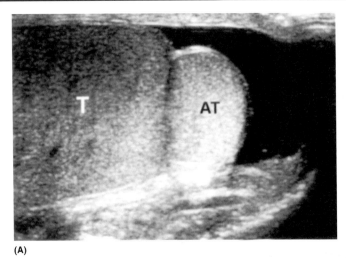
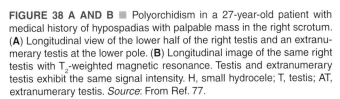
(A)

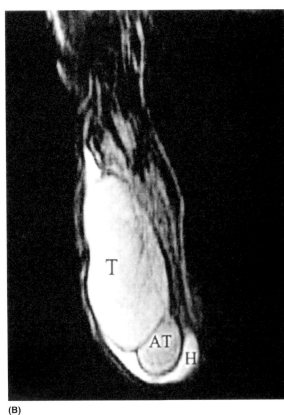
(B)

FIGURE 38 A AND B ■ Polyorchidism in a 27-year-old patient with medical history of hypospadias with palpable mass in the right scrotum. (**A**) Longitudinal view of the lower half of the right testis and an extranumerary testis at the lower pole. (**B**) Longitudinal image of the same right testis with T$_2$-weighted magnetic resonance. Testis and extranumerary testis exhibit the same signal intensity. H, small hydrocele; T, testis; AT, extranumerary testis. *Source*: From Ref. 77.

frequently associated with cysts (Fig. 41). In the literature, tubular ectasia of the rete testis has been associated with a history of previous surgery, infection, or tumor (79,80), but often, in our practice, we have seen this finding with no relevant prior history. It is not associated with urological abnormalities and should not be confused with the next described cystic dysplasia of the testis, which has associated findings.

Cystic dysplasia of the testis is a rare congenital malformation, usually found in children and occasionally

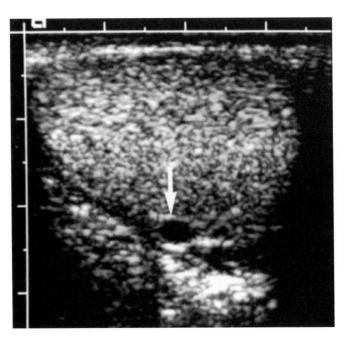

FIGURE 39 ■ Cyst (*arrow*) of the tunica albuginea in a 71-year-old patient with a palpable finding.

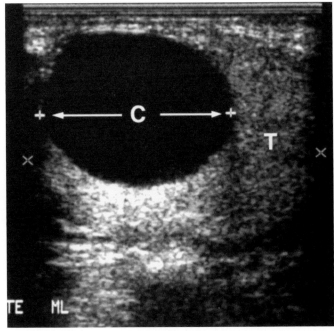

FIGURE 40 ■ Testicular cyst (*calipers*) as an incidental finding in a 65-year-old patient with a history of alcohol abuse. C, cyst; T, testis. *Source*: From Ref. 23.

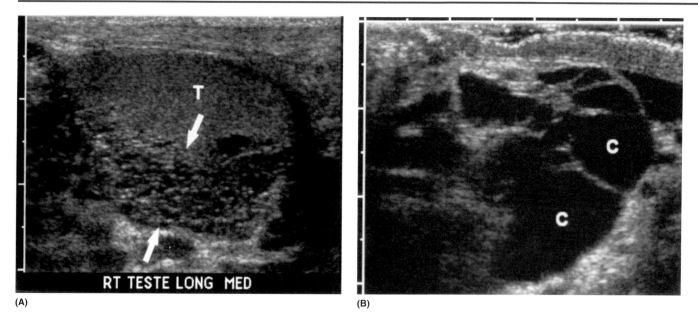

(A)

(B)

FIGURE 41 A AND B ■ Bilateral tubular ectasia of the rete testis on a 77-year-old patient with bilateral inguinal hernias. (**A**) Longitudinal view of the right testis showing microtubular dilation (*arrows*) involving the posterior aspect. (**B**) Axial view of the epididymis showing multiple cysts. T, testis; C, cysts.

in young adults, that consists of multiple small cysts, affecting part or the whole testis and originating in the mediastinal area. This disorder results in enlargement of the testis and atrophy of the remaining parenchyma (81,82). The dysplasia has been explained on the basis of an embryologic defect that prevented connection of the tubules of the rete testis with the efferent ducts. Of interest is the association of cystic dysplasia with renal agenesis,

bilateral renal dysplasia (82), and duplication of the renal collecting systems. On ultrasound, it appears as an enlarged testis with multiple irregular anechoic areas measuring a few millimeters each (Fig. 42).

Neoplastic Cysts ■ Neoplastic cysts of the testis are mostly found in association with teratomas, which are prone to cyst formation in the tumor. Cysts are less frequently

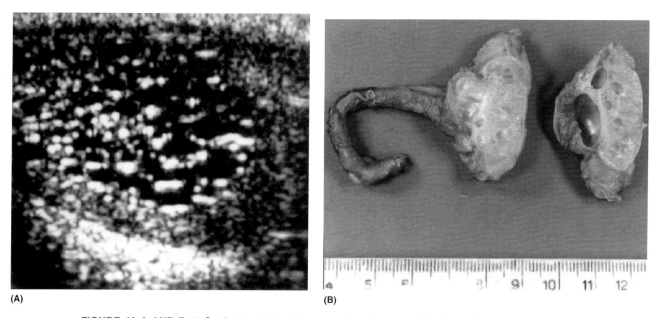

(A)

(B)

FIGURE 42 A AND B ■ Cystic dysplasia of the testes in a nine-year-old patient with one-year history of left scrotal enlargement. The patient had a solitary hypertrophied right kidney and absent left kidney. (**A**) Longitudinal view of the left testis showing replacement of the normal parenchyma by multiple small cysts. (**B**) Longitudinal section of the pathology specimen showing multiple cysts. *Source*: From Ref. 83.

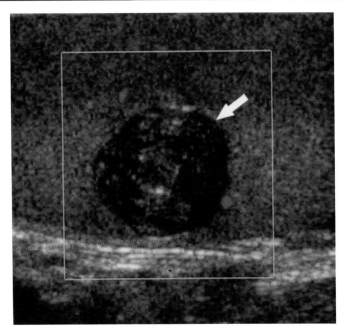

FIGURE 43 ■ Epidermoid cyst of the testis in a 21-year-old patient with palpable, nontender mass in the left scrotum. Magnified view of hypoechoic avascular lesion (*arrow*) with well-defined margins and "onion-skin" internal structure. *Source*: From Ref. 85.

found in other tumors such as seminoma in which the presence of the cysts is explained by extensive tumor infiltration of the rete testis, with resulting cyst formation by necrosis. Granulosa cell tumor is rare and is usually cystic (84). The mechanism of cyst formation in tumors of the testis may differ. Most of these cysts are associated with solid components of the tumor that expand the testis, resulting in palpatory findings, except teratomas, which may appear as an isolated cyst.

Epidermoid cysts are thought to represent monolayer teratomas. Solitary and palpable, the cysts are surrounded by a thick wall of keratinized epithelium (Fig. 43). They account for 1% of all testicular tumors. Although unusual, they may exhibit calcification of the walls that results in a sonographic appearance difficult to distinguish from other diagnoses such as teratoma and parenchymal scars (86). These cysts are more often seen in white men during the second to fourth decades of life. On ultrasound, a variable sonolucent cystic component is surrounded by a thick echogenic wall with variable posterior shadowing. A correct diagnosis is important because of the recommendation of enucleation as treatment.

A summary of cystic lesions of the scrotum is given in Table 11.

TABLE 11 ■ Cystic Lesions of the Scrotum

Structure	Diagnosis		Patient age	Ultrasound findings
Tunica vaginalis	Hydrocele, hematocele		Any age	Sonolucency with possible echogenicity (debris) and septa (organization) surrounding the testis
	Pyocele		Any age, peak in adolescence and middle age	
Epididymis	Simple cyst		Any age	"Classic" appearance
	Spermatocele		Postpubertal	"Classic" appearance; may contain sediment
	Tubular ectasia		Postvasectomy	Thickened epididymis with tubular dilation
Testis	Simple cysts	Intraparenchymal	Older adults	"Classic" appearance, single, peripheral, variable size (mm–cm)
		Tunica albuginea	Middle age	"Classic" appearance, single, peripheral, posterior, size: mm
	Cystic dysplasia		Children	Multiple small cysts extending from the mediastinum testis; parenchymal atrophy; associated with renal agenesis and bilateral renal dysplasia
	Complex cysts	Epidermoid cyst (benign tumor)	2nd–4th decades	Hypoechoic center, echogenic wall, variable attenuation
		Teratoma, adults (strong malignant potential)	2nd–4th decades	Large, heterogeneous (soft tissue, bone, cartilage); multiple cystic areas; rarely a single cyst
		Large seminoma with invasion of rete testis or necrosis	4th–5th decades	Large mass with cystic components

Extratesticular Lesions

Extratesticular Solid Lesions

As discussed previously, epididymitis and epididymo-orchitis are common clinical problems usually involving the extratesticular content of the scrotum. These entities are explained in detail in the previous section.

Ninety percent of extratesticular scrotal tumors are derived from the funiculus (spermatic cord), and 70% of them are benign (87). Epididymal tumors are rare and account for only 5% of all scrotal masses.

Adenomatoid tumors account for one-third of all paratesticular lesions and are the most common neoplasms of the epididymis. They are benign and slow-growing and most commonly arise from the epididymis, but they may also arise from the tunica albuginea and spermatic cord. Most of the tumors are small, under 2 cm. The tail of the epididymis is a common location. They are well marginated and solitary. This tumor is usually found in patients from the second to the fourth decades of life. On ultrasound, these tumors are well defined and have an echogenicity similar to or slightly higher than that of the testis (Fig. 44) (5).

Lipomas of the spermatic cord, the most common tumors of this structure, are benign. They may be difficult to differentiate on ultrasound from the adjacent inguinal adipose tissue. They exhibit from medium to low echogenicity. Infarcted lipomas have an ultrasound appearance similar to those that are not complicated (88). They are most commonly seen in men 40 to 60 years old.

Rhabdomyosarcomas are the most common malignant lesions of the spermatic cord in infants and children. They are most often seen in the first two decades of life. These highly aggressive tumors exhibit metastatic spread to the retroperitoneal lymph nodes. On ultrasound, they have been described as a large extratesticular mass of homogeneous hypoechogenicity or as a heterogeneous echo pattern (Fig. 45). Color Doppler imaging of rhabdomyosarcoma in a case report (89) demonstrated increased vascularity of the mass. This case demonstrates the difficulty found in differentiating this extratesticular, highly

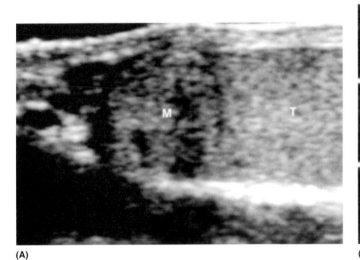

(A)

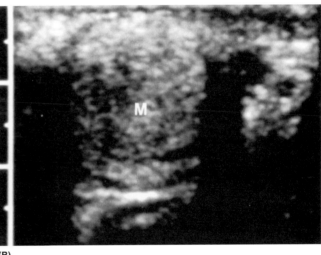

(B)

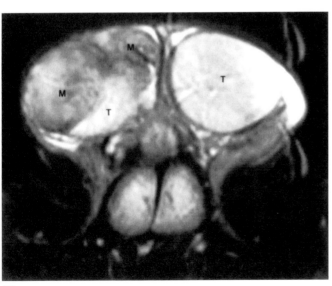

(C)

FIGURE 44 A–C ▓ Adenomatoid tumor in the head of the right epididymis of a 39-year-old patient. (**A**) Longitudinal view with the mass deforming the upper pole of the testis. (**B**) Axial view through the mass. (**C**) Magnetic resonance imaging, T_2-weighted, axial view. M, mass (adenomatoid tumor); T, testes. *Source*: Courtesy of Dr. Raymond Dougherty, Department of Radiology, David Grant USAF Medical Center, Travis Air Force Base, California.

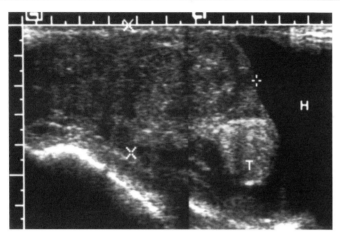

FIGURE 45 ■ Embryonal rhabdomyosarcoma (*calipers*) of the cord in a 20-year-old patient who had had scrotal and abdominal masses for six months. T, testis; H, hydrocele. *Source*: From Ref. 58.

malignant tumor from severe epididymitis. Liposarcomas are the most frequent malignant tumors of the spermatic cord in adults. They are slow-growing and usually multilobular. On ultrasound, a reported tumor demonstrated hyperechogenicity (90).

Multiple other tumors have been described in isolated cases. Among the malignant extratesticular tumors are neuroblastoma and leiomyosarcoma. Among the benign tumors are hemangioma, lymphangioma, fibroma, neurofibroma, and leiomyoma.

Important in the differential diagnosis is the possibility of polyorchidism, a rare condition in which more than two testes are present. The extra testis may be scrotal, inguinal, or retroperitoneal. Each testis has its own epididymis with a single shared vas deferens. When located in the scrotum, the extra testis should not be confused with an extratesticular mass (Fig. 38) (91).

A summary of the most frequent extratesticular tumors is provided in Table 12.

Extratesticular Cystic Lesions

Hydrocele ■ Hydrocele is an abnormal accumulation of fluid in the sac of the tunica vaginalis. Normally, only a few drops of serous fluid are present between the visceral and parietal layers. This lesion has received more specific names depending on the type of fluid content: hematocele when containing blood, pyocele when containing pus. As mentioned before, in rare cases of urethral rupture, the fluid may represent urine. Hydrocele is the most common cause of scrotal swelling and may be unilateral or bilateral (5). Most hydroceles are idiopathic and serous, and clinically they are significant to the patient when they become large and to the physician because they limit the evaluation of the testes in the enlarged scrotum (92). Small hydroceles may be found in utero, and they are common in newborns and infants. They usually resolve by 18 months (5). Incomplete closure of the processus vaginalis connects the peritoneum to the tunica vaginalis. Hydroceles may be associated with inguinal hernias. Occasionally, cystic fluid collections in the spermatic cord may persist into adulthood. Reactive or secondary hydroceles are associated with inflammatory disease, trauma (up to 50% of acquired hydroceles are traumatic), neoplasia, infarction, or rheumatic disease (46).

Ultrasound study of a simple hydrocele shows sonolucency surrounding the testis on the anterior and lateral aspects where the tunica vaginalis is located (the testes are attached to the scrotal wall on the posterior aspect) (Fig. 46). Sometimes, a large epididymal cyst may mimic a hydrocele, but a knowledgeable examiner will see that the cyst does not wrap around the testis, as a hydrocele does. Homogeneous low-level echoes may be observed in the fluid, indicating an increased cholesterol crystal content. Simple hydroceles may be unilocular or septated and multilocular (Fig. 47). Hydroceles may demonstrate color flow from acoustic streaming and should not be misinterpreted as true blood flow (Fig. 3).

Hematocele results from trauma, surgery, tumor, diabetes, and coagulopathies. On ultrasound, the fresh clot looks mildly echogenic, and lucent when lysed. Intermediate stages show variable amounts of fluid with internal echoes (93). When hematocele does not resolve and becomes chronic, ultrasound may show thickening and septation of the tunica vaginalis (94).

Pyocele may result from epididymitis, epididymoorchitis, extension of adjacent infection such as perianal abscess, hematogenous spread of distant infection, trauma, surgery, diabetes, and immunosuppression.

TABLE 12 ■ Most Frequent Extratesticular Tumors

Type	Diagnosis	Patient age	Site of origin	Ultrasound findings
Benign	Adenomatoid tumor	2nd–4th decades	Epididymis (tail + +)	Well marginated, isoechoic to the testis, size: <2 cm
			Spermatic cord	
			Tunica albuginea	
Malignant	Lipoma	4th–6th decades	Spermatic cord	Echogenic
	Rhabdomyosarcoma	2–20 yr	Spermatic cord	Large, hypoechoic
	Liposarcoma	Adults	Spermatic cord	Hyperechoic

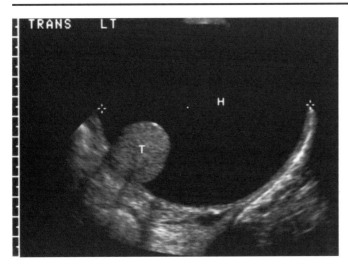

FIGURE 46 ■ Large hydrocele (*calipers*) following a recent inguinal hernia repair in a 27-year-old patient. T, testis; H, hydrocele.

Ultrasound in the early stages demonstrates lucency with variable level of echogenicity secondary to the presence of debris. In the chronic stage, findings are similar to those seen in chronic hematocele. They are difficult to differentiate by imaging.

Varicocele and Infertility ■ Varicoceles are a dilation (over 2–3 mm) and tortuosity of the pampiniform plexus veins in the spermatic cord or the epididymis (14). Most varicoceles are primary and affect adolescents and young adults. They usually involve the left side, a finding attributed to the drainage pattern of the more tortuous left internal spermatic vein into the left renal vein. Bilateral varicoceles have been reported with an incidence varying from 10% to 70%. Secondary varicoceles result from increased intra-abdominal pressure such as from hepatosplenomegaly and abdominal masses. They are less frequent. An acute onset on either side, a right varicocele, or a varicocele in a mature man raises the possibility of an abdominal or pelvic mass. A right varicocele has been associated with situs inversus (95). Varicocele is the most common single, correctable cause of male infertility, and it is found in 37% of patients with this problem. Histologic examination of the testes of infertile males with a varicocele reveals hypospermatogenesis, maturation arrest, complete germ cell aplasia, and tubular fibrosis of variable degree. Varicocele increases the temperature on the affected hemiscrotum, as demonstrated by thermography. The degree of hyperthermia is not related to the size of the varicocele but to its location. When located in the spermatic cord, it results in circumscribed hyperthermia, whereas even a small varicocele in a paratesticular location results in hyperthermia of the entire hemiscrotum (96). Varicocele does not completely explain the mechanism of infertility because only 20% of cases are bilateral. Whereas approximately one-fourth of all males have varicosity of the spermatic veins, only a few develop infertility. On the other hand, improvement of sperm quality has been documented in 70% to 80% of surgically treated patients. The degree of fertility depends on the extent of the preexisting damage to the testes.

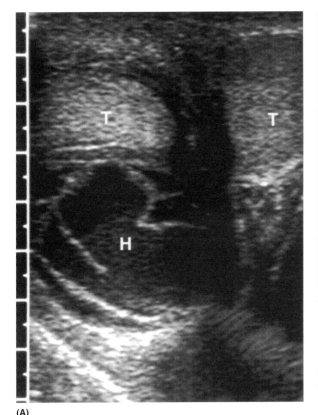

(A)

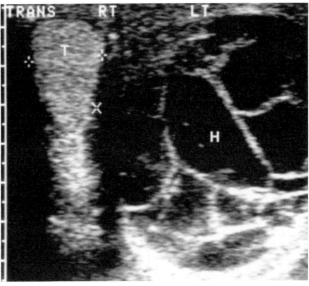

(B)

FIGURE 47 A AND B ■ Organized (septated) right hydrocele with resolution and recurrence on the left side in a 60-year-old patient. (**A**) *December, 1993*: Axial view of both testes shows an organized right hydrocele. (**B**) *December, 1994*: Axial view of both testes shows resolution of the right hydrocele (*calipers*) with conservative treatment and development of a similar problem on the left side. T, testes; H, hydrocele.

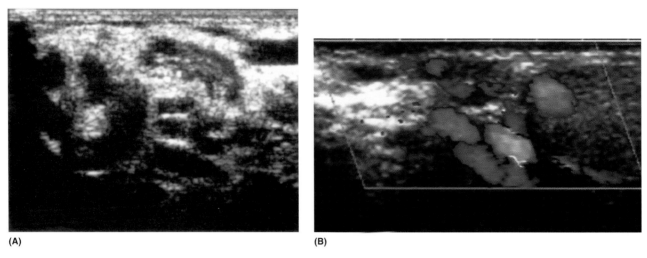

(A)   **(B)**

FIGURE 48 A AND B ■ Varicocele in a 37-year-old man. **(A)** Gray-scale ultrasound demonstrates multiple 4 to 5 mm hypoechoic tubular structures superior to the testis. **(B)** Color Doppler demonstrates flow within these tubes representing dilated and tortuous veins.

On ultrasound, gray-scale and color Doppler studies do not usually identify veins in the epididymis and spermatic cord in healthy patients. Two or more tortuous, sonolucent tubular structures with a caliber of 2 mm or more are seen as the hallmark findings in varicoceles (Fig. 48). These venous channels dilate during the Valsalva maneuver or when the patient is upright (97). Color Doppler imaging reveals flow unless thrombosis has occurred. Pulsed Doppler imaging reveals typical continuous nonpulsatile flow. Doppler ultrasound and percutaneous retrograde venography demonstrate retrograde flow in the pampiniform plexus and testicular veins. On the basis of the Doppler tracing during a Valsalva maneuver, varicoceles have been classified in two types. The stop type shows only retrograde blood in the internal spermatic vein. An explanation for this situation is the presence of competent valves in the pampiniform plexus. Small and subclinical varicoceles are usually of this type. The shunt type shows both retrograde and antegrade (physiologic) blood flow in the same vein. This phenomenon is explained by the presence of incompetent valves in the pampiniform plexus that allow communication and collateral circulation by way of the deferential and cremasteric veins. Moderate-to-large varicoceles display this pattern (98). Color Doppler imaging has a sensitivity of 93% in the detection of venographically diagnosed varicoceles as compared with 71% using physical examination (99). Ultrasound was found to have a 95% sensitivity in the detection of subclinical varicocele (100). Rarely, and in cases of thrombosed varicocele, phleboliths have been seen on ultrasound as intraluminal areas of echogenicity with posterior shadowing (101).

Ultrasound demonstrated scrotal lesions in 40% of 658 consecutive patients in an infertility clinic. In decreasing order of incidence, they were varicocele, hydrocele, epididymal abnormalities, spermatoceles, increased or decreased echogenicity of the testes, intratesticular cysts, tumors, and carcinoma in situ (102). On scrotal ultrasound studies of 200 men studied for infertility, 57% were found to have some detectable abnormality (signs of infection in 19.5%, varicocele in 14%, atrophic testis in 13%, hydrocele in 12%, and spermatocele and undescended testes in 1.5% each) (103).

Cysts ■ Epididymal cysts can be seen in 20% to 40% of asymptomatic males. They are not as common in children as in adults. They may be single or multiple and are more common in the epididymal head. They may be simple or septated and measure from several millimeters up to several centimeters (5). They contain serous fluid. *Spermatoceles* are cysts that contain spermatic elements, are most commonly located in the head of the epididymis, and represent 25% of the epididymal cysts. Multiple cysts of the epididymis have been described after vasectomy, in cystic dysplasia of the testes, and in patients exposed to diethylstilbestrol in utero (104).

On ultrasound, all epididymal cysts have a similar appearance with typical sonolucency, solid back wall, and through transmission (Fig. 49). Occasionally, spermatoceles contain internal echoes (Fig. 50).

Epidermoid inclusion cysts of the scrotal wall are special kinds of cysts (Fig. 51). They contain sebaceous material and exhibit a medium echogenicity similar to that of the testis. For this reason, they resemble solid masses. Important features for the diagnosis are the superficial location, separate from testes and epididymides, and absence of blood flow (105).

Postvasectomy Epididymal Changes ■ Postvasectomy lesions can be divided into two groups. The first group corresponds to acute complications of vasectomy in the immediate postoperative period. The most common are hematoma and infection. The second group corresponds to chronic complications found months after surgery. In a study of 31 men, an ultrasound examination was performed at two months and at 12 months after vasectomy;

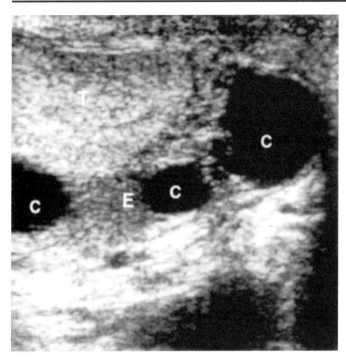

FIGURE 49 ■ Multiple epididymal cysts in a 70-year-old patient. Axial view of the testis and epididymis. C, cysts; T, testis; E, epididymis.

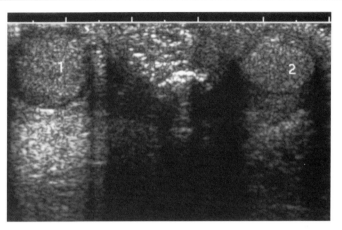

FIGURE 51 ■ Epidermoid inclusion cysts of the scrotal wall in a 46-year-old patient with palpable scrotal masses. Magnified view of part of the scrotal wall showing two well-circumscribed round masses with medium echogenicity and through transmission (1 and 2), which demonstrated no blood flow. Observe the echogenic intraluminal content of the cyst.

the authors found that 45% of these men had persistent changes in the epididymis that consisted of enlargement, development of cysts, and heterogeneous echo pattern. The changes are explained by congestion and dilation of the epididymal tubules seen on pathologic examination; 4.3% of patients who had undergone vasectomy had clinical findings five to seven years later, the late postvasectomy syndrome (106). These patients suffered from constant scrotal pain that was exacerbated by sexual or physical activity. The epididymides were swollen, indurated, and tender. These patients were thought to have

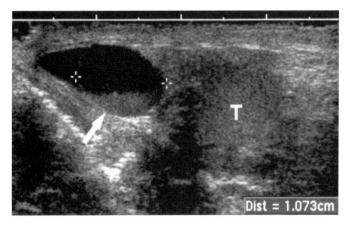

FIGURE 50 ■ Spermatocele in a 27-year-old patient with right groin pain with this incidental finding. Axial view at the upper pole of the right testis showing a cyst in the adjacent epididymal head (*calipers*) with sediment at the most dependent portion (*arrow*). Small amount of free fluid adjacent to the lateral aspect of the cyst. T, testis.

infectious epididymitis despite negative bacterial studies and lack of response to repeated antibiotic treatment. Epididymo-vasectomy was performed with immediate improvement of the symptoms. Pathologic study demonstrated dilation of the ductus deferens and tubules of the epididymis. The dilation was occasionally cystic, resulting in the formation of spermatoceles. Rupture of tubules with extravasation of sperm produces varying histologic appearances. Chronic inflammatory changes lead to a swollen nodular epididymis containing microscopic or macroscopic granulomas, which may be single or multiple. On ultrasound, the epididymides are thickened and with tubular dilation (Fig. 52). These findings may be uni- or bilateral. Spermatic granuloma results from invasion of spermatozoa into the stroma of the epididymis and testis that causes a secondary inflammatory reaction. It may be the result of trauma, inflammation, or following vasectomy. Histologically, these lesions represent a necrotizing granulomatous response to the extravasation, with resulting lesions ranging in size from a few millimeters up to 3 cm. Clinically, these lesions manifest as painless masses. On ultrasound, they appear as a solid mass with variable beam attenuation and hypovascularity (Fig. 53) (5).

Calcifications

Testicular Calcifications

Testicular calcifications are of different types. Isolated calcifications with no associated findings are common and may represent benign phleboliths, fibrosed-calcified spermatic granulomas, the end result of previous epididymo-orchitis, or trauma. They are of no clinical significance (107). A different situation arises when the calcifications are multiple, minute, and grouped. They should be considered highly suggestive of malignancy. Necrotic or hemorrhagic areas in germ cell tumors may calcify. Embryonal carcinoma is the most common tumor to present with

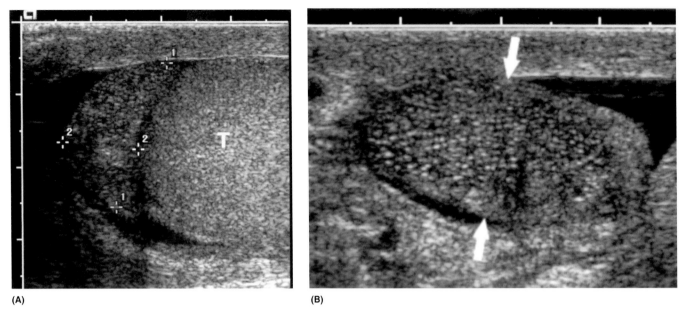

(A)   (B)

FIGURE 52 A AND B ■ Tubular ectasia of the epididymis in a 68-year-old patient who had a vasectomy 30 years before and complained of intermittent swelling and tenderness of the scrotum. (**A**) Longitudinal view of the upper pole of the testis and epididymis (*calipers*) showing slight enlargement of the last one with microtubular dilation which is better seen on **B**. (**B**) Longitudinal view of the body of the epididymis (*arrows*) showing enlargement and microtubular dilation with no blood flow seen on Doppler. T, testis.

necrosis and hemorrhage, whereas seminomas rarely necrose and calcify. Calcifications may also be seen with teratoma, but in this case they represent calcified cartilage or bone fragments. A discrete, small calcification in a testis that is normal in size or atrophic in a young person should lead the examiner to consider the possibility of a

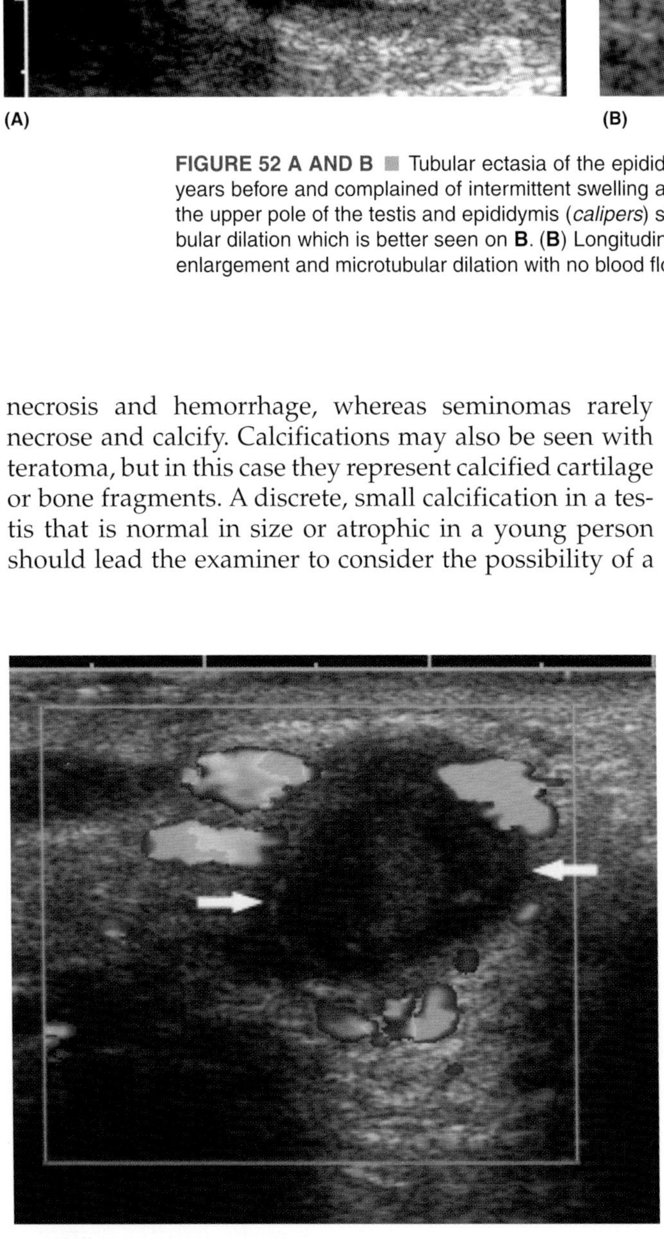

FIGURE 53 ■ Sperm granuloma in a 40-year-old patient with a palpable left scrotal mass above the left testis and history of vasectomy two years before. Axial view with color Doppler above the left testis showing a fairly well-marginated, hypoechoic, and avascular mass (*arrows*) in the region of the spermatic cord.

calcified scar in a "burned-out" primary testicular germ cell tumor. This diagnosis should be considered if retroperitoneal or mediastinal mass is the indication to perform the scrotal ultrasound study (Fig. 29). Testicular calcifications are not specific for malignancy and may be seen in tuberculosis and sarcoidosis. Calcified granuloma of the tunica albuginea is rare. The wall of an epidermoid cyst may calcify (86).

Testicular microlithiasis is an uncommon, usually incidental, finding. It is caused by the formation of microliths from degenerating cells in the seminiferous tubules (Fig. 54) (108). Microlithiasis may occur in healthy patients, but it has also been found in nonneoplastic conditions such as Klinefelter's syndrome, Peutz-Jeghers syndrome, cryptorchidism, postorchiopexy testis, testicular infarcts, granulomas, subfertility, infertility, male pseudohermaphroditism, Down's syndrome, and pulmonary alveolar microlithiasis (109). Testicular microlithiasis has been associated with germ cell tumors: seminomas, seminoteratoma (110), and intratubular germ cell neoplasia (111). In cases of seminoma with pathologic correlation, the area of microlithiasis was confined to the nontumoral portion of the testis (Fig. 55). Because of the described association of microlithiasis with neoplasia, the ultrasound diagnosis of microlithiasis should warrant more aggressive follow-up. We recommend monthly self-examination, six months ultrasound for several years, and then yearly.

On ultrasound, microliths that measure an average of 0.2 mm in diameter are seen as multiple, punctate, hyperechoic areas with no discrete individual shadowing and possible mild global attenuation behind the testes (112).

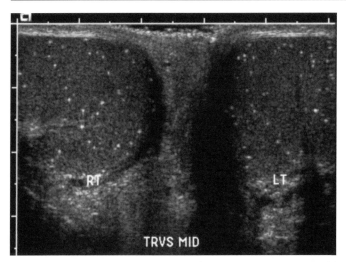

FIGURE 54 ■ Bilateral microlithiasis of the testes in a 15-year-old patient with findings of mild epididymitis. This finding was incidental.

Extratesticular Calcifications

Extratesticular calcifications are mostly benign. Frequently, they are solitary, large, and found in the epididymis, which is usually not enlarged. These calcifications are usually due to chronic epididymitis with fibrosis and secondary calcification. Other possible causes are tuberculosis and gonorrhea in which calcification is due to necrosis. Infrequently, parasitic diseases, especially filariasis, should be considered in patients from areas where these diseases are endemic. In filariasis, epididymal calcification is related to the dead parasite (113).

The most common calcification of the tunica vaginalis is in the form of loose bodies (calculi, "pearls"). They are

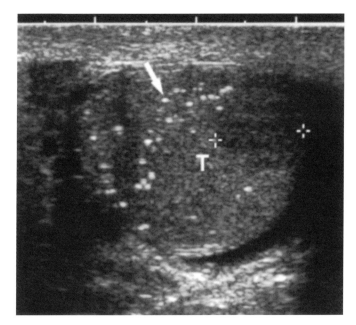

FIGURE 55 ■ Seminoma (*calipers*) in a patient with testicular microlithiasis (*arrow*) in a 30-year-old patient who presented with acute scrotal pain. T, testis.

located between the two layers of the tunica vaginalis. They are thought to originate from fibrinous debris of an inflamed tunica vaginalis or from torsion of the appendix testis or of the appendix epididymidis, which then becomes detached and calcified (114). These calcifications may be palpable. On ultrasound, the loose body is visualized as a discrete, coarse echogenic focus with shadowing, which moves freely within the tunica vaginalis (Fig. 56). It is easier to see with a concomitant hydrocele.

Rarely, one sees calcification of the parietal layer of the tunica vaginalis and scrotal wall, thought to be related to previous trauma or inflammation. When multiple painless calcified nodules are observed in this location, the diagnosis of idiopathic scrotal calcinosis has been suggested. This condition is thought to represent dystrophic calcification of inflamed epidermoid cysts of the scrotal wall (115).

Meconium peritonitis results from in utero perforation of the gastrointestinal tract with peritoneal leakage of its contents. Perforation may result from volvulus, atresia, intussusception, or congenital megacolon, or it may be idiopathic (116). The processus vaginalis (which connects the peritoneum and the tunica vaginalis) forms by the sixth fetal month and enters the scrotum in the seventh month. It remains patent until birth. For this reason, chemical peritonitis equally affects the abdomen and the scrotum. On ultrasound of the neonate, the scrotum shows complex masses with shadowing resulting from calcifications. The diagnosis is facilitated if similar findings are observed in the abdomen. A radiograph of the same area is also helpful.

A main pitfall to consider is a technical artifact produced by the thumb or fingers of the operator beneath the scrotal sac that causes an arciform shadow posterior to the testes (113). An inguinal hernia with bowel in the scrotum may result in areas of echogenicity with pseudoshadowing (117). A dense foreign body may also mimic an area of calcification, but the patient's history of penetrating trauma should help (92). On ultrasound, the calcifications are discrete and echogenic, and they have posterior shadowing.

A summary of scrotal calcifications is given in Table 13.

Undescended Testis (Cryptorchidism)

The gonads of both sexes are identical in appearance until the seventh week after conception. At that time, under the influence of the Y chromosome, the differentiation into testes begins. In turn, the newly differentiating gonads determine the sexual differentiation of the genital ducts and external genitalia by secretion of testosterone, genital duct inducer, and suppressor substances produced by the interstitial cells of Leydig. A ligament called gubernaculum descends from the inferior pole of the gonads into the developing inguinal canals and attaches to a labioscrotal swelling to become the scrotum. This change is followed by an evagination of the peritoneum, the processus vaginalis that surrounds the gubernaculum and follows the same path. Later on, it is obliterated in the inguinal canal and remains in the scrotum as the tunica

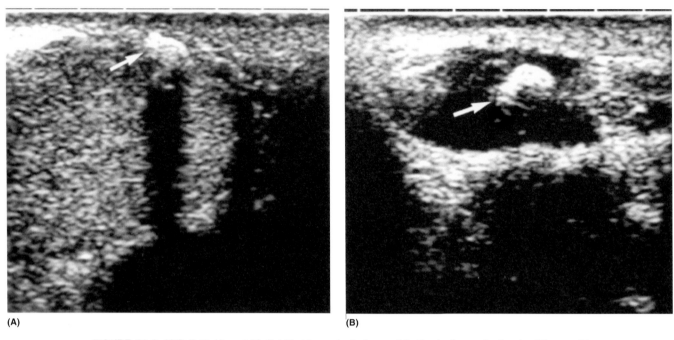

(A)　　　　　　　　　　　　　　　　　　**(B)**

FIGURE 56 A AND B ■ (**A** and **B**) Calcified loose body (*arrows*) in the tunica vaginalis of a 37-year-old patient with a history of scrotal trauma three months before the ultrasound examination and current point tenderness in the scrotum. The loose body is displaced by the examiner's hand from one position in (**A**) to a new position in (**B**).

vaginalis. Because the gubernaculum does not grow as rapidly as the body wall, the testis descends (beginning in the 28th week and reaching the scrotum at 32 weeks). Approximately 97% of full-term newborns have both testes in the scrotum. An additional small percentage of testes descends into the scrotum in the first few months of life. Several problems may occur during the descent of the testes.

Cryptorchidism is the arrest in the descent of the testis somewhere in its normal path. Its incidence is 100% in premature infants weighing less than 900 g and approximately 3% in full-term infants. This condition is one of the most common disorders of the genitourinary system in male infants and children. In 25% of infants, the finding is bilateral. Approximately 80% of undescended testes are found at or below the level of the inguinal canal (5).

TABLE 13 ■ Scrotal Calcifications

			Location		Form of calcification	
		Diagnosis	Testis	Epididymis	Focal	Stippled
Testis and epididymis	Benign	Spermatic granuloma	✓	✓	✓	–
		Phlebolith	✓	✓	✓	–
		Scar	✓		✓	–
		Chronic epididymitis		✓	✓	–
		Tuberculosis	✓	✓	✓	–
		Microlithiasis	✓	–	–	✓
	Malignant	Embryonal cell carcinoma	✓	–	–	✓
		Tumor, posttherapy	✓	–	–	✓
		Metastatic neuroblastoma	✓	–	–	✓
		Teratoma	✓	–	✓	–
		"Burned-out" germ cell tumor	✓	–	✓	–
Tunica vaginalis	Benign	Postinflammatory, posttrauma, postappendix torsion (attached or mobile)	–	–	✓	–
		Meconium peritonitis	–	–	✓ (possible mass)	–

Possible causes of cryptorchidism are impairment in the hypothalamus-pituitary-gonadal axis, short spermatic vessels, adhesions to the peritoneum, poor development of the inguinal canal or superficial abdominal ring, and maldevelopment of the scrotum or cremaster muscles. Abdominal undescended testes are found in the Prune-Belly syndrome. Undescended testes have also been associated with other congenital anomalies such as Beckwith's, Prader-Willi, and Fanconi's syndromes, imperforate anus, intersex disorders, congenital rubella, cystic fibrosis, and in utero exposure to diethylstilbestrol. Associated abnormalities of the epididymis, vas deferens, and spermatic vessels are common. Almost all patients with untreated bilateral cryptorchidism are infertile. This percentage is reduced to 20% in patients with unilateral cryptorchidism and 75% in patients with bilateral cryptorchidism after orchiopexy (118). A serious problem is the multifold increase in the risk of germ cell neoplasms. Approximately 10% of patients with testicular tumors have a history of cryptorchidism. The contralateral and normally descended testis also carries an increased risk of malignancy. Seminoma is the most common tumor, accounting for 60% of cases (107). The incidence of malignancy is higher when the testis is located in the abdomen. The abnormally placed testis is more prone to injury by trauma. In addition, undescended testes are prone to torsion because of the lack of normal attachments (5). Undescended testes are palpable in 80% of the cases (119).

Most nonpalpable testes are located in the inguinal canal, where they can be easily found by ultrasound (Fig. 57). In infants, the diameter of the testis is in the range of 1 cm, and thus it is important to use high-resolution transducers in the range of 10–15 MHz. The echogenicity of the undescended testis is similar to that of the normal testis. The technical parameters of the equipment should be set on the normal testis as recommended for all scrotal examinations. Scanning begins inferiorly and slowly moves upward to the base of the scrotum and inguinal canal. Most testes are found in this region. Care should be paid to avoid confusing a testis with a lymph node or gubernaculum. Some authors have recommended the use of the echogenic mediastinum testis for reliable identification (120), but other authors indicate that this structure is not so easily seen (121). Our experience supports the latter opinion. Ultrasound detection of the undescended testis is effective up to the internal inguinal ring. In the older child and adult, the undescended testis may be atrophic. Abnormal echo texture may indicate torsion and infarction or malignant degeneration (122). The sensitivity of ultrasound in the detection of palpable undescended testes in children is reported at 97%, and at 75% of nonpalpable testes. Three undescended testes missed by ultrasound were found to be atrophic at surgery, and one was ectopic in the femoral canal (123). When ultrasound fails to visualize the absent testis, other modalities are indicated. Each technique has advantages and disadvantages. In infants, CT and MRI require sedation of the patient. CT has the additional drawbacks of exposure to ionizing radiation and difficult visualization of the testis because of the small amount of retroperitoneal fat in infants (124). MRI with a T_2-weighted sequence in the axial and coronal planes is helpful, but failure to localize the testis does not exclude its presence and requires other studies (125). Ultrasound plays an important role after orchiopexy in the early detection of developing tumors in the testis.

Ectopic testis occurs about one-fifth as frequently as cryptorchidism and is not usually associated with a hernia sac. It results when a portion of the gubernaculum passes to an abnormal location after traversing the inguinal canal. The testis may be found in different abnormal locations, most commonly external to the aponeurosis of the

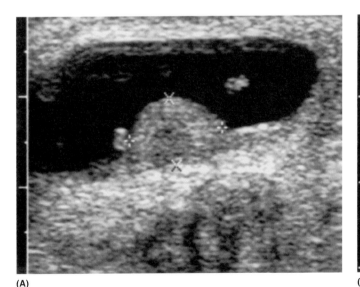
(A)

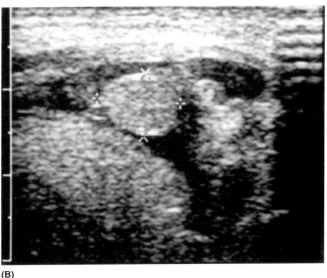
(B)

FIGURE 57 A AND B ■ Undescended testis in a newborn. (**A**) Left testis (*calipers*) in the scrotum and surrounded by a hydrocele. (**B**) Right testis (*calipers*) in the inguinal canal.

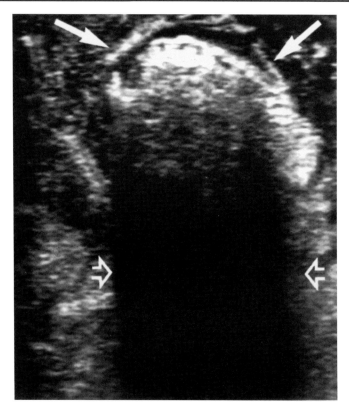

FIGURE 58 ■ Inguinal hernia containing bowel (*arrows*) presenting as a scrotal mass in a 49-year-old patient. Beam attenuation posterior to the mass.

external oblique muscle (interstitial), but also in the femoral triangle of the thigh, dorsal to the penis, or on the opposite side of the patient (crossed ectopia) (126).

Congenital inguinal hernia is often associated with cryptorchidism on the same side and is due to failure of the processus vaginalis to close. This situation allows the descent of bowel loops into the scrotum.

Congenital hydrocele is also due to a persistently open processus vaginalis, with an opening too small to permit herniation. Only peritoneal fluid is allowed into the scrotum. If only a small portion of the processus vaginalis remains open in the middle of the inguinal canal, fluid may accumulate and may give rise to a hydrocele of the spermatic cord (126).

Complications of Inguinal Herniorrhaphy

After inguinal hernia repair, acute findings over the groin and scrotum may develop. Local complications are in the range of 5% to 10% and include hernia recurrence, edema, hematoma, epididymo-orchitis, and ischemic orchitis (94).

On ultrasound, recurrence of the hernia has the typical appearance of an echogenic mass representing omentum, or peristalsis and reverberation (gas) if bowel is present (Fig. 58). The mass is in continuity with the abdominal content and cannot be separated from the abdominal wall. A Valsalva maneuver or scanning while the patient is standing may show descent or enlargement of the mass. A reactive hydrocele may be seen.

Hematoma may occur in the inguinal canal and may extend to the scrotum. Depending on the size, it may displace the testes posteroinferiorly.

Epididymitis with acute pain and swelling may be related to hemorrhage, extension of an existing subclinical infection, trauma, or ischemic epididymitis (127).

Ischemic orchitis, a rare complication of primary inguinal herniorrhaphy, is seen in 0.3% to 0.5% of patients and is 10 times more common in patients who have undergone recurrent hernia repairs. Under these circumstances, interpretation of gray-scale and color Doppler findings is difficult because of the coexistence

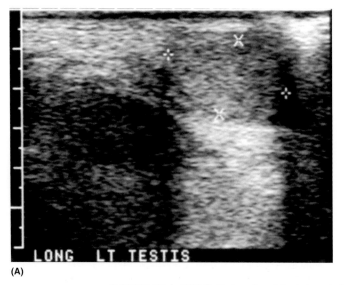

(A)

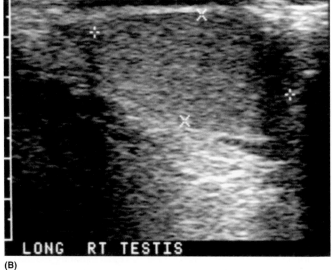

(B)

FIGURE 59 A AND B ■ Atrophy of the left testis in a 32-year-old patient with a history of epididymectomy. (**A**) Longitudinal view shows a small and isoechoic left testis (*calipers*) measuring 19 × 32 mm. (**B**) Longitudinal view of the normal right testis (*calipers*), for comparison, measures 26 × 51 mm.

of other scrotal findings such as extratesticular hemorrhage (128).

Atrophy of the Testes

Atrophy of the testes may be congenital or acquired in association with multiple conditions such as mumps, senility, infertility, prolonged hyperpyrexia, avitaminosis, hepatic cirrhosis, hypothyroidism, schizophrenia, estrogen therapy, and hormonal imbalance. Painful acute atrophy has been described as a complication of renal transplantation (46). The condition is usually bilateral, but it may also be unilateral. Clinically, it manifests as a small and soft testis. On ultrasound, clinicians diagnose testicular atrophy in the adult when the testis is significantly smaller than its opposite or when it is less than 3 cm in length and 2 cm in transverse diameter (Fig. 59). The echo pattern is variable and may be diffusely isoechoic, hypoechoic, or hyperechoic. Atrophy after torsion may give the testis a heterogeneous echo pattern (129). Atrophy of the testis is significant not only because of infertility, but also because of its reported association with an increased incidence of testicular malignancy.

REFERENCES

1. Miskin M, Bain J. B-mode ultrasonic examination of the testes. J Clin Ultrasound 1974; 2:307.
2. Grunberger I, Suhrland MJ, Greco MA, et al. Effects of ultrasound on ultrastructure of human testes. Urology 1987; 30:201.
3. Sunden B. The biological effects of ultrasound. Acta Obstet Gynecol Scand 1964; 43(suppl 6):46–80.
4. Gerscovich EO, Kurzrock EA. Acoustic streaming versus venous pseudoaneurysm in a scrotal mass. J Clin Ultrasound 2002; 30(9):569–570.
5. Krone KD, Carroll BA. Scrotal ultrasound. Radiol Clin North Am 1985; 23(1):121–139.
6. Middleton WD, Thorne DA, Melson GL. Color Doppler ultrasound of the normal testis. AJR Am J Roentgenol 1989; 152(2):293–297.
7. Middleton WD, Bell MW. Analysis of intratesticular arterial anatomy with emphasis on transmediastinal arteries. Radiology 1993; 189(1):157–160.
8. Dewire DM, Begun FP, Lawson RK, et al. Color Doppler ultrasonography in the evaluation of the acute scrotum. J Urol 1992; 147(1):89–91.
9. Burks D, Markey BJ, Burkhard TK, et al. Suspected testicular torsion and ischemia: evaluation with color Doppler sonography. Radiology 1990; 175(3):815–821.
10. Mittemeyer BT, Lennox KW, Borski AA. Epididymitis: a review of 610 cases. J Urol 1966; 95(3):390–392.
11. Lewis AG, Bukowski TP, Jarvis PD, et al. Evaluation of acute scrotom in the emergency department. J Pediatr Surg 1995; 30(2):277–281; discussion 281–282.
12. Petrack EM, Hafeez W. Testicular torsion vs. epididymitis: a diagnostic challenge. Pediatr Emerg Care 1992; 8(6):347–350.
13. Horstman WG, Middleton WD, Melson GL. Scrotal inflammatory disease: color Doppler ultrasound findings. Radiology 1991; 179(1):55–59.
14. Rifkin MD. Ultrasonography of the lower genitourinary tract. Urol Clin North Am 1985; 12(4):645–656.
15. Rifkin MD, Kurtz AB, Pasto ME, et al. The sonographic diagnosis of focal and diffuse infiltrative intrascrotal lesions. Urol Radiol 1984; 6(1):20–26.
16. Eisner DJ, Goldman SM, Petronis J, et al. Bilateral testicular infarction caused by epididymitis. AJR Am J Roentgenol 1991; 157(3):517–519.
17. Sanders LM, Haber S, Dembner A, et al. Significance of reversal of diastolic flow in the acute scrotum. J Ultrasound Med 1994; 13(2):137–139.
18. Begley MG, Shawker TH, Robertson CN, et al. Fournier gangrene: diagnosis with scrotal US. Radiology 1988; 169(2):387–389.
19. Wolfson K, Sudakoff GS. Ultrasonography and color Doppler imaging of the scrotal phlegmon in acute necrotizing pancreatitis. J Ultrasound Med 1994; 13(7):565–568.
20. Holden A, List A. Extratesticular lesions: a radiological and pathological correlation. Australas Radiol 1994; 38(2):99–105.
21. Lattimer JK, Colmore HP, Sanger G, et al. Transmission of genital tuberculosis from husband to wife via semen. Am Rev Tuberc 1954; 69(4):618–624.
22. Drudi FM, Di Nardo R, Burrai L, et al. Le flogosi tubercolari del testicolo: quadri caratteristici in ecografia. Radiol Med 1991; 81(3):293–296.
23. Gerscovich EO. High-resolution ultrasonography in the diagnosis of scrotal pathology. I. Normal scrotum and benign disease. J Clin Ultrasound 1993; 21:355.
24. Wolf JS Jr, McAninch JW. Tuberculous epididymo-orchitis: diagnosis by fine needle aspiration. J Urol 1991; 145(4):836–838.
25. Amenta PS, Gonick P, Katz SM. Sarcoidosis of the testis and epididymis. Urology 1981; 17(6):616–617.
26. Luker GD, Siegel MJ. Color Doppler sonography of the scrotum in children. AJR Am J Roentgenol 1994; 163(3):649–655.
27. Ransler CW, Allen TD. Torsion of the spermatic cord. Urol Clin North Am 1982; 9:245.
28. Williamson RCN. Torsion of the testis and allied conditions. Br J Surg 1976; 63(6):465–476.
29. Donohue RE, Utley WL. Torsion of spermatic cord. Urology 1978; 11(1):33–36.
30. Haynes BE, Bessen HA, Haynes VE. The diagnosis of testicular torsion. JAMA 1983; 249(18):2522–2527.
31. Hadziselimovic F, Geneto R, Emmons LR. Increased apoptosis in the contralateral testes of patients with testicular torsion as a factor for infertility. J Urol 1998; 160(3 Pt 2):1158–1160.
32. Bird K, Rosenfield AT, Taylor KJ. Ultrasonography in testicular torsion. Radiology 1983; 147(2):527–534.
33. Ralls PW, Larsen D, Johnson MB, et al. Color Doppler sonography of the scrotum. Semin Ultrasound CT MR 1991; 12(2):109–114.
34. Middleton WD, Siegel BA, Melson GL, et al. Acute scrotal disorders: prospective comparison of color Doppler ultrasound and testicular scintigraphy. Radiology 1990; 177(1):177–181.
35. Sheldon CA. Symposium on pediatric surgery. I. Undescended testes and testicular torsion. Surg Clin North Am 1985; 65:1303–1329.
36. Knight PJ, Vassy LE. The diagnosis and treatment of the acute scrotum in children and adolescents. Ann Surg 1984; 200(5):664–673.
37. Yang DM, Lim JW, Kim JE, Kim JH, Cho H. Torsed appendix testis: gray scale and color Doppler sonographic findings compared with normal appendix testis. J Ultrasound Med 2005; 24(1):87–91.
38. Lerner RM, Mevorach RA, Hulbert WC. Color Doppler ultrasound in the evaluation of acute scrotal disease. Radiology 1990; 176(2):355–368.
39. Feld R, Middleton WD. Recent advances in sonography of the testis and scrotum. Radiol Clin North Am 1992; 30:1033.
40. Horstman WG, Middleton WD, Melson GL, et al. Color Doppler ultrasound of the scrotum. Radiographics 1991; 11(6):941–957; discussion 958.
41. Cass A, Luxenberg M. Testicular injuries. Urology 1991; 37(6):528–530.
42. Gross M. Rupture of the testicle: the importance of early surgical treatment. J Urol 1969; 101(2):196–197.
43. Lupetin AR, King W III, Rich PJ, et al. The traumatized scrotum: ultrasound evaluation. Radiology 1983; 148(1):203–207.
44. Paredes Esteban RM, Ramirez Chamond R, Carracedo Anon J, et al. Apoptosis of the contralateral testis after unilateral testicular injury. Experimental study. Cir Pediatr 2000; 13(1):3–6.
45. Kukadia AN, Ercole CJ, Gleich P, et al. Testicular trauma: potential impact on reproductive function. J Urol 1996; 156(5):1643–1646.
46. Hricak H, Filly RA. Sonography of the scrotum. Invest Radiol 1983; 18:112.

47. Cooper SG, Sherman SB, Gross RI, et al. Ultrasound diagnosis of acute scrotal hemorrhage in Henoch-Schönlein purpura. J Clin Ultrasound 1988; 16(5):353–357.

48. Pottern LM, Brown LM, Hoover RN, et al. Testicular cancer risk among young men: the role of cryptorchidism and inguinal hernia. J Natl Cancer Inst 1985; 74(2):377–381.

49. Tollerud DJ, Blattner WA, Fraser MC, et al. Familial testicular cancer and urogenital developmental anomalies. Cancer 1985; 55(8):1849–1854.

50. Kaldor JM, Day NE, Band P, et al. Second malignancies following testicular cancer, ovarian cancer, and Hodgkin's disease: an international collaborative study among cancer registries. Int J Cancer 1987; 39(5):571–585.

51. Martin B, Conte J. Ultrasonography of the acute scrotum. J Clin Ultrasound 1987; 15(1):37–44.

52. Glazer HS, Lee JK, Melson GL, et al. Sonographic detection of occult testicular neoplasms. AJR Am J Roentgenol 1982; 138(4):673–675.

53. Mostofi FK. Proceedings: testicular tumors. Epidemiologic, etiologic, and pathologic features. Cancer 1973; 32(5):1186–1201.

54. Mostofi FK, Sesterhenn IA, Davis CJ Jr. Immunopathology of germ cell tumors of the testis. Semin Diagn Pathol 1987; 4(4):320–341.

55. Polák V, Hornák M. The value of scrotal ultrasound in patients with suspected testicular tumour. Int Urol Nephrol 1990; 22(5):467–473.

56. Mostofi FK, Davis CJ Jr. Male reproductive system and prostate. In: Kissane JM, ed. Anderson's Pathology. 8th ed. St Louis: CV Mosby, 1985:791–832.

57. Schwerk WB, Schwerk WN, Rodeck G. Testicular tumors: prospective analysis of real-time US patterns and abdominal staging. Radiology 1987; 164(2):369–374.

58. Gerscovich EO. High-resolution ultrasonography in the diagnosis of scrotal pathology. II. Tumors. J Clin Ultrasound 1993; 21:375.

59. Azzopardi JG, Mostofi FK, Theiss EA. Lesions of testes observed in certain patients with widespread choriocarcinoma and related tumors. Am J Pathol 1961; 38:207–225.

60. Givler RL. Testicular involvement in leukemia and lymphoma. Cancer 1969; 23(6):1290–1295.

61. Phillips G, Kumari-Subaiya S, Sawitsky A. Ultrasonic evaluation of the scrotum in lymphoproliferative disease. J Ultrasound Med 1987; 6(4):169–175.

62. Haupt HM, Mann RB, Trump DL, et al. Metastatic carcinoma involving the testis: clinical and pathological distinction from primary testicular neoplasms. Cancer 1984; 54(4):709–714.

63. Carroll BA, Gross DM. High-frequency scrotal sonography. AJR Am J Roentgenol 1983; 140(3):511–515.

64. Finkelstein MS, Rosenberg HK, Snyder HM III, et al. Ultrasound evaluation of the scrotum in pediatrics. Urology 1986; 27(1):1–9.

65. Mostofi FK, Sobin LH. Histological typing of testis tumours. In: International Histological Classification of Tumors #16. Geneva: World Health Organization, 1977:1–39.

66. Bercovici JP, Nahoul K, Tater D, et al. Hormonal profile of Leydig cell tumors with gynecomastia. J Clin Endocrinol Metab 1984; 59(4):625–630.

67. Dehner LP. The male reproductive system. In: Pediatric Surgical Pathology. 2nd ed. St. Louis: CV Mosby, 1987:712–742.

68. Cunningham JJ. Echographic findings in Sertoli cell tumor of the testis. J Clin Ultrasound 1981; 9(6):341–342.

69. McAlister WH, Sisler CL. Scrotal sonography in infants and children. Curr Probl Diagn Radiol 1990; 19(6):201–242.

70. Uehling DT, Smith JE, Logan R, et al. Newborn granulosa cell tumor of the testis. J Urol 1987; 138(2):385–386.

71. Chapman WH, Plymyer MR, Dresner ML. Gonadoblastoma in an anatomically normal man: a case report and literature review. J Urol 1990; 144(6):1472–1474.

72. Arenson AM, Hamilton P, Silverberg J, et al. Ultrasound diagnosis of testicular masses secondary to hyperplastic adrenal rest in a patient with adrenal insufficiency. J Clin Ultrasound 1991; 19(7):430–433.

73. Seidenwurm D, Smathers RL, Kan P, et al. Intratesticular adrenal rests diagnosed by ultrasound. Radiology 1985; 155(2):479–481.

74. Wright LF, Bicknell SL. Systemic necrotizing vasculitis presenting as epididymitis. J Urol 1986; 136(5):1094.

75. Huisman TK, Collins WT Jr, Voulgarakis JR. Polyarteritis nodosa masquerading as a primary testicular neoplasm: a case report and review of the literature. J Urol 1990; 144(5):1236–1238.

76. Weingärtner K, Gerharz EW, Kohl U, et al. Focal necrotizing vasculitis of the testis. Urologe A 1994; 33(4):320–324.

77. Amodio JB et al. Polyorchidism. Report of three cases and review of the literature. J Ultrasound Med 2004; 23:951–957.

78. Gooding GA, Leonhardt W, Stein R. Testicular cysts: US findings. Radiology 1987; 163(2):537–538.

79. Nistal M, Mate A, Paniagua R. Cystic transformation of rete testis. Am J Surg Pathol 1996; 20(10):1231–1239.

80. Ortega Herrera R, Medina Benitez A, Lopez Milena G. Tubular ectasia of the rete testis: ultrasonography findings in 19 patients. Arch Esp Urol 2000; 53(5):455–459.

81. Cho CS, Kosek J. Cystic dysplasia of the testes: sonographic and pathologic findings. Radiology 1985; 156(3):777–778.

82. Fisher JE, Jewett TC, Nelson SJ, et al. Ectasia of the rete testis with ipsilateral renal agenesis. J Urol 1982; 128(5):1040–1043.

83. Piotto Lino et al. Congenital cystic dysplasia of the rete testes. Pediatr Radiol 2001; 31:724–726.

84. Hamm B, Fobbe F, Loy V. Testicular cysts: differentiation with ultrasound and clinical findings. Radiology 1988; 168(1):19–23.

85. Cittadini G et al. Bilateral epidermoid cysts of the testis: sonographic and MRI findings. J Clin Ultrasound 2004; 32(7): 370–372.

86. Meiches MD, Nurenberg P. Sonographic appearance of a calcified simple epidermoid cyst of the testis. J Clin Ultrasound 1991; 19(8):498–500.

87. Sogani PC, Grabstald H, Whitmore WF. Spermatic cord sarcoma in adults. J Urol 1978; 120(3):301–305.

88. Gooding GA. Sonography of the spermatic cord. AJR Am J Roentgenol 1988; 151(4):721–724.

89. Wood A, Dewbury KC. Case report: paratesticular rhabdomyosarcoma—colour Doppler appearances. Clin Radiol 1995; 50(2): 130–131.

90. Haller J, Tscholakoff D, Gundry C, et al. Sonography of unusual extratesticular lesions. Urol Radiol 1989; 11(3):190–193.

91. Goldberg RM, Chilcote W, Kay R, et al. Sonographic findings in polyorchidism. J Clin Ultrasound 1987; 15(6):412–415.

92. Rifkin MD. Diagnostic imaging of the lower genitourinary tract. New York, Raven Press, 1985:241–324.

93. Fowler RC, Chennells PM, Ewing R. Scrotal ultrasonography: a clinical evaluation. Br J Radiol 1987; 60(715):649–654.

94. Cunningham JJ. Sonographic findings in clinically unsuspected acute and chronic scrotal hematoceles. AJR Am J Roentgenol 1983; 140(4):749–752.

95. Rifkin MD, Kurtz AB, Pasto ME, et al. Diagnostic capabilities of high-resolution scrotal ultrasonography: prospective evaluation. J Ultrasound Med 1985; 4(1):13–19.

96. Hamm B, Fobbe F, Sorensen R, et al. Varicoceles: combined sonography and thermography in diagnosis and posttherapeutic evaluation. Radiology 1986; 160(2):419–424.

97. Demas BE, Hricak H, McClure RD. Varicoceles: radiologic diagnosis and treatment. Radiol Clin North Am 1991; 29(3): 619–627.

98. Sigmund G, Gall H, Bahren W. Stop-type and shunt-type varicoceles: venographic findings. Radiology 1987; 163(1):105–110.

99. Petros JA, Andriole GL, Middleton WD, et al. Correlation of testicular color Doppler ultrasonography, physical examination and venography in the detection of left varicoceles in men with infertility. J Urol 1991; 145(4):785–788.

100. Gonda RL Jr, Karo JJ, Forte RA, et al. Diagnosis of subclinical varicocele in infertility. AJR Am J Roentgenol 1987; 148(1): 71–75.

101. Gottlieb RH, Poster R, Subudhi MK. Computed tomographic, ultrasound, and plain film appearance of phleboliths in varicoceles. J Ultrasound Med 1989; 8(6):329–331.

102. Nashan D, Behre HM, Grunert JH, et al. Diagnostic value of scrotal sonography in infertile men: report on 658 cases. Andrologia 1990; 22(5):387–395.

103. Patel PJ, Pareek S. Scrotal ultrasound in male infertility. Eur Urol 1989; 16(6):423–425.

104. Bibbo M, Gill WB, Azizi F, et al. Follow-up study of male and female offspring of DES-exposed mothers. Obstet Gynecol 1977; 49(1):1–8.

105. Gerscovich EO, Reid MH. Unusual appearance of an extratesticular epidermal inclusion cyst of the scrotum. Clin Radiol Extra 2003; 58:1–2.

106. Chen TF, Ball RY. Epididymectomy for post-vasectomy pain: histological review. Br J Urol 1991; 68(4):407–413.

107. Doherty FJ. Ultrasound of the nonacute scrotum. Semin Ultrasound CT MR 1991; 12(2):131–156.

108. Smith WS, Brammer HM, Henry M, et al. Testicular microlithiasis: sonographic features with patholgical relation. AJR Am J Roentgenol 1991; 157(5):1003–1004.

109. Janzen DL, Mathieson JR, Marsh JI, et al. Testicular microlithiasis: sonographic and clinical features. AJR Am J Roentgenol 1992; 158(5):1057–1060.

110. Hobarth K, Susani M, Szabo N, et al. Incidence of testicular microlithiasis. Urology 1992; 40(5):464–467.

111. Kragel PJ, Delvecchio D, Orlando R, et al. Ultrasonographic findings of testicular microlithiasis associated with intratubular germ cell neoplasia. Urology 1991; 37(1):66–68.

112. Doherty FJ, Mullins TL, Sant GR, et al. Testicular microlithiasis: a unique sonographic appearance. J Ultrasound Med 1987; 6(7): 389–392.

113. Martin B, Tubiana JM. Significance of scrotal calcifications detected by sonography. J Clin Ultrasound 1988; 16(8):545–552.

114. Linkowski GD, Avellone A, Gooding GA. Scrotal calculi: sonographic detection. Radiology 1985; 156(2):484.

115. Sarma DP, Weilbaecher TG. Scrotal calcinosis: calcification of epidermal cysts. J Surg Oncol 1984; 27(2):76–79.

116. Kenney PJ, Spirt BA, Ellis DA, et al. Scrotal masses caused by meconium peritonitis: prenatal sonographic diagnosis. Radiology 1985; 154(2):362.

117. Hricak H, Jeffrey RB. Sonography of acute scrotal abnormalities. Radiol Clin North Am 1983; 21(3):595–603.

118. Gilhooly PE, Meyers F, Lattimer JK. Fertility prospects for children with cryptorchidism. Am J Dis Child 1984; 138(10):940–943.

119. Friedland GW, Chang P. The role of imaging in the management of the impalpable undescended testis. AJR Am J Roentgenol 1988; 151(6):1107–1111.

120. Weiss RM, Carter AR, Rosenfield AT. High resolution real-time ultrasonography in the localization of the undescended testis. J Urol 1986; 135(3):936–938.

121. Johansen TE, Larmo A. Ultrasonography in undescended testes. Acta Radiol 1988; 29(2):159–163.

122. Dudiak CM, Venta LA, Olson MC, et al. Ultrasound of the scrotum. Crit Rev Diagn Imaging 1992; 33(4):369–406.

123. Graif M, Czerniak A, Avigad I, et al. High-resolution sonography of the undescended testis in childhood: an analysis of 45 cases. Isr J Med Sci 1990; 26(7):382–385.

124. Lee JK, Glazer HS. Computed tomography in the localization of the nonpalpable testis. Urol Clin North Am 1982; 9(3):397–404.

125. Kier R, McCarthy S, Rosenfield AT, et al. Nonpalpable testes in young boys: evaluation with MR imaging. Radiology 1988; 169(2):429–433.

126. Moore KL. The developing human, clinically oriented embryology. Philadelphia: WB Saunders, 1982:255–297.

127. Pintauro WL, Klein FA, Vick CW III, et al. The use of ultrasound for evaluating subacute unilateral scrotal swelling. J Urol 1985; 133(5):799–802.

128. Vick CW, Bird K, Rosenfield AT, et al. Extratesticular hemorrhage associated with torsion of the spermatic cord: sonographic demonstration. Radiology 1986; 158(2):401–404.

129. van Dijk R, Hitge-Boetes C, Debruyne FM, et al. Sonographic detection of a nonpalpable regressed germ cell tumor in an atrophic testis. J Clin Ultrasound 1989; 8(17):594–597.

The Penis ● *Vikram S. Dogra,*
Ercan Kocakoc, and Shweta Bhatt

36

INTRODUCTION

The development of high-frequency broadband transducers has improved the quality of ultrasound imaging, particularly of superficial tissues such as those of the penis. Sonography is the preferred imaging technique for evaluation of the penile anatomy and vascularity because of its improved spatial resolution and increased color Doppler sensitivity for low-flow states (1). Ultrasonography using a high-frequency transducer helps to characterize penile anatomy and penile blood flow and in many circumstances allows specific diagnoses such as erectile dysfunction (ED) (2). Sonography plays a definite role in the diagnosis and followup of patients with ED. Other penile disorders such as priapism, Peyronie's disease, penile trauma, and penile masses can be evaluated using the penile gray-scale and color-flow Doppler sonography.

ANATOMY OF THE PENIS

The penis is composed of two dorsal corpora cavernosa (CC) and one ventral corpus spongiosum (CS). The two CC are enclosed in a fibrous sheath, the tunica albuginea, which partially covers the CS. The tunica albuginea is composed of elastic fibers that form an irregular, latticed network on which collagen fibers rest. The septum between the two CC is complete proximally and is incomplete in its distal two-thirds. The CC join beneath the pubis (penile hilum) to form the major portion of the body of the penis. The CC is composed of sinusoidal spaces lined by smooth muscles (erectile tissue) and endothelium. The glans penis is formed by expansion of the CS (3).

The CS is traversed throughout its length by the anterior urethra, which begins at the perineal membrane. The CS provides support to the urethra and helps with the expulsion of semen from the urethra. Buck's fascia surrounds both the CC and the CS external to the tunica albuginea (Fig. 1).

The penile blood vessels arise from the internal pudendal artery, a branch of the internal iliac artery. Occasionally, accessory arteries exist, arising from the external iliac, obturator, vesicle, and femoral arteries; these vessels may occasionally become the dominant or only arterial supply to the corpus cavernosum (5). Injury to these accessory arteries during radical prostatectomy or cystectomy may result in vasculogenic ED following the surgery (6,7). The common penile artery continues in the Alcock's canal above the perineal membrane and terminates in three branches to supply the erectile bodies. The three branches of the penile artery are the bulbourethral artery, the cavernosal artery, and the dorsal penile arteries. The bulbourethral artery supplies the urethra, the spongiosum, and the glans (3). The cavernosal artery enters the corpus cavernosum on the superomedial surface of the penis. The cavernosal artery travels in the center of each corporal body. The branches of this artery are called the helicine arteries; they subsequently divide into smaller vessels that communicate with the lacunae of the corpus cavernosum (Fig. 1) (2). The cavernosal artery branches dilate and bring extra blood to the erectile tissue during erection. The dorsal artery of the penis passes between the crus of the penis and the pubis to reach the dorsal surface of the corporal bodies. The

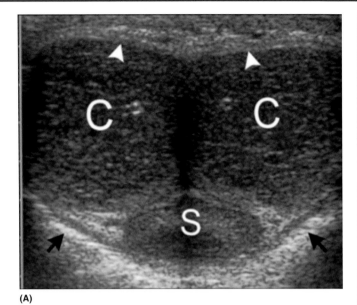

(A)

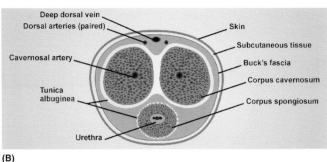

(B)

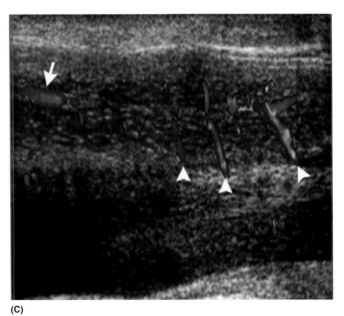

(C)

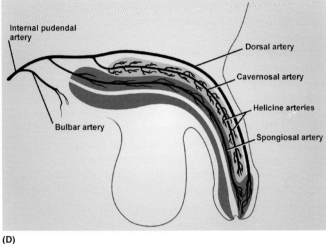

(D)

FIGURE 1 A–D ■ Sonogram of the normal penis. (**A**) Transverse gray-scale ultrasound of the penis demonstrates the two corpora cavernosa surrounded by the tunica albuginea (*arrowheads*). The corpus spongiosum is seen inferior to the corpora cavernosa. All three corpora are surrounded by the Buck's fascia (*arrows*). (**B**) Corresponding diagrammatic representation. (**C**) Longitudinal color-flow image of the normal penis shows the cavernosal artery (*arrow*) with its helicine branches (*arrowheads*) radiating into the corpus. (**D**) Corresponding diagrammatic representation. C, corpora cavernosa; S, corpus spongiosum. *Source*: From Ref. 4.

dorsal artery runs between the paired dorsal veins and primarily supplies blood to the glans penis (3,8).

The penile veins comprise the superficial dorsal veins, the intermediate venous system, and the deep system (5). The superficial dorsal veins are small venous channels in the subcutaneous layer of the skin and subcutaneous tissue of the penis. The superficial dorsal veins of the penis drain into the superficial external pudendal vein. The intermediate system includes the venae circumflexae and the deep dorsal veins; it is formed from the sinusoids of the CC, which empty into small venules under the tunica albuginea (5,8,9). Small venules then form subtunic venular plexuses that perforate the tunica albuginea as the emissary veins. The emissary veins course obliquely through the tunica albuginea to join the deep dorsal vein (2,3). The deep system includes the cavernous and crural veins. The proximal third of the penis is drained by the cavernous

veins, which arise from the penile hilum. The crural veins arise on the dorsomedial surface of each corpus cavernosum and drain into the internal pudendal vein (5,8,9).

The penis is innervated by autonomic (parasympathetic and sympathetic) and somatic (sensory and motor) nerves. Parasympathetic nerve fibers originate from sacral segments (S2–S4) of the spinal cord, whereas sympathetic nerves originate from lower thoracic and upper lumbar segments (T11–T12, L1–L2) (10). Somatic, sensory, and motor fibers enter and leave the sacral cord (S2–S4) and innervate the penis and the perineum via the pudendal nerve (10,11). The cavernosal nerves are branches of the pelvic plexus that innervate the CC of the penis.

The lymph drainage system from the penile skin runs proximally toward the presymphyseal plexus and then divides into the right and left trunks to join the lymphatics from the scrotum and the perineum. These lymphatic